Coercion
as
Cure

Coercion as Cure

A Critical History of Psychiatry

Thomas Szasz

Transaction Publishers
New Brunswick (U.S.A.) and London (U.K.)

Second paperback edition 2010
Copyright © 2007 by Transaction Publishers, New Brunswick, New Jersey.

This book is printed on acid-free paper that meets the American National Standard for Permanence of Paper for Printed Library Materials.

Library of Congress Catalog Number: 2006050465
ISBN: 978-0-7658-0379-5 (cloth); 978-1-4128-1050-0 (paper)
Printed in the United States of America

Library of Congress Cataloging-in-Publication Data

Szasz, Thomas Stephen, 1920-
Coercion as cure : a critical history of psychiatry / Thomas Szasz.
    p. cm.
Includes bibliographical references and index.
ISBN-13: 978-0-7658-0379-5 (alk. paper)
ISBN-10: 0-7658-0379-8 (alk. paper)
    1. Psychiatry—History. 2. Involuntary treatment—History.
3. Insane—Commitment and detention—History. I. Title.

RC438.S915 2007
616.89009—dc22   2006050465

For my grandson
Andrew

This is the great, the uncanny problem which I have been pursuing the longest: the psychology of the "improvers" of mankind. A small, and at bottom modest, fact—that of the so-called *pia fraus* [holy lie]--offered me the first approach to this problem: the *pia fraus*, the heirloom of all philosophers and priests who "improved" mankind. Neither Manu nor Plato nor Confucius nor the Jewish and Christian teachers have ever doubted their *right* to lie.

—Friedrich Nietzsche (1895)[1]

Contents

Preface

All modern history, as learnt and taught and accepted, is purely conventional. For sufficient reasons, all persons in authority combined, by a happy union of deceit and concealment, to promote falsehood.
—*Lord Acton[1]*

Silvano Arieti's three-volume *American Handbook of Psychiatry* opens with this statement: "Perhaps no other field of human endeavor is so…difficult to define as that of psychiatry."[2] Eighty years earlier, Emil Kraepelin, considered the greatest psychiatrist of his age, made almost exactly the same observation. "Our science," he declared in 1886, "has not arrived at a consensus on even its most fundamental principles, let alone on appropriate ends or even on the means to those ends."[3]

None of this is true. Contrary to Arieti's and Kraepelin's assertions, it is easy to define psychiatry. The problem is that defining it truthfully—acknowledging its self-evident ends and the means used to achieve them—is socially unacceptable and professionally suicidal. Psychiatric tradition, social expectation, and the law—both criminal and civil—identify coercion as the profession's determining characteristic.

Accordingly, I regard *psychiatry as the theory and practice of coercion, rationalized as the diagnosis of mental illness and justified as medical treatment aimed at protecting the patient from himself and society from the patient.*[4] The history of psychiatry I present thus resembles, say, a critical history of missionary Christianity.

The heathen savage does not suffer from lack of insight into the divinity of Jesus, does not lack theological help, and does not seek the services of missionaries. Just so, the psychotic does not suffer from lack of insight into being mentally ill, does not lack psychiatric treatment, and does not seek the services of psychiatrists. This is why the missionary tends to have contempt for the heathen, why the psychiatrist tends to have contempt for the psychotic, and why both conceal their true sentiments behind a facade of caring and compassion. Each meddler believes that he is in possession of the "truth," each harbors a passionate desire to improve the

Other, each feels a deep sense of entitlement to intrude into the life of the Other, and each is intolerant of those who dismiss his precious insights and benevolent interventions as worthless and harmful.

Non-acknowledgment of the fact that coercion is a characteristic and potentially ever-present element of so-called psychiatric treatments is intrinsic to the standard dictionary definitions of psychiatry. According to the *Unabridged Webster's*, psychiatry is "A branch of medicine that deals with the science and practice of treating mental, emotional, and behavioral disorders." The entry in the *Wikipedia Encyclopedia* is similar: "Psychiatry refers to the practice of medicine relating to the mind and behavior.... It is a subspecialty of medical practice.... While all clinicians encounter patients with mental illnesses and any of them may treat it, psychiatrists specialize in these areas."[5]

Plainly, voluntary psychiatric relations differ from involuntary psychiatric interventions the same way as, say, sexual relations between consenting adults differ from the sexual assaults we call "rape." Sometimes, to be sure, psychiatrists deal with voluntary patients. As I explain and illustrate throughout this volume, it is necessary, however, not merely to distinguish between coerced and consensual psychiatric relations, but to contrast them. The term "psychiatry" ought to be applied to one or the other, but not both. As long as psychiatrists and society refuse to recognize this, there can be no real psychiatric historiography.

The writings of historians, physicians, journalists, and others addressing the history of psychiatry rest on three erroneous premises: that so-called mental diseases exist, that they are diseases of the brain, and that the incarceration of "dangerous" mental patients is medically rational and morally just. The problems so created are then compounded by failure—purposeful or inadvertent—to distinguish between *two radically different kinds of psychiatric practices, consensual and coerced, voluntarily sought and forcibly imposed.*

In free societies, ordinary social relations between adults are consensual. Such relations—in business, medicine, religion, and psychiatry—pose no special legal or political problems. By contrast, coercive relations—one person authorized by the state to forcibly compel another person to do or abstain from certain actions of his choice—are inherently political in nature and are always morally problematic.

Mental disease is fictitious disease. Psychiatric diagnosis is disguised disdain. Psychiatric treatment is coercion disguised as care, typically carried out in prisons called "hospitals." Formerly, the social function of psychiatry was more apparent than it is now. The asylum inmate was incarcerated against his will. Insanity was synonymous with unfitness for liberty. Toward the end of the nineteenth century, a new type of psychiatric relationship entered the medical scene: persons experiencing so-called "nervous symptoms" began to seek medical help, typically from the family physician or a specialist in "nervous disorders." This led psychiatrists to distinguish between two kinds of mental diseases, neuroses and psychoses: Persons who complained of their own behavior were classified as neurotic, whereas persons about whose behavior others complained were classified as psychotic. The legal, medical, psychiatric, and social denial of this simple distinction and its far-reaching implications undergirds the house of cards that is modern psychiatry.

The American Psychiatric Association, founded in 1844, was first called the Association of Medical Superintendents of American Institutions for the Insane. In 1892, it was renamed the American Medico-Psychological Association, and in 1921, the American Psychiatric Association (APA). In its first official resolution, the Association declared: "Resolved, that it is the unanimous sense of this convention that the attempt to abandon entirely the use of all means of personal restraint is not sanctioned by the true interests of the insane."[6] The APA has never rejected its commitment to the twin claims that insanity is a medical illness and that coercion is care and cure. In 2005, Steven S. Sharfstein, president of the APA, reiterated his and his profession's commitment to coercion. Lamenting "our [the psychiatrists'] reluctance to use caring, coercive approaches," he declared: " A person suffering from paranoid schizophrenia with a history of multiple rehospitalizations for dangerousness and a reluctance to abide by outpatient treatment, including medications, is a perfect example of someone who would benefit from these [forcibly imposed] approaches. We must balance individual rights and freedom with policies aimed at caring coercion."[7] Seven months later, Sharfstein conveniently forgot having recently bracketed caring and coercion into a single act, "caring coercion." Defending "assisted treatment"—a euphemism for psychiatric coercion—he stated: "In assisted treatment, such as Kendra's Law in New York, psychiatrists' primary role is to foster patient improvement and help restore the patient to health."[8]

Psychiatry and society face a paradox. The more progress scientific psychiatry is said to make, the more intolerable becomes the idea that mental illness is a myth and that the effort to treat it a will-o'-the-wisp. The more progress scientific medicine actually makes, the more undeniable it becomes that "chemical imbalances" and "hard wiring" are fashionable clichés, not evidence that problems in living are medical diseases justifiably "treated" without patient consent. And the more often psychiatrists play the roles of juries, judges, and prison guards, the more uncomfortable they feel about being in fact pseudomedical coercers—society's well-paid patsies. The whole conundrum is too horrible to face. Better to continue calling unwanted behaviors "diseases" and disturbing persons "sick," and compel them to submit to psychiatric "care." It is easy to see, then, why the right-thinking person considers it inconceivable that there might be no such thing as mental health or mental illness. Where would that leave the history of psychiatry portrayed as the drama of heroic physicians combating horrible diseases?

Alexander Solzhenitsyn is right: "Violence can only be concealed by a lie, and the lie can only be maintained by violence. Any man who has once proclaimed violence as his method is inevitably forced to take the lie as his principle."[9]

Scientific discourse is predicated on intellectual honesty. Psychiatric discourse rests on intellectual dishonesty. The psychiatrist's basic social mandate is the coercive-paternalistic protection of the mental patient from himself and the public from the mental patient. *Yet, in the professional literature as well as the popular media, this is the least noted feature of psychiatry as a medical specialty.* Pointing it out is considered to be in bad taste. It would be difficult to exaggerate the extent to which historians of psychiatry as well as mental health professionals and journalists ignore, deny, and rationalize the involuntary, coerced, forcibly imposed nature of psychiatric treatments. This denial is rooted in language. Psychiatrists, lawyers, journalists, and medical ethicists routinely call incarceration in a psychiatric prison "hospitalization," and torture forcibly imposed on the inmate "treatment." Resting their reasoning on the same faulty premises, psychiatric historians trace alleged advances in the diagnosis and treatment of mental illnesses to "progress in neuroscience." In contrast, I focus on what psychiatrists have done to persons who have rejected their "help" and on how they have rationalized their "therapeutic" violations of the dignity and liberty of their ostensible beneficiaries.

I regard consensual human relations, however misguided by either or both parties, as radically different, morally as well as politically, from human relations in which one party, empowered by the state, deprives another of liberty. The history of medicine, no less than the history of psychiatry, abounds in interventions by physicians that have harmed rather than helped their patients. Bloodletting is the most obvious example. Nevertheless, physicians have, at least until now, abstained from using state-sanctioned force to systematically impose injurious treatments on medically ill people. Misguided by fashion and lack of knowledge, sick people have often sought and willingly submitted to such interventions. In contrast, the history of psychiatry is, *au fond*, the story of the forcible imposition of injurious "medical" interventions on persons called "mental patients."

In short, where psychiatric historians see stories about terrible illnesses and heroic treatments, I see stories about people marching to the beats of different drummers or perhaps failing to march at all, and the terrible injustices committed against them, rationalized by hollow "therapeutic" justifications. Faced with vexing personal problems, the "truth" people crave is a simple, fashionable falsehood. That is an important, albeit bitter, lesson the history of psychiatry teaches us.

One of the melancholy truths of the story I have set out to tell is that, stripped of its pseudomedical ornamentation, it is not a particularly interesting tale. To make it interesting, I have tried to do what, according to Walt Whitman (1819-1892), the "greatest poet" does: He "drags the dead out of their coffins and stands them again on their feet.... He says to the past, Rise and walk before me that I may realize you."[10] To this end, I have, where possible, cited the exact words psychiatrists have used to justify their stubborn insistence, over a period of nearly three centuries, that psychiatric coercion is medical care.

Largely because psychiatric slavery has been so successfully misrepresented as therapeutic liberation, the result of the struggle against it, so far, has been inconsequential, if not counterproductive. This has not deterred me. I believe, with Whitman, that

> Liberty is poorly served by men whose good intent is quelled from one failure or two failures or any number of failures, or from the casual indifference or ingratitude of the people, or from the sharp show of the tushes of power, or the bringing to bear soldiers and cannon or any penal statutes. Liberty relies upon itself, invites no one, promises nothing, sits in calmness and light, is positive and composed, and knows no discouragement.... How beautiful is candor!... Henceforth let no man of us lie.[11]

Introduction: Force and Freedom

"The myth of mental illness": No phrase has had as profound an impact on public attitudes toward the mentally ill as this provocative title of a 1960 [sic] book by maverick psychiatrist Thomas Szasz."

—*Paul S. Appelbaum*[*]

1

Coercion may be virtuous or wicked, prescribed, permitted, or prohibited by religion, law, society, and the actor's own conscience. Coercing a child to submit to a painful but necessary medical intervention is virtuous, but coercing it to submit to a sexual act is wicked. These are judgments, not facts. Judgments issue from and reflect the values of the judge and, more generally, the values of his culture. In the judgment of our contemporary American culture, psychiatric coercion is virtuous provided its purpose is to protect the subject—defined as a "dangerous mentally ill patient"—from harming himself or society. This is a distinctly modern, post-Enlightenment secular view.

It is often said that people love liberty. It would be more accurate to say that people do not like to *feel* coerced. It is easy to confuse our quasi-instinctive aversion to being in the power of another person with love of liberty. But they are not the same. No duties are attached to the desire to be free of coercion. Liberty, in contrast, entails self-control, self-responsibility, and respect for the rights of others.

Peaceful social existence depends on cooperation. The preference for cooperation over coercion is rooted in our biological nature and is reinforced by religious and moral codes. At an early stage of civilization, acts experienced as wrongs were punished—more precisely, avenged—by the wronged person or his kin. Eventually, this "primitive" arrangement was replaced by the transformation of revenge by the offended party into punishment of the offender by an impartial, "higher" authority, a chief or king or judge. "Dearly beloved, avenge not yourselves...for it is written,

---

* Appelbaum is professor of psychiatry and director, Division of Psychiatry, Law, and Ethics, Department of Psychiatry, College of Physicians and Surgeons of Columbia University. He is a past president of the American Psychiatric Association (2002-2003).

Vengeance is mine" (*Romans* 12:19), commands the Bible. From the idea that the right to punish wrongdoing belongs to God we move, by easy steps, to the idea that it belongs to the sovereign, the state, the law. Avenging a wrong and punishing a wrongdoer requires the use of force to restrain and punish him. *However, it is one thing to use force to harm a person, and it is quite another thing to use force to help him.* A person qua individual cannot coerce another in the name of helping him. Why should a person as agent of the state be able to do so?

As a rule, helping others does not require force. The person in need of help asks for and secures the goods or services he desires, typically by offering goods or services, or at least gratitude, in return. Such exchanges form the warp and woof of everyday human relations, especially trade. The situation of the person who needs help but is too immature or too impaired to be able to ask for it, or to offer anything in return, is an exception. Is it our duty, as "our brother's keeper," to help him, on his terms? Is it our duty to help him, on our terms, even if to do so requires coercing him "in his own best interest"? John Locke's philosophy of liberty explicitly enjoins and justifies such coercive paternalism. In his *Second Treatise on Government*, he wrote:

> Though I have said above "That all men by nature are equal," I cannot be supposed to understand all sorts of "equality".... Children, I confess, are not born in this full state of equality, though they are born to it. Their parents have a sort of rule and jurisdiction over them when they come into the world, and for some time after, but it is but a temporary one. The bonds of this subjection are like the swaddling clothes they are wrapt up in and supported by in the weakness of their infancy. Age and reason as they grow up loosen them, till at length they drop quite off, and leave a man at his own free disposal.... For law, in its true notion, is not so much the limitation as the direction of a free and intelligent agent to his proper interest, and prescribes no farther than is for the general good of those under that law.... The end of law is not to abolish or restrain, but to preserve and enlarge freedom. For in all the states of created beings, capable of laws, where there is no law there is no freedom. For liberty is to be free from restraint and violence from others, which cannot be where there is no law; and is not, as we are told, *"a liberty for every man to do what he lists."* For who could be free, when every other man's humour might domineer over him? But a liberty to dispose and order freely as he lists his person, actions, possessions, and his whole property within the allowance of those laws under which he is, and therein not to be subject to the arbitrary will of another, but freely follow his own.... The power, then, that parents have over their children arises from that duty which is incumbent on them, to take care of their offspring during the imperfect state of childhood. ... But if through defects that may happen out of the ordinary course of Nature, any one comes not to such a degree of reason wherein he might be supposed capable of knowing the law, and so living within the rules of it, he is never capable of being a free man, he is never let loose to the disposure of his own will; *And so lunatics and idiots are never set free from the government of their parents:* "Children who are not as yet come

unto those years whereat they may have, and innocents, which are excluded by a natural defect from ever having.... Madmen, which, for the present, cannot possibly have the use of right reason to guide themselves, have, for their guide, the reason that guideth other men which are tutors over them, to seek and procure their good for them," says Hooker (*Eccl. Pol., lib. I., s. 7*). The freedom then of man, and liberty of acting according to his own will, is grounded on his having reason, which is able to instruct him in that law he is to govern himself by, and make him know how far he is left to the freedom of his own will. To turn him loose to an unrestrained liberty, before he has reason to guide him, is not allowing him the privilege of his nature to be free, but to thrust him out amongst brutes, and abandon him to a state as wretched and as much beneath that of a man as theirs. This is that which puts the authority into the parents' hands to govern the minority of their children.[2]*

The analogy between the infant-parent relationship and the madman-psychiatrist relationship lies at the heart of the justifications for coercive treatment in psychiatry. There are serious problems with this comparison.[3] The infant's needs for food and protection mesh with the parent's biologically rooted need to nourish and support its offspring, a reciprocity manifested by the affectionate bond between them. No similar bond binds the needy adult to the stranger on whose kindness he depends. The non-reciprocity is especially intense and troublesome when the dependent's behavior offends the moral values of the stranger ostensibly charged with caring for him, as is the case in the relationship between the typical "psychotic" and his psychiatrist.

Furthermore, neither Lockean philosophers, nor psychiatrists, nor mental health laws distinguish between individuals so impaired from birth that they never reach the age of reason, and individuals who have reached that stage but are deemed to have become impaired and lost their reason. Persons in both groups require guardians, not psychiatrists. Those impaired from birth must have guardians appointed for them. Those not necessarily permanently impaired ought to have the option, while in a "state of reason," to appoint guardians of their own choice. In no case is the psychiatrist a fit guardian for his own patient.

Lastly, it is important to scrutinize how a person considered mentally healthy becomes defined as mentally ill. Who "accuses" Harry of having lost his mind and why? Who benefits from Harry's psychiatric invalidation, Harry or his accuser(s)? What is the nature of the legal and psychiatric process by means of which Harry is deprived of his liberties and rights?[4] The hypocrisy of the psychiatric enterprise is painfully obvious. It is also obvious that the liberty interests of persons threatened with

---

* Locke was, inter alia, a physician.

psychiatric invalidation could be better protected than they are at present by letting them execute psychiatric advance directives similar to the familiar medical advance directives. Not surprisingly—since psychiatric advance directives are incompatible with mental health laws—they have been bitterly opposed by psychiatrists and ignored by lawmakers.[5] Rejection of the psychiatric advance directive, in a medical-social milieu that strongly supports the use of the medical advance directive, is evidence that our society is eager to leave the established legal-psychiatric order undisturbed.

2

The use of force vis-à-vis adults is a privilege reserved to the modern state, that is, to its duly authorized agents. In the eyes of the law, confinement, regardless of how it is justified, is deprivation of liberty. It may be just or unjust, but it is loss of liberty. This is what makes coerced psychiatric "care" similar to law enforcement and punishment for crime, and different from medical care and treatment for disease. At the same time, the psychiatrist's legally and socially validated claim that *his* coercion is treatment, not punishment, makes psychiatric coercion appear to be similar to health care and unlike imprisonment for crime.

The history of liberty teaches us that attempts to define the limits of power go hand in hand with the legitimation of power. Religion, Politics, and Law, each protects liberty, and each also justifies limiting it. Religious coercion poses no moral or political problems for members of a community who share the view that the religious beliefs and practices are matters of the utmost concern for its safety and well-being. In such a group, the practice of coercion in the name of God is legitimate, a virtue. Only in a community that shares the view that religious beliefs and practices are matters of private conscience, provided they do not violate the criminal laws, does religious coercion become a problem, indeed a crime. As Jefferson memorably put it: "The legitimate powers of government extend to such acts only as are injurious to others. But it does me no injury for my neighbor to say there are twenty gods, or no God. It neither picks my pocket nor breaks my leg."[6] It also does me no injury for my neighbor to say that he is God or that God is talking to him.[7] Religious tolerance is a virtue. "Psychiatric tolerance" is the opposite—a callous disregard of the mental patient's need for involuntary treatment. Indeed, in a therapeutic society such tolerance may be redefined as reprehensible neglect and dereliction of the duty to provide "life-saving treatment for mental illness."

Locke and the Founders understood that social cooperation requires a measure of maturity, of personal and moral development, and of self-restraint, and that infants and idiots lack these qualities, necessary for full membership in society. Accordingly, they placed "Lunaticks" and "Madmen" in the same category as infants, individuals unable to survive without care. It is our task to remedy their facile and erroneous categorization. In the twenty-first century, the typical person classified as mentally ill is not like a helpless infant. If he were, he would not protest his confinement and would not present the social problems he often presents. It behooves persons unable to tolerate behaviors our society defines as symptoms of mental illness to reject psychiatric coercions and develop methods of controlling persons who exhibit them more in harmony with modern ideas of personal autonomy, individual liberty, and the right to substantive due process. Such *emancipation of the mentally ill from psychiatric slavery*—respecting their right to liberty and privacy and their responsibility for legal and social transgressions—may appear unrealistic and uncompassionate to many people today. They ought to remember John Stuart Mill's wise observation of nearly one hundred fifty years ago:

> The entire history of social improvement has been a series of transitions, by which one custom or institution after another, from being a supposed primary necessity of social existence, has passed into the rank of a universally stigmatized injustice and tyranny. So it has been with the distinctions of slaves and freemen, nobles and serfs, patricians and plebeian; and so it will be, and in part already is, with the aristocracies of color, race, and sex.[8]

And so it has been with drapetomania, masturbatory insanity, nymphomania, and homosexuality, and so it ought to be with depression, schizophrenia, attention deficit hyperactivity disorder, and all the other "mental disorders."

3

Ida Macalpine (1899-1974) and her son, Richard Hunter (1923-1981), both psychiatrists, are two of the most important twentieth-century historians of psychiatry. In 1963, in their monumental *Three Hundred Years of Psychiatry, 1535-1860: A History Presented in Selected English Texts,* they observe: "There can as yet be no definitive history of the subject since psychiatry is still too little differentiated from its past."[9] This is a remarkable statement, the more so because psychiatry is much older than other medical specialties, such as neurology or nephrology.

How do present psychiatric principles and practices resemble seemingly different psychiatric principles and practices in the past? Hunter and

Macalpine answer: "Rather than a chronicle of feats, facts, and discoveries, the history of psychiatry presents a record of perennial problems, recurrent ideas, disputes and treatments, trailing in the wake of medicine and exhibiting…a mixture of as many false facts as false theories."[10] In other words, the ruling principle in the history of psychiatry is: *plus ça change, plus c'est la même chose.* Why is this so? Hunter and Macalpine neither raise nor answer the question. I will: it is so because psychiatry masquerades as a medical specialty. The truth is that mad-doctoring, unlike medicine, came into being as an arm of the coercive, social-control apparatus of the state and has continued to perform that function to this day. What distinguishes psychiatrists from other physicians and indeed other professionals is their legally authorized power to impose their "services" on individuals without their consent, indeed against their will. This reality, a source of both pride and shame for psychiatrists, accounts for the mutual antagonism between psychiatrists and mental patients (especially if they are incarcerated), and is the reason for the violence endemic to mental hospitals and other so-called mental-health facilities.

Ironically, Hunter and Macalpine themselves present a wealth of evidence that compels the conclusion that psychiatry is not a bona fide branch of medicine. Yet they cannot accept this view. No psychiatrist or historian of psychiatry can do so, without jeopardizing his good standing with the profession and the public. Like Jefferson, who recognized the horrors of slavery but, eager to be an American patriot, was unwilling to publicly denounce that institution, Macalpine and Hunter, eager to be psychiatric patriots, were unwilling to denounce the psychiatric slavery their work documented.

4

The typical relationship between doctor and patient rests, and has always rested, on consent. In contrast, the typical relationship between mad-doctor and madman rests, and has always rested, on coercion. The paradigmatic psychiatric act is the use of force, which takes two forms. One is involuntary mental hospitalization, called "civil commitment," the alleged justification for this deprivation of liberty being the need to protect the patient from himself (his illness), and the public from the patient (his dangerousness). The other intervention is the excusing of the person guilty of a crime by attributing his unlawful behavior to mental illness, a practice called the "insanity defense." The alleged justification for this deprivation of liberty is that it "humanizes" the criminal law by sentencing the mentally ill offender to treatment instead of punishment.

In both cases, the result is the subject's incarceration, called "hospitalization." Once we recognize these facts, and the self-evidently fictitious nature of mental illnesses, the barriers identified by Hunter and Macalpine against writing a definitive history of psychiatry disappear. Perforce, such a history must differ radically from conventional hagiographies of mad-doctoring modeled on histories of medicine.

Faced with a long series of inconvenient facts, Hunter and Macalpine avert their eyes from the evidence and declare their loyalty to psychiatry: "The historian of the contemporary scene must work from a viewpoint. Ours is that psychiatry is foremost a branch of medicine.... Patients suffer from mental symptoms which like bodily symptoms are caused by disease."[11] *Ipse dixit.*

Are psychiatrists deceiving themselves or the public? Are priests deceiving themselves or the public? These are poorly framed questions. "It is not miracles that generate faith, but faith that generates miracles," observed Fyodor Dostoevsky (1821-1881). Priests and pious persons alike believe in God, the beliefs of each party validating and supporting the beliefs of the other. Similarly, psychiatrists and educated persons believe in mental illness, the beliefs of each party validating and supporting the beliefs of the other. People believe in religion and psychiatry because they prefer the consequences of holding such beliefs to the consequences of rejecting them. That is why people do not like to be un-deceived or dis-illusioned, especially by others, and why exposing naked emperors is an unrewarding enterprise. *Disillusion, like illusion, must come from within.* So long as the illusion remains, it is the individual's and the culture's reality. In modern Western societies, the view that mental illness is an illness "like any other" and that mental hospitalization is therapeutic is considered an important humanitarian-scientific insight, not an illusion. This reality has framed and continues to frame the context for psychiatric historiography.

"You cannot judge a book by its cover," says the proverb. Nor can you judge what psychiatrists do by *what they say they do.* What psychiatrists in fact do is self-evident: they stigmatize people, deprive them of liberty, injure their bodies and minds by means of forcibly imposed physical and chemical agents and interventions, and call their actions the "diagnosis and treatment of disease." They do not, of course, do this all by themselves. In the ordinary course of events, the "prepatients"—to use Erving Goffman's felicitous term—are first stigmatized by their families or peers.[12] The psychiatrist makes the unofficial stigma official by pinning a psychiatric diagnosis on the subject. The diagnosis is a double stigma, identifying the subject as both deranged and dangerous.

I reject the disease-categorization of behaviors called "mental illnesses." Hence, I shall not be concerned with the alleged therapeutic effectiveness or ineffectiveness of psychiatric treatments. In a free society, providing products and services intended to help people is legitimized by the buyer's informed consent based on the seller's non-fraudulent representation, not by the "proven" helpfulness of the product or service. In psychiatry, providing products and services ostensibly intended to help mental patients is legitimized by the supposedly scientifically demonstrated effectiveness of the intervention, not the subject's informed consent to it. Hence the endless controversies—ironically themselves the sources of immense existential benefit and economic profit to psychiatrists—about whether one or another treatment for mental illness "works."

Language, law, medicine, and tradition define psychiatry as a medical specialty: we speak and write about psychiatric "illnesses," "patients," "symptoms," "diagnoses," and "treatments." Accordingly, that is how psychiatric historians view psychiatry and why they perceive psychiatrists as combating diseases of the mind on the model of physicians combating diseases of the body.

The military metaphor—the microbe hunter "waging war" against illness-as-enemy, seeking out and destroying the spirochete of syphilis or the bacillus of tuberculosis—fits contagious diseases well enough to be useful for understanding medical efforts to conquer them. However, the military metaphor does not fit the struggle against mental illnesses, and is worse than useless for understanding the history of psychiatry. The psychiatrist *says* that he fights against mental illness, that mental illness is the enemy. But if there is no mental illness, this cannot be true. What, then, does the psychiatrist fight against? Against freedom! Consider the correct parallel. The medical doctor fights against the microbes that make the patient dangerously ill: he engages in *bactericide*. The psychiatric doctor fights against the freedom that makes the mental patient "dangerous to himself and others": he engages in *liberticide*.

The phenomena we call "mental illnesses" are not external to, or separate from, "mental patients." So-called mental illnesses are unwanted behaviors, not diseases. The forcible control of persons is coercion, not cure. Conventional psychiatric historiography rests on a monstrous mendacity, the claim that *the psychiatric use of force is care and cure, not coercion.* In 1817, John Haslam (1764-1844), then one of the leading alienists in England, stated: "Abundant experience teaches us that restraint is not only necessary as a protection to the patient and those about him, but that it also contributes to the cure of insanity."[13] In modern, intellectually respectable circles, this mendacious mantra has hardened into sacred dogma: the insane person has no voice, hence he cannot be dispossessed of one. The following letter in the *New York Review of Books* is illustrative. Replying to a review by prominent British historian J. H. Plumb (1911-2001), Ian R. Christie, Professor Emeritus of British History at the University of London, writes: "I disagree wholly with Jack Plumb's discussion of George III's illness in his recent review.... Plumb refers to George III's fears of losing his sanity; *but any competent alienist would point out that the insane never recognize that they are in such a condition. George III's self-knowledge on this subject is in fact one of the clearest proofs that he was perfectly sane.*"[14]

This premise—"that the insane never recognize that they are in such a condition" and that this requires and justifies a coercive-paternalistic posture toward them—is intrinsic to the concept of "the insane," the practice of psychiatry, and the proper style of writing about psychiatry. Thus, psychotherapy is not a dialogue but an operation the surgeon-doctor performs on the patient. "Far better results may then be achieved by a combination of psychotherapy with one or another of the newly introduced modern shock treatments, or with operations on the brain."[15]

5

Long before I entered medical school, I suspected that mental illness was a medical fiction. By the time I graduated, I had no doubt about it. When I discontinued my postgraduate training in internal medicine and decided to become credentialed as a psychiatrist, I did so, in part, because I wanted to critique psychiatric fictions and state-sponsored psychiatric violence, much the way Voltaire critiqued *l'infame*, "that infamous thing," his term for theological fictions and the violence intrinsic to the alliance of church and state.

The problem we face is not a matter of ideas or words; it is a problem of justifying and legitimating the use of force. The exercise of legitimated force, a prerogative of the (modern) state, makes coercion virtuous, not wicked. There is a long historical tradition according to which the dispossessing, imprisoning, and killing of the other in the name of religion/God makes those deeds virtuous, not wicked. In truly revolutionary spirit, the Founders rejected the religious-theological sanctification of violence. They separated church and state. They did not anticipate, nor could they have anticipated, that the idea of mental health and the alliance of psychiatry and the state might one day replace the idea of salvation and the alliance of church and state, in short, that the therapeutic state might supplant the theological state.[16]

Most scientists in fields having to do with mental health—from evolutionary psychologists to cognitive scientists and psychiatrists—affirm the doctrine that mind is brain and that brain is mind. The operative term in the formal definition of psychiatry is "mental disease." The psychiatrist's power to persecute and punish rests on *mental health laws*, not *brain health laws*. If mental disease is brain disease in the same sense that the Eucharist is the body and blood of Jesus Christ, what then is psychiatry? It is a pseudoscientific statist religion, the study and teaching of psychiatric fictions authoritatively acclaimed as scientific truths, and the enforcement of social controls rationalized by pseudo-medical diagnoses and defined as treatments.

Without exception, historians of psychiatry treat Freud and psychoanalysis as integral parts of psychiatric history. Frank Heynick, a physician and would-be psychiatric historian states:

> Freud and Kraepelin, the two great pillars of modern psychiatry, were both born in 1856, only three months and 300 miles apart. But whatever the conjunction of planets, the time and place of their appearance on the medical scene were ideal. For the late 19th century, especially in the German-speaking lands of Europe, was an era of breathtaking advances in medicine.... They shared a strong scientific interest in language and in dreams (albeit for different reasons) and also broad cultural interests in ancient civilizations, theater, and humor. But the focus of their respective work was so very different—Freud on neuroses and the psychological, Kraepelin on psychoses and the somatic—that they made virtually no reference to one another. They never met or corresponded. To return to our astrology metaphor: The lifelines of Freud and Kraepelin were destined never to cross.[17]

Freud was not a psychiatrist. Freud's and Kraepelin's lives never crossed because the objects of their study were radically different. One of my aims in this critical history of psychiatry is to demonstrate the folly of commixing psychoanalysis and psychiatry—contract and coercion—and treating them as a single subject, a type of medical practice devoted to remedying the same diseases, or even, *horribile dictu*, the same "science." Notwithstanding his vigorous defense of coerced treatment, even the president of the American Psychiatric Association feels compelled to acknowledge the incompatibility of consent and coercion. In an editorial titled "Caring versus Coercion: Differences are Clear," Steven S. Sharfstein writes: "Fortunately, the overwhelming majority of encounters between psychiatrists and patients involve our provision of treatment of voluntary, help-seeking patients."[18] I maintain that as long as psychiatrists cling to caring by coercion, all of psychiatry is tainted by coercion.

Furthermore, virtually all histories of psychiatry are Whig interpretations, painting pictures of unrelenting psychiatric progress, a steady scientific advance in the *diagnosis and treatment of mental illnesses*. This should not surprise us. Rejecting the reality of mental illness and the benevolence of psychiatry is scientific heresy. It automatically brands the heretic as ignorant of "breakthroughs" in modern neuroscience and of the humane "treatment of severe mental illnesses." For example, historian Norman Dain recognizes the cogency of my insistence that the core problem of psychiatry is the psychiatrist's privilege and power to deprive his patient of liberty, but he is so hostile to this view that he distorts and dismisses it. Dain writes: "The most influential ideologist of the 'new' anti-psychiatry of the 1960s and 1970s was himself a medical psychoanalyst, Thomas Szasz, *whose position was a replay of the issues raised by moral treatment in the early nineteenth century.* Szasz was so attractive to many critics of psychiatry because he rejected the right of psychiatrists forcibly to institutionalize and treat people *who he said were as a rule not really mentally ill.*"[19] Dain's brief summary is long on malice and misrepresentation:

- Writers who support psychiatric fraud and force call themselves "academics" and "psychiatric historians." I oppose such practices and psychiatric historians call me an "ideologist" and "anti-psychiatrist."
- The term "moral treatment" was virtually synonymous with therapeutic coercion. The advocates of moral treatment opposed somatic treatments, not the use of force. Dain says my "position was *a replay of the issues raised by moral treatment.*"
- Dain states that I oppose depriving innocent persons of liberty and adds, *"who he said were as a rule not really mentally ill."* This qualification implies that I oppose only so-called "false commitment"—an absurd distortion of my views.

Psychiatric historian Gerald Grob, though no more sympathetic to my views, is more truthful than Dain. He writes: "[Szasz] was committed to nineteenth-century liberalism that made individual liberty the paramount value. His work emphasized two distinct but interrelated themes: 'the myth of mental illness,' and the role of psychiatry in suppressing noncomformity.... Commitment laws, ostensibly intended to promote the welfare of patients, actually enhanced what Szasz called the Therapeutic State.... As such, it [psychiatry] constituted a threat to individual liberty in a free society precisely because of its rejection of such values as personal autonomy, volition, liberty, and responsibility."[20]

6

In the days of the insane asylum, the nature of psychiatry was clear: the madhouse was a snake pit and snake pits could be found only in insane asylums. Today, the nature of psychiatry is unclear: "snake pits" are everywhere, from the kindergarten to the hospice, and the reality of psychiatric coercions and dehumanizations is camouflaged by a facade of fake diagnoses, outpatient commitment, the renaming of insane asylums as "health care facilities," and a lexicon of euphemisms concealing the exploitation and injury of so-called mental patients as "treatments."

I have never harbored any patriotic sentiments toward psychiatry. My aim has been to abolish psychiatric slavery, not reform it. In 1994, Roy Porter (1946-2002) and Mark Micale, both noted historians, summarized my approach to the history of psychiatry as follows:

> Szasz began from the premise that institutional psychiatry is an unsupportable enterprise because it is based on a notion of mental illness that is itself fictitious. Accordingly, Szasz viewed the history of "compulsory psychiatry" as a gigantic error, if not a gigantic evil.... In his view, the entire history of psychiatry is the obdurate and pitiless defense of a fantasy.... Szasz has offered fundamental rereadings of exemplary episodes and topics in the history of mental medicine, such as the role of doctors in the European witch-hunts, the medical practices of Benjamin Rush, the eighteenth- and nineteenth-century medical literature on masturbatory insanity, and past scientific writings about homosexuality. A time line appended to Szasz's *The Manufacture of Madness* (1970) enumerates with ironic commentary the landmark dates of the triumphalist Whig version of psychiatric history.[21]

If psychiatry remains undifferentiated from its past, it is because psychiatrists and mental patients alike are caught in a web of violence and counter-violence, oppression and rebellion: psychiatrists, patients, and the public continue to be fixated on the hopeless effort to "conquer" mental illness as if it were a disease like polio and feel unable to abandon the idea that the management of the (mis)behavior they mistake for a malady requires the use of state-sanctioned force. As prolegomenon to the systematic account of what I regard as the truth about the history of psychiatry presented in this book, I offer Roy Porter's restatement of the premises that underlie my writings on this subject:

> Perhaps most radically...Thomas Szasz deemed mental illness a mythic and monstrous beast, and proclaimed that "mental illness" was a fiction. Insanity, he has continued ever since to claim, is not a real disease, whose nature has been progressively scientifically unveiled; mental illness is rather a myth, forged by psychiatrists for their own greater glory. Over the centuries, medical men and their supporters have been involved, argues Szasz, in a self-serving "manufacture of madness." In this, he indicts both the pretensions of organic psychiatry and the psychodynamic followers of Freud, whose notion of the "unconscious" in effect breathed new life into the obsolete metaphysical Cartesian dualism. For Szasz, any expectation of finding the etiology of mental illness in body or mind—above all in some mental underworld—must be a lost cause, a dead-end, a linguistic error, and even an exercise in bad faith. "Mental illness" or the "unconscious" are not realities but at best metaphors. In promoting

such ideas, psychiatrists have either been involved in improper cognitive imperialism or have rather naively pictorialized the psyche—reifying the fictive substance behind the substantive. Properly speaking, contends Szasz, insanity is not a disease with origins to be excavated, but a behavior with meanings to be decoded. Social existence is a rule-governed game-playing ritual in which the mad person bends the rules and exploits the loopholes. Since the mad person is engaged in social performances that obey certain expectations so as to defy others, the pertinent questions are not about the origins, but about the conventions, of insanity. In this light, Szasz dismisses traditional approaches to the history of madness, as questions mal posés, and aims to reformulate them.[22]

Psychiatry, like religion, is a belief-system impregnated with rules and values, permissions and prohibitions. Psychiatric principles and practices are irrefutable and inviolable not because they are true or good, but because it is taboo to deny or reject them. Asserting that a respected social institution, such as religion or psychiatry, rests on a farrago of fables supported by force and rejecting it is disrespectful of received opinion and personally risky. Yet, embracing coercive social policies championed by custom and rationalized by fictions-as-facts is inimical to individual liberty, personal responsibility, and justice. We reject coercion in the name of religion and condemn persons who embrace violence in the name of God.[23] We ought also to reject coercion in the name of psychiatry and condemn persons who embrace violence in the name of mental health or psychiatric treatment.

Many people recognize that psychiatrists deal with human problems, not diseases of the brain, which fall in the domain of neurologists and neurosurgeons. However, it is one thing privately to recognize a "forbidden fact," another to accept its moral and social implications, and still another to proclaim publicly that the psychiatrist-emperor is not merely naked but a liar and an abuser of his fellow man, unworthy of being considered a member of a healing profession. Despite seemingly radical changes in psychiatric principles and practices during the past half century, I contend that the truth about this *mala fide* medical specialty remains so terrible that it invites disbelief.

1

Mental Hospitalization:
Therapeutic Imprisonment

Every confinement of the person is an "imprisonment," whether it be in a common prison, or in a private house, or in the stocks, or even by forcibly detaining one in the public streets.

—*Black's Law Dictionary*[1]

1

Although psychiatric illness is a fiction, psychiatric coercion is not. In this chapter, I examine how this practice came into being and offer some remarks about its present status.

Incarcerating people is what psychiatrists do. This is why mental illness is rightly considered a stigmatizing term and stigmatized condition, and psychiatry rightly considered a stigmatizing and stigmatized profession. Tennessee Williams was well aware of this when he wrote, "Confinement [in a mental hospital] has always been the greatest dread of my life."[2]

Consensual relations—religious, psychiatric, sexual—pose no special moral or political problems. Coercive relations do. We recognize this with respect to religious and sexual coercion, but not with respect to psychiatric coercion. American law prohibits involuntary religious practices and protects voluntary religious worship. In contrast, American law forcibly compels persons to submit to psychiatric practices and does not protect voluntary psychiatric relations. This development is emblematic of the transformation of traditional theological societies into modern therapeutic states.

For millennia, religious affiliations, beliefs, and practices were forcibly imposed on people and they, in turn, generally accepted this arrangement as the natural order of things. In many parts of the world, this is still the case. Children still "inherit" the religious status of their parents. It requires deliberate effort on the part of an adult to reject the religious affiliation ascribed to him by birth, and his effort is more likely to fail than succeed.

15

In the modern world, psychiatric identities ("diagnoses") and psychiatric interventions ("treatments") are routinely imposed on millions of persons, and they, in turn, often accept this arrangement without protest. It requires great effort on the part of a "diagnosed mental patient" to reject the psychiatric affiliation ascribed to him, and his effort is more likely to fail than succeed.

Despite these seemingly self-evident caveats, psychiatrists and writers on the history of psychiatry refuse to distinguish between voluntary and involuntary psychiatry, as if doing so were a kind of heresy. *In fact, it is heresy: a violation of the taboo against rejecting the analogy between bodily illness and mental illness.* By definition, there are no mental illnesses the presence of which can be detected by objective methods such as those used in the detection of microbial diseases. If there were such methods, the conditions would not be called or considered mental illnesses and could not be treated against the patient's will.[3]

A person infected with a microbial disease responsive to appropriate antibiotic treatment can be cured of his illness regardless of whether he voluntarily submits to treatment or is forcibly injected with the therapeutic agent. If we accept that mental illness is that kind of disease and if we also accept that mental patients, like infants, have no insight into their needs, then the forcible treatment of mental patients becomes just as beneficial and permissible as is the forcible treatment of sick infants.[4] Virtually all psychiatric historiography reflects blind adherence to this *pediatric model* of mental health care. The professionally correct approach to psychiatry does not merely fail to distinguish between voluntary and involuntary interventions, it refuses to acknowledge the difference between them.[5]

This refusal pervades the writings of the experts on modern psychiatric ethics. Paul R. McHugh, long-time professor and chairman of the Department of Psychiatry at the Johns Hopkins University Medical School, simply denies that psychiatrists deprive their hospitalized patients of liberty. He cites my book, *Schizophrenia: The Sacred Symbol of Psychiatry,* in which I write, "In other words, the identity of an individual with schizophrenia depends on the existence of the social system of [institutional] psychiatry," and he continues: "The only reply to such commentary is to know the patients for *what* they are—in schizophrenia, people disabled by delusions, hallucinations, and disruptions of thinking capacities—and *to reject an approach that would ... deny them their frequent need for hospital care.*"[6] McHugh, a prominent figure in American medical and psychiatric ethics, speaks of knowing mental patients for *what* they are, not for *who* they are, and describes the desire of relatives and psychiatrists to imprison them as the denominated patients' "need" for hospital care.

Sidney Bloch, professor of psychiatry at the University of Melbourne, Australia, and another prominent psychiatric ethicist, writes: "Ethical concerns about the psychiatrist's role and function have dogged the profession for at least three centuries. Moral harms have emerged from the misuse of asylum as a 'custodial warehouse,' misunderstanding of the transference relationship, the gruesome effects of physical treatments such as leucotomy [lobotomy] and insulin coma."[7] Lobotomy causes *physical harms*, not just moral harms. Note Bloch's silence about the neurological damage caused by ECT and psychotropic drugs, and his bracketing of involuntary psychiatric interventions with voluntary psychiatric relationships. He lists, as if they were the same kinds of harms, the physical and civil liberties injuries inflicted on mental patients by incarceration, coerced lobotomy and insulin shock on the one hand, and the harm the patient suffers as a result of "misunderstanding of the transference relationship," on the other hand. This is to equate rape with marital misunderstanding, violent crime with inevitable contingency.

2

In his classic, *The Mentally Ill in America: A History of Their Care and Treatment from Colonial Times,* journalist and psychiatric historian Albert Deutsch (1905-1961) declares, "It is safe to assume that mental disease has always existed among mankind."[8] Gregory Zilboorg, author of the standard *History of Medical Psychology,* begins the story of psychiatry with remarks about tuberculosis in the Stone Age, as if mental illnesses were similar to infectious diseases. Yet, even he acknowledges that "until the very end of the eighteenth century there were no real hospitals for the mentally sick.... Bedlam and Bicêtre were no more hospitals than a trench on a battlefield is a retreat and shelter of safety."[9] Franz Alexander and Sheldon Selesnick subtitle their *History of Psychiatry: An Evaluation of Psychiatric Thought and Practice from Prehistoric Times to the Present,* glibly pretending that there was, in ancient times, such a thing as "psychiatric thought and practice."[10] The truth is that the idea of mental illness and the incarceration of the mentally ill are recent historical phenomena. Nevertheless, psychiatrists maintain, and historians of psychiatry assume, that mental illnesses have existed at all times and in all cultures, but that people called them by different names, for example madness or possession. This is a facile and self-serving view, which, for reasons I have set forth in detail elsewhere, I reject.[11] Suffice it to say that people exhibiting odd and offensive behaviors have, of course, always existed. But the idea that such behaviors are the symptoms of medical, that is, "mental," illnesses is a modern idea, inseparably connected with the practice of incarcerating or otherwise coercing the persons exhibiting them. The only analogous medical practice is the segregation of individuals with contagious diseases, intended to protect the healthy members of society, not cure the patients.[12]

Historian Edward Shorter begins his *History of Psychiatry* by correctly stating, "Before the end of the eighteenth century, there was no such thing as psychiatry."[13] *Mutatis mutandis*, there was also no such thing as mental illness. This view Shorter emphatically rejects. Instead, he proclaims his belief in the existence of psychiatric illness as a disease entity outside of culture and history: "Having a partly biological and genetic basis, psychiatric illness is as old as the human condition.... It follows then that *human society has always known psychiatric illness*, and has always had ways of coping with it."[14] Shorter doesn't say what psychiatric illness is, or which part is "biological and genetic," and how he knows that.

David J. Rothman, professor of social medicine at Columbia University College of Physicians and Surgeons, is one of the rare historians of psychiatry sensitive to the role of coercion in so-called psychiatric hospital treatment. He notes that in the asylums one of the problems was "violence between patients, with staffs either too small or too uninterested to interfere,"[15] and cogently criticizes Clifford Beers's famous psychiatric autobiography, *A Mind That Found Itself* (1908).[16] Although Beers (1876-1943) felt abused during the three years he spent incarcerated in a mental hospital, he became a zealous mental health crusader and a founder of the American mental hygiene movement. Comparing mental illness to typhoid fever, Beers declared: "Most insane persons are better off in an institution than out of one.... I have criticized with considerable, yet merited, severity, our State Hospitals for the Insane. Nevertheless, these two hundred and odd hospitals, erected at a cost to the Nation of over one hundred millions of dollars, constitute the nucleus of what will, in time—if rightly managed—become *the most perfect hospital system in the world*."[17]

Skeptically, Rothman juxtaposes Beers's enthusiasm with the candid remark of an anonymous state mental hospital superintendent in 1920: "Is it not a confession of weakness to commit an act of grand larceny by assuming a name which we have not earned and thus take a short cut to popular favor? There is nothing to gain by masquerading in borrowed plumage."[18] Citing a Massachusetts asylum superintendent's boast about the hospital's "various industries and kinds of employment...[in] the daily routine work of the hospital, the farm, kitchen, laundry, stable, engineer's department, domestic work of all kind, etc., in all of which patients take an active part," Rothman disdainfully comments: "It remains very doubtful that inmate labor was more a mode of therapy than of institutional peonage, more a matter of treatment than of exploitation.... In hospital economy employment established a blessed circle: work is good for the patient and the patient is good for work."[19] Rothman flirts with the idea that the whole business of defining psychiatric coercion as medical treatment may be a hoax, but stops short of reaching that conclusion:

> [T]o confuse menial labor with therapy indicates just how crude the state of treatment was.... It may well be, with all the advantages that hindsight allows, that reformers made a fateful mistake in helping to justify a custodial role for the state hospitals.... As the performance of the state hospitals over these decades makes amply clear, institutional survival, not patient welfare, was the ultimate consideration."[20]

Having said this, I must add that Rothman's psychiatric historiography displays many of the same flaws as do those that I have surveyed, plus one: he overemphasizes the similarities among the juvenile justice system, the criminal justice system, and the mental health system. To be sure, there are some similarities. However, no one believes that children who fall into the net of the juvenile justice system or adults into the net of the criminal justice system suffer, *ipso facto*, from brain diseases and need psychiatric treatment for their brain-mind disorder, whereas this is what psychiatrists now preach, and most people now believe, about persons who fall into the net of the mental health system. The so-called medical model of mental illness—there is no other model of it, nor can there be—requires either regarding the mental health system as fundamentally different from the criminal justice system or rejecting mental illness as a misleading metaphor. Rothman does neither. Instead, he protects himself from being branded as an "antipsychiatrist" by assuming the stance of a psychiatric apologist: "However disappointing the outcome of Progressive [sic] efforts, *the analysis here is far more favorable to the prospects of constructive change within the systems of criminal justice and mental health care than might be at first imagined.*"[21] Rothman does not say what a system of psychiatric coercions reformed by the "constructive changes" to which he alludes would look like. In the Foreword to the revised edition of Rothman's *Conscience and Convenience*, Thomas G. Blomberg, professor of criminology at Florida State University, writes: "In communicating the story of these progressive reforms, Rothman reveals an unbroken pattern of good intentions leading to bad consequences."[22]

3

Samuel Johnson's remark, "Hell is paved with good intentions," has become a cliché. Nevertheless, we accept every new psychiatric brutality called "reform" as if we had never been warned. But we have been warned, time and again, as for example by Daniel Webster: "Good intentions will always be pleaded for every assumption of authority. It is hardly too strong to say that the Constitution was made to guard the people against the dangers of good intentions."[23] With his customary acuity, Gilbert K. Chesterton (1874-1936) observed: "The business of Progressives is to go on making mistakes. The business of Conservatives is to prevent mistakes from being corrected."[24]

The terms "reform" and "progressive" prejudge the phenomena to be explained and preempt debate. "Progressive reform," a pleonasm, accomplishes this even more effectively. Not surprisingly, persons who propose new social policies invariably call them "reforms" and "progressive." The truth is that liberals and conservatives, Democrats and Republicans, have outdone one another in their vigor in waging the war on mental illness. This has not prevented some experts on mental health policy from casting conservatives as psychiatric slave holders, and liberals as psychiatric abolitionists. In *Back to the Asylum* (1992), John Q. La Fond and Mary L. Durham—one a law professor, the other a medical sociologist—write:

> There has recently been a clear pendulum swing in how society perceives and treats the mentally ill. From about 1960 to about 1980—a period we will call the Liberal Era—law and mental health policy strongly emphasized fairness to mentally ill offenders...and permitted most other mentally ill individuals to live in the community, largely free of government interference. From about 1980 on—a period we will call the Neoconservative Era—there has been a noticeable reversal in these policies. ...there was growing pressure to return the mentally ill to the "asylum" of prisons and mental hospitals, a trend that continues to this day.... The Liberal Era toleration of personal differences and protection of individual rights gave way in the 1980s.... Tolerance for those who were different or dangerous evaporated almost overnight.[25]

This is a wholly imaginary story. For two centuries—ever since Pinel's iconic striking off the chains of lunatics—persons incarcerated by psychiatrists have been the beneficiaries of one well-intentioned reform after another, each leaving them worse off than before. I believe we ought to consider the possibility that persons whose passion is to devise novel coercive mental health measures are badly intentioned and the consequences of their policies are the punishments the "reformers" believe the mentally ill deserve. No mainstream psychiatric historian has proposed abolishing psychiatric coercion. Because I have done so, Gerald N. Grob calls my historical analysis of psychiatry "ostensibly historical" and dismisses it as an "attack on psychiatry from the libertarian right."[26] He writes:

> "To maintain that a social institution suffers from certain 'abuses,'" he [Szasz] wrote in an ostensibly historical work [*The Manufacture of Madness*], "is to imply that it has certain desirable or good uses. This, in my opinion, has been the fatal weakness of the countless exposés—old and recent, literary and professional—of private and public mental hospitals. My thesis is quite different. Simply put, it is that there are, and can be, no abuses of Institutional [coercive] Psychiatry, because Institutional Psychiatry *is,* itself, an abuse."[27]

I wrote these words in the late 1960s and have had no reason to change my opinion. Since then, we have witnessed more psychiatric "good intentions leading to bad consequences," such as outpatient commitment and the indefinite psychiatric incarceration of so-called sex offenders who have completed their prison sentences, each reform imposed on its beneficiaries by force, each in turn denounced in new exposés. Never at a loss for new reforms, "progressive" psychiatrists, such as Steven S. Sharfstein and E. Fuller Torrey, now propose to remedy the system by "caring coercion" combined with forced treatment to overcome "anosognosia," the long-sought brain lesion that causes the patient to lack insight into his need for the psychiatric treatment *de jour.*[28] Attributing anosognosia to anyone who resists the psychiatrist's offer of help eliminates, once and for all, the troublesome concept of liberty from the psychiatric vocabulary.

The Treatment Advocacy Center (TAC)—Torrey's influential lobby for psychiatric coercion—recommends the widest possible use of outpatient commitment because it is a form of coercion the coerced person supposedly does not perceive as coercion. Calling it "leverage," not coercion, Mary T. Zdanowicz, the Executive Director of TAC, states: "Outpatient commitment is preferable to other forms of leverage because the level of perceived coercion is comparable to voluntary care..."[29] Regarding the matter of anosognosia, a TAC "Briefing Paper" explains:

> Anosognosia (impaired awareness of illness)...is the single largest reason why individuals with schizophrenia and bipolar disorder do not take their medications. This impaired awareness of illness is caused by damage to specific parts of the brain, and affects approximately 50 percent of individuals with schizophrenia and 40 percent of individuals with bipolar disorder.... People with impaired awareness of illness may not recognize that they are ill. Instead, they believe their delusions are real...and that

their hallucinations are real.... Impaired awareness of illness is the same thing as lack of insight. The term used by neurologists is "anosognosia," which comes from the Greek word for disease (*nosos*) and knowledge (*gnosis*).[30]

Xavier Amador, professor of psychology in the Department of Psychiatry at Columbia University College of Physicians and Surgeons, is another anosognosia enthusiast. Among his credentials he lists having "a brother, Henry, who has schizophrenia."[31] Amador evidently believes that such personal information is relevant to his ostensibly neurological argument and that his brother's privacy is of no consequence. He explains:

> Anosognosia bears a striking resemblance to the type of poor insight we have been discussing [such as occurs in some patients with strokes].... Like neurological patients with anosognosia, they [seriously mentally ill patients] appear rigid in their unawareness, ... The bottom line to all of this research is that more likely than not, a broken brain is creating barriers to insight and acceptance of treatment in mentally ill persons you're trying to help. There are two immediate ways in which you can use this knowledge to benefit your loved one and yourself. First, when faced with the frustration of trying to convince her to get help, remember *the enemy is brain dysfunction*, not the person.[32]

Such "research"—by a professor in one of America's leading medical institutions, endorsed by leading mental health professionals—is an embarrassment that will be hard to expiate or expunge. To sum up, we are told that the brain damage called "anosognosia" converts a legally competent person who rejects psychiatric help into a psychiatrically disabled patient who needs coerced treatment for his own benefit.

In *The Old Régime and the French Revolution* (1856), Alexis de Tocqueville (1805-1859) observed that the Revolution went astray because "the desire for reforms took precedence of the desire for freedom."[33] True liberty for the mental patient was never on the psychiatric reformers' agenda. The refusal to recognize this accounts for the failure of the potted and Whiggish histories of psychiatry.

My critique of the psychiatrist's passionate commitment to coercion has left a mark on at least one prominent psychiatrist. Karl Menninger (1893-1990), co-founder of the famous Menninger Clinic and a major player in the madhousing business, reigned as the undisputed leader of his profession during the postwar years. He and I were on friendly terms. In 1988, Menninger wrote me: "Dear Dr. Szasz: / I am holding your new book, *Insanity: The Idea and Its Consequences,* in my hands.... I think I understand better what has disturbed you these years and, in fact, it disturbs me, too, now. We don't like the situation that prevails whereby a fellow human being is put aside, outcast as it were, ignored, labeled, and said to be 'sick in his mind.'"[34] In a language at once touching and melancholy, Menninger briefly reviewed the history of psychiatry, the tenor of his remarks illustrated by the following sentence: "Added to the beatings and chainings and baths and massages came treatments that were even more ferocious: gouging out parts of the brain, producing convulsions with electric shocks, starving, surgical removal of teeth, tonsils, uteri, etc."[35] Unfortunately, Menninger expressed this view only at the end of his long life.[36]

4

At the beginning of the seventeenth century, when Shakespeare wrote his immortal plays, there were neither psychiatrists nor mental hospitals.* A century later, there were "mad-doctors" who plied their "trade in lunacy," which is what the business of operating private madhouses was called.[37] How did this happen? How did psychiatry, composed of the idea of mental illness, the institution of the insane asylum, and the practice of incarcerating individuals deemed to be insane, come into being?

As a healing art or practice, medicine is as old as mankind. Its source lies in the sick person's suffering and seeking relief from it. That is not how psychiatry began. The existence of madness or mental illness as abnormal behavior is intrinsic to society, to people living together governing themselves and one another by sets of rules called custom, religion, and law. It is inherent in the concept of abnormal behavior that it is conduct that displeases others and causes them to suffer. As a rule, the person said to be having a mental illness does not suffer and does not seek psychiatric help. He makes others suffer, and it is they who seek psychiatric help for their suffering by removing its source, that is, by imprisoning the disturbing person. In 1800, the mad-doctor "treated" persons who did not want to be his patients, for behaviors that embarrassed and upset their relatives or society. Typically, today's psychiatrist does the same.[38]

By calling persons subjected to psychiatric coercion "patients," psychiatrists and psychiatric historians misrepresent the simple fact that such persons are not patients in the usual sense of the term. Typically, physically ill persons accept the patient role and are cared for without being subjected to coercive social control. In contrast, many mentally ill persons reject, or would like to reject, the role of mental patient; this is one of the main reasons why they are subjected to coercive social control.

---

*There were a few facilities—such as Bethlehem Hospital, better known as Bedlam—for confining a small number of paupers deemed insane.

Madness and its synonyms are fuzzy terms. It is clear, however, that mad persons are unwanted persons and that we use the term broadly to refer to abnormal, unwanted behavior.[39] As a rule, a person behaves "madly" for reasons of his own, that is, because of the particular adaptation he has made to the events that comprise his life. Examples abound, especially instructively in literature. King Lear goes mad because of his poor choice of a retirement plan. Lady Macbeth is driven mad by guilt and remorse over a criminal career. Hamlet breaks down under the stress of discovering that his mother and uncle murdered his father. Yet, none of these persons is relocated in a madhouse. Why? Because there are as yet no madhouses. A century later, the practice of resolving similar family problems by the stronger party's forcible rehousing of the weaker one in a private madhouse was well on its way to becoming accepted in principle, established in practice, ratified by law, and embraced by the public. *Pari passu*, the retrospective falsification of psychiatric history quickly goes into high gear.

For example, when Sir John Bucknill (1817-1897), one of the founders of British psychiatry, looked at the protagonists of Shakespeare's great tragedies, he saw nothing but madness—an illness in the literal, medical sense of the term.[40] He knew, of course, that there were no insane asylums in England in 1600. In *The Mad Folk of Shakespeare* (1859), Bucknill wrote, "In his [Shakespeare's] time the insane members of society were not secluded from the world as they are now."[41] Instead of interpreting the absence of mental hospitals in Shakespeare's time as a sign that there was more tolerance for personal eccentricity in Elizabethan than in Victorian England, Bucknill continued: "The consistency of Shakespeare is in no characters more close and true, than in those most difficult ones wherein he portrays the development of mental unsoundness, as in Hamlet, Macbeth, and Lear;... It is on the development of insanity ... that the great dramatist delights to dwell."[42]

In Bucknill's view, Shakespeare describes the development of mental diseases. In my view, Shakespeare paints imperishable literary portraits of grand moral dilemmas and moral failures. Consider the case of Lady Macbeth's madness. After a long, bloody struggle, Macbeth destroys his rivals and reaches the pinnacle of political power. Unable to relish the role she so hungrily coveted, Lady Macbeth becomes unhinged by guilt. She is tormented by anguish, cannot rest or sleep, and "hallucinates" blood on her hands that she cannot wash away. Macbeth summons a doctor to cure her. He does not ask the doctor to discover what ails Lady Macbeth; he just wants him to restore her to her "premorbid" condition. However, the doctor, quickly grasping the meaning of Lady Macbeth's madness and her husband's desire to deny its meaning, tells Macbeth that his wife is "Not so sick, my lord / As she is troubled with thick-coming fancies / That keep her from her rest."[43] Macbeth is not satisfied. He presses the doctor with these immortal words: "Cure her of that: / Canst thou not minister to a mind disease'd, / Pluck from the memory a rooted sorrow, / Raze out the written troubles of the brain, / and with some sweet oblivious antidote / Cleanse the stuff'd bosom of that perilous stuff / Which weighs upon her heart?"[44]

The doctor, conscientious and wise, remains unmoved. His exemplary reply is, "Therein the patient / Must minister to himself."[45] This answer leaves the disturbed and disturbing persons to their own devices, to cope with their problematic lives as best they can. In my reading of this play, part of its message is that personal misconduct is not a disease; that the troubling consequences of moral failure do not constitute a treatable medical condition; that the mad person needs moral, not medical, guidance; and that, in the final analysis, the patient must "cure" himself. When this formula is inverted—when madness is accepted as a disease over which the patient has no control, and when the mad-doctor is empowered to control him by force and fraud—*then, and only then,* can mad-doctoring as a profession arise and coercion begin to masquerade as cure.

Soon after psychiatry as a profession begins, some psychiatrists note that psychiatric progress poses a threat to individual liberty. In his *Clinical Psychiatry in Imperial Germany*, historian Eric J. Engstrom cogently observes: "Wernicke noted that the medical treatment of [mental] patients began with the infringement of their personal freedom. Given the high premium placed upon personal freedom, Wernicke therefore reasoned that the responsibility of psychiatrists was enormous. In other words, by virtue of their carceral authority, psychiatrists had become the true guarantors of individual rights and the rule of law."[46]* Thus was the fox put in charge of guarding the rights of the chickens. And thus, too, did socialism as statist medicine put its foot in the door of Western capitalist societies. Wrote Albert Deutsch:

> Psychiatry, historically considered, occupies a rather unique place in the development of American medicine. From an institutional viewpoint, it has been practiced for decades as "state medicine" in a very literal sense. While heated debates still rage

---

*Karl Wernicke (1848-1904) was a famous Polish-born, German neuropathologist and neuropsychiatrist. He was the first to describe many neurological abnormalities, some of which are identified by his name, for example, Wernicke's aphasia and Wernicke's dementia.

around the general issue of "state medicine," it was a widely accepted principle in the care and treatment of the mentally sick a century or more ago.[47]

Deutsch alone, among psychiatric historians, recognized and emphasized the socialist-statist character of psychiatry, a basic feature of the mental-health professions that even contemporary libertarians tend to overlook.

5

The practice of psychiatry as we know it began in England in the eighteenth century when members of the upper classes began to "outsource" the care and coercion of certain embarrassing and troublesome relatives. In what ways did English men or women of means embarrass and offend their relatives, prompting them to take such action? They did so by deviant personal habits, for example by improvidence or self-neglect, behaviors that provided a convenient conceptual bridge between the old idea of incompetence and the new idea of insanity.[48] The law has long recognized imbecility or mental retardation as a justification for placing the mentally deficient person under guardianship. Now the law was asked to do the same for the "mentally deranged" person. Long before pauper lunatics were exiled to madhouses, propertied persons considered to be mad were managed in a manner that presaged the practice of present-day mad-doctoring: "Physical supervision and care of the disabled party was commonly handled by retaining a live-in servant, the so-called "lunatics keeper," a person usually of the same gender as the disabled individual.... Boarding out the lunatic or idiot at a private dwelling, in the company of a servant, was also commonplace; this practice in some respects anticipated the development of private madhouses in the eighteenth century."[49]

The nub of the history of psychiatry is the story of involuntary mental hospitalization: that is, *the removal of the unwanted person from his family or home, presented and publicly perceived as the treatment of the mentally ill person by psychiatrists struggling to cure mental illness.** Forcibly removed from his home, the mad person was forcibly re-housed in the home of a surrogate caretaker. The first such domiciles for housing the mentally ill, later called "mental hospitals," were the private homes of so-called asylum keepers, mainly clergymen or apothecaries.

---

*Here and elsewhere I omit scare quotes around the terms "mad," "sane," "insane," and "mentally ill." It is to be understood that these terms refer to roles, not conditions. The roles may be assumed or attributed.

Today, we associate mental illness with homelessness and poverty. In the eighteenth century, the typical person denominated as mad had a home and was well to do. The problem that commitment then posed was how to justify forcibly expelling such a person from his home and relocating him in someone else's home. Mad-doctors and laws regulating the management of private madhouses provided the justification. The practice of incarcerating rich persons in private madhouses was later extended to the incarceration of poor persons in public insane asylums.

Before the middle of the nineteenth century, when mass construction of lunatic asylums began, the practice of psychiatric confinement involved relatively few persons. Medical historian Roy Porter emphasizes that early psychiatry was *not* "a discipline for controlling the rabble.... Provision of public asylums did not become mandatory until 1845.... Even at the close of the eighteenth century, the tally of the confined mad poor in Bristol, a town of some 30,000, was only twenty... [Whereas] about 400 people a year were being admitted to private asylums."[50] In this connection, it should be noted that the conjoining of the terms "insane" and "asylum" results in an ironic inversion of the root meaning of asylum as a place of protection or refuge. For the asylum inmate, the insane asylum is a *place of imprisonment, not freedom.*

The creation of a system of private madhouses and the forcible rehousing of people in them entailed depriving the inmates of their basic right to liberty and required a persuasive justification. This was accomplished by analogizing the outsourcing of the care of mad persons to the outsourcing of the care of infants. Once society advances beyond the stage of subsistence economy, the role of the mother, in families able to afford domestic help, is often taken by surrogates—wet-nurses, governesses, and tutors. This arrangement served as the template for transferring the care of mad persons from family members to hired help. Delegating the care of an insane adult, however—especially if he resists being cared for—presents a problem very different from that of delegating the care of a child. Children have neither the physical strength nor the political power to resist being controlled by their parents and the parents' deputies. Adults do. Before an adult deemed to be insane can be treated as a madman, he must first be divested of his rights.[51] Reframing the political status of the insane adult as similar to that of a child accomplishes this task.

Consider the predicament of an upper-class person in England living with a spouse, elderly parent, or adult child who had flaunted convention and perhaps neglected her or his health, but was endowed by law and social status with the right to liberty and property. No longer could such persons be treated as they had been in earlier times—as members of the clan, devoid of individual rights, responsible to the group. The post-Enlightenment view of the rule of law destroyed the autocratic prerogatives of elders or the family vis-à-vis deviant adults. Increasingly, adult members of families were held together by cooperation and compromise, rather than coercion and domination. However, cooperation, as the term implies, requires a willingness to cooperate by at least two persons. One person's willingness to cooperate is useless vis-à-vis another person who is unable or unwilling to do so. Embarrassed or victimized by his (mad) kinsman, the (sane) relative lacked means by which to control him. The sane, or perhaps merely scheming, family member needed a socially acceptable legal method for gaining control over his troublesome, unwanted relative. Mental illness as medical disease, coercion as care, and mental health laws turning these fictions into facts, resolved this dilemma.

To establish themselves as respected medical professionals, mad-doctors had to medicalize madness and define it as a disease that deprives the patient of his mental faculties. It is the duty of the parent to control and care for the incompetent infant. Based on this model, it became the duty of the responsible family member to control and care for the relative rendered *non compos mentis* by his mental illness. Both elements, that is, the medicalization of madness and the infantilization of the insane, were needed to reconcile people's devotion to individual liberty and responsibility with their desire to relieve themselves of certain (troublesome) individuals by means other than those provided by the criminal law.

6

The disease model of derangement originated from, and was based on, a particular illness that is now, thanks to modern antibiotics, virtually extinct: general paralysis of the insane, paresis, a form of neurosyphilis. Some mad people suffered from syphilis, some did not. The paucity of medical knowledge in the eighteenth century made it virtually impossible to know whether a particular person's abnormal behavior was or was not due to a brain disease. I should add, however, that even then there was a simple and reliable method for distinguishing the person whose brain was being destroyed by syphilis from the person who was mad for other reasons: the syphilitic madman died, usually within a year or two after admission to hospital, whereas the healthy madman often outlived his sane mad-doctors.

The historical record is clear. When the trade in lunacy began, the asylums were privately owned and operated, and the individuals incarcerated in them were members of the propertied classes. This did not stop French philosopher and social critic Michel Foucault (1926-1984) from tracing the origin of the practice of incarcerating madmen to the large-scale confinement of urban indigents in France in the seventeenth century.[52] This thesis—that psychiatry was a new type of warfare between the haves and have-nots, the former labeling the latter as insane in order to remove them to the madhouse—is, as we have seen, false. And so, too, is the view that he rejected the concept of mental illness. In *Mental Illness and Psychology* (1954), Foucault stated: "The structural description of mental illness, therefore, would have to analyze the positive and negative signs for each syndrome.... The science of mental pathology cannot but be the science of the sick personality."[53] Nevertheless, many intellectuals who shared Foucault's anticapitalist-Marxist political sympathies embraced his version of psychiatric history. The truth is that the imprisonment of the Parisian rabble in *Hôpitaux Général* under the rule of Louis XIII had nothing to do with madness or medicine or hospitalization. The seventeenth-century French *Hôpital Général* had no doctors, nurses, or medical treatments and did not pretend to be a medical or therapeutic establishment. It was a prison-home for paupers and vagrants, the aged and the disabled. Translating *Hôpital Général* into General Hospital without explanation is to misname it and mislead the reader.*

Historian Edward Shorter states: "In England, it would be nonsense to speak, as the French philosopher Michel Foucault does, of any kind of 'grand confinement.'"[54] The incarceration of propertied persons in private madhouses came first and was followed, considerably later, by the incarceration of poor persons in public insane asylums.

Except for some historians of psychiatry, few people realize that the early madhouses were not hospitals, but the keepers' homes into which they took a few, often only one or two, madmen or mad women as involuntary boarders. As previously noted, the keepers who owned and operated these private madhouses were principally clergymen, not physicians. Once again, we touch here on the close connections between religion as the cure of souls, and psychiatry as the cure of minds. The practice of healing began as an undifferentiated religious-medical enterprise. Later, as the social world split into sacred and profane parts, the practice of healing also split, one part remaining a sacred, religious activity, the other becoming the secular profession of medicine. In the West, this separation occurred twice: First, with respect to the body, in

---

*The root meaning of hospital is a "place of hospitality" or "refuge." Before the modern age, the term "hospital" denoted a hospice, a charitable institution—for a pilgrim, traveler, or other person in need of a roof over his head and some sustenance—maintained by the church.

Greece, two and a half millennia ago; second, with respect to the mind, in England, less than four hundred years ago. Since the Enlightenment, spiritual and scientific healing have become, and have been perceived to be, distinct and separate enterprises.

There was a long-standing Western tradition of interpreting insanity in religious terms, attributing it to demonic possession, and treating it by means of exorcism. Viewed from that perspective, clerical coercion was a morally laudable and politically legitimate intervention, justified by both religion and law, church and state. When people believed that eternal life in the hereafter was more important than a brief sojourn on earth, torturing the possessed person to improve the quality of his life after death was regarded as an act of beneficence. Hence the long history of lawful clerical coercion.

In contrast, in the West, neither tradition nor law justified the use of force by physicians. The doctor of medicine, unlike the doctor of divinity, had no right to imprison and torture his patients. In fact, when Englishmen first tried to enlist the doctor in the diagnosis and disposition of their problematic relatives, the physician, as Shakespeare so magnificently showed, declined the invitation.

7

The physician's traditional avoidance of the use of force was consistent with his historical role. From ancient times, the medical healer's help was sought by suffering persons on their own behalf, or by healthy persons on behalf of relatives too disabled to seek help for themselves. The clergyman labored under no such tradition, which explains his role as pioneer mad-doctor and madhouse keeper. Subsequently, as the clergyman's power diminished and the mad-doctor's increased, theological coercion was replaced by psychiatric coercion.

The trade in lunatics must be understood in economic and social terms, rather than in medical terms. The enterprise satisfied the existential needs of the lunatics' relatives, and the economic needs of the entrepreneurs who supplied the required services.[55] The madhouse keeper's typical customers were socially prominent, wealthy individuals or families, able and willing to pay a servant able and willing to relieve them of the company of their unwanted relatives. The keepers were relatively impecunious, eager to please their paymasters.*

---

*Outsourcing the torture of suspected Muslim terrorists by the American government to the governments of certain Third-World countries is an example of a similar kind of collusion today.

The collusion between the madhouse keepers and their paymasters was an open secret. In 1815, Thomas Bakewell, the proprietor of a madhouse, observed, "The pecuniary interest of the proprietor and the secret wishes of the lunatics' relatives, led not only to the neglect of all means of cure, but also to the prevention and delay of recovery."[56] In 1825, another madhouse keeper wrote, "If a man comes in here mad, we'll keep him so; if he is in his senses, we'll soon drive him out of them."[57] The practice of involuntary mental hospitalization—the foundation of psychiatric slavery—thus began as a private, capitalist enterprise. Like chattel slavery, psychiatric slavery had of course to be sanctioned by the state, turning mad-doctors and psychiatrists into coercive agents of the state.[58]

The entrepreneurial origin of psychiatry as a form of private imprisonment needs to be reemphasized because, in the nineteenth century, madhousing became transformed into an essentially statist program of confining troublesome people, poor and rich alike. In the seventeenth century, England was a two-class society, consisting of those who owned property and those who did not. Because wealth, especially land, generated income, members of the propertied classes did not have to work to procure a livelihood for themselves and their families. The poor, whose only property was their labor, had to work or face destitution. Hence, their relatives had nothing to gain, and much to lose, by having them declared mad: *the poverty of the poor protected them from the "care" of the early mad-doctors.*

Ironically, long before the misery of poorly paid factory workers generated denunciations of private profit, the critics of private madhouses blamed the abuses of the trade in lunacy on the profit motive. It was an important factor, to be sure, but it was merely a symptom. Forbes Benignus Winslow (1810-1874), the proprietor of two private asylums, denounced the practice of patients' being "brought into the market and offered for sale, like a flock of sheep, to the highest bidder."[59] He was referring to the practice of madhouse keepers' advertising for "guests." A typical advertisement ran as follows: "Insanity. Twenty per cent annually on the receipts will be guaranteed to any medical man recommending a quiet patient of either sex, to a first class asylum, with highest testimonials."[60] Today, private mental hospitals not only advertise their services but encourage their staff to double as psychiatric bounty hunters. It hardly needs to be added that the contemporary psychiatrist hawks his wares not to the so-called patients but to their relatives who are eager to get rid of them. Since government and insurance programs now pick up the tab, this tactic has become more tempting and more popular than ever.[61]

Unfortunately, the early critics of the madhouse business aimed their fire at the wrong target. The root problem was power, not profit, the mad-doctor's state-sanctioned power to lawfully transform a sovereign British subject from a person into a mental patient and thus deprive him of liberty. My thesis that mad-doctoring, like limited government, the free market, and the workhouse, was an English invention is supported by the writings of seventeenth- and eighteenth-century English physicians, who maintained that mental illness was a peculiarly English malady. For example, in 1672, Gideon Harvey (1637-1700), physician to King Charles II, wrote a treatise titled, *Morbus Anglicus,* a term he used for the "hypochondriacal melancholy" he believed affected mainly English men and women.[62] In 1733, George Cheyne (1671-1743) popularized this notion in his classic, *The English Malady.*[63]

8

The madhousing of unwanted family members was a novel method for coping with certain age-old familial and social problems. Since every solution of a human problem creates a new set of problems, protests against the novel practice, usually called "reform," typically arise in the same cultural milieu as does the new practice. The Industrial Revolution and the Luddite revolt against the machine both began in England. So did the protests against what we now term "psychiatric abuses."

Official determination that an individual is insane, like official determination that he is guilty of a felony, justifies depriving him of liberty. The risks inherent in both practices are similar. In each case, a person might be wrongfully identified and wrongfully deprived of liberty. However, the analogy between crime and mental illness can easily mislead: it implies that depriving individuals correctly identified as mentally ill or as lawbreakers is right and proper. I disagree. This inference may be valid for criminals, but is invalid for mental patients. Nevertheless, preoccupation with the wrongful confinement of sane persons in insane asylums, called "false commitment," runs through the history of psychiatry like a red thread. It is characterized by the stereotypical claim of the incarcerated mental patient that he is sane and has been misdiagnosed as insane, maintaining, at the same time, that others incarcerated as insane are diagnosed correctly and confined properly. For centuries, the mad, no less than the sane, have accepted the principle that the illness called insanity justifies incarcerating the patient.

Madhouse inmates who claimed to be sane were, however, not the only critics of the early madhouse system. Their pleas were supported by journalists and men of letters who sought to alert the public to the fact that individuals were often committed not because they were insane but because they were victims of scheming relatives and greedy madhouse keepers. Unfortunately, obsession with false commitment reinforced the belief that incarcerating the "truly insane" was in the best interests of both the patient and society. The madhouse critique of Daniel Defoe (1660-1731), author of *Robinson Crusoe,* falls into this class. Like other madhouse reformers, Defoe objected only to the confinement of sane persons, an abuse he attributed partly to the selfishness of the relatives instigating the commitment process, and partly to the rapacity of the madhouse keepers:

> This leads me to exclaim against the vile Practice now so much in vogue among the better Sort, as they are called, but the worst sort in fact, namely, the sending their Wives to Mad-Houses at every Whim or Dislike, that they may be more secure and undisturb'd in their Debaucheries.... This is the height of Barbarity and Injustice in a Christian Country, it is a clandestine Inquisition, nay worse.... Is it not enough to make any one mad to be suddenly clap'd up, stripp'd, whipp'd, ill fed, and worse us'd? To have no Reason assign'd for such Treatment, no Crime alledg'd or accusers to confront?... In my humble Opinion all private Mad-Houses should be suppress'd at once.[64]

Note that Defoe is speaking, in 1728, *only* of the psychiatric incarceration of persons of "the better Sort," as he called members of the propertied class. The large-scale psychiatric incarceration of persons of "the worst sort," that is, the poor, did not begin in earnest until a century later. Defoe was not alone. In 1816, John Reid (1776-1822), a British mad-doctor, warned:

> A heavy responsibility presses upon those who preside or officiate in the asylums of lunacy. Little is known how much injustice is committed, and how much useless and wantonly inflicted misery is endured in these infirmaries for disordered, or rather cemeteries for deceased intellect.... Many of the depots for the captivity of intellectual invalids may be regarded only as nurseries for and manufactories of madness.[65]

Because the critics of false commitment never questioned the idea of mental illness or the morality of depriving individuals diagnosed as insane of liberty, their efforts were counterproductive. By shaming the madhouse keepers and society into prettifying the psychiatric plantations, the critics helped to preserve and strengthen the system of psychiatric slavery. The result was that psychiatrists became more adept at concealing their tortures as treatments and more shameless in their justifications of the use of force.[66] In 1890, the English psychiatrist Charles Mercier explained:

[T]he distinguishing feature of the insane is, not their dangerous aggressiveness, but their revolting indecency and obscenity.... It is not merely that the public must be protected from such conduct as this. They have a right, also, to be prevented from witnessing it, to be protected from the danger of witnessing it; and it is for this reason, more than for any other, that the seclusion of the insane in asylums is necessary and right.[67]

From then until past the end of World War II, the more the seclusion of the insane changed, the more it remained the same. The following vignette is illustrative. In 1952, Humphry Osmond (1917-2004), a British-born psychiatrist who coined the term "psychedelic," had accepted a job in the Canadian province of Saskatchewan, as clinical director of Saskatchewan Hospital.* "The place was touted as the finest mental hospital on the prairies.... Actually the place was so rank, so depressingly nineteenth-century-madhouse, that when Osmond and his colleagues received the APA's Silver Plaque award for most improved mental hospital, American customs declared the 'before' pictures to be obscene and special dispensation had to be obtained before they were allowed into the country."[68]

Unwilling and unable to come to grips with the misleading notion of mental illness, psychiatry needed a new "explanation" for the intrinsically intractable problems created by psychiatric slavery. It chose the large state mental hospitals. In 1958, Harry Solomon, president of the American Psychiatric Association, declared: "I do not see how any reasonably objective view of our mental hospitals today can fail to conclude that they are bankrupt beyond remedy."[69] It was time to get rid of the "obscene" state mental hospitals by diffusing the obscenity inherent in the practice of psychiatric coercion into society at large. This was the goal the architects of "deinstitutionalization" had set themselves. They quickly accomplished it.

9

Deinstitutionalization, that is, the policy and practice of transferring homeless, involuntarily hospitalized mental patients from state mental hospitals into many different kinds of *de facto* psychiatric institutions funded largely by the federal government, began in the United States and was quickly adopted by most Western governments. The plan was set in motion by the Mental Health Study Act, passed by Congress in 1955, mandating the appointment of a Commission to make recommendations for "combating mental illness in the United States."[70] The Act proclaimed:

---

*For a discussion of Osmond's work, see chapter 7.

"It is declared to be the policy of the Congress to [undertake an] *objective analysis of mental illness...*[and] *promote mental health.*"[71] In effect, the Act recast the nature and purpose of the American government, from protecting individual liberty and personal property to protecting the mental health of each citizen and of the community as a whole.

Looking to the Manhattan Project as a model of what the national government could accomplish, the American people and their political-psychiatric leaders assumed that victory in the War on Mental Illness was inevitable and imminent. It was just a matter of investing enough federal dollars in "psychiatric research." No one with political influence or media visibility pointed out the folly inherent in the project.

Mental diseases and antipsychotic drugs resemble infectious diseases and antibiotic drugs in name only. Psychiatry, allied with the state, was once again rushing headlong down a dead-end road. The taboo against scrutinizing the concept of mental illness and expressing misgivings about the legal compulsions intrinsic to the practice of psychiatry was intensified. It was a time for action, not caution. It was also a time of unparalleled opportunity for psychiatric opportunism. Vast amounts of federal moneys were made available for psychiatric research and training. The going joke was, "While you are up, get me a grant." The result is that today more Americans are mentally ill than ever, more are on drugs than ever, more patients are more personally disabled and socially destructive than ever, more people than ever live under the threat that their relatives, together with their psychiatrists, will incarcerate them to prevent their suicide—and the cost of caring for mental patients is far greater than ever.[72] In the 1950s, the cost of caring for a patient in a state mental hospital was as little in some areas as $1 per day. Now, the cost is $600 per day or more. To understand how we have arrived at this situation, it is not enough to understand the history of psychiatric drug use. It is necessary also to understand the story of the Joint Commission on Mental Illness and Health and its role in the reductionist-statist definition of mental illness as brain disease and in the reign of drugs-and-deinstitutionalization it sponsored and legitimized.

In 1962, the Joint Commission published its "Final Report" to Congress, entitled *Action for Mental Health*.[73] This was the document that informed President Kennedy's declaration about the dawn of a glorious new era in psychiatry and formed the basis of the Community Mental Health Centers program. The centerpiece of the *Report* was mental illness, authoritatively defined as brain disease, its frequency and severity dramatized by suitably sensational case histories. Thenceforth, the psychiatrically correct and compassionate concept of mental illness has been that it is a "no-fault" disease. Morally, the doctrine means that if a person succeeds in life, he deserves credit for his achievement; if he fails, he must not be blamed because he is a victim of mental illness. Medically, it means bracketing mental diseases with bodily diseases and declaring them "no-fault diseases." This is doubly foolish: a bodily disease—for example, diabetes or lung cancer—may be life-style related, but, in any particular case, it is often impossible to know whether it is or is not.

The ideas that inspired the authors of the *Report* were the familiar materialist-reductionist clichés of modern psychiatric scientism such as, "Human behavior is caused."[74] This premise negates the presumption that persons are moral agents responsible for their behavior and entails the authors' conclusions that mental illnesses have *material causes* and *material cures:* "These [antipsychotic] drugs have revolutionized the management of the psychotic patient." Supported by politicians and journalists, psychiatrists managed to convince the public that the care of mental patients had been revolutionized by antipsychotic drugs, much as the care of patients with infectious diseases had been revolutionized by antibiotic drugs. This latest psychiatric "revolution," however, is just a hugely successful public-relations scam. It helps psychiatrists to bury more deeply than ever the true nature of mental illnesses as public health/social problems, namely, that the typical chronic mental patient is unemployed and unemployable, homeless, economically dependent on his family or society, and inclined to violate marginal or not-so marginal social rules.

Carried away by the daring sweep of their grandiose lies, the writers of the *Report* contradict themselves, stating that "the [antipsychotic] drugs might be described as *moral treatment* in pill form."[75] Never mind that material causes and chemical cures are neither moral nor immoral. The *Report* enthusiastically endorses the policy of mandating a reduction of the patient population of state mental hospitals, that is, relocating chronic mental patients to different domiciles. Mental patients were discharged not because the new drugs cured their diseases, nor because they relieved their disability, nor because the patients wanted to leave, but because the federal government ordered it. Trying to conceal this, the members of the Joint Commission got so carried away by their rhetoric that they appeared to condemn involuntary mental hospitalization itself: "To be rejected by one's family, removed by the police, and *placed behind locked doors can only be interpreted, sanely, as punishment and imprisonment, rather than hospitalization.*"[76] Did official American psychiatry suddenly embrace

my views? Not exactly. I had advocated the abolition of psychiatric coercions and excuses. The Joint Commission advocated the expansion of
psychiatric coercions: to traditional civil commitment it added coerced
deinstitutionalization and coerced outpatient psychiatric drugging, and
it urged the federal government to relieve the states of the burden of
funding psychiatric services, training, and research.

In 1961, when *Action for Mental Health* appeared, I was a professor
of psychiatry at the SUNY Health Science Center in Syracuse, New
York,* and had just published *The Myth of Mental Illness*.[77] It seemed to
me then—and I have had no reason to change my opinion—that there
was something ominous about the Congress of the United States of
America's removing mental illness from the nether regions of psychiatry,
law, journalism, and popular prejudice, and placing it, with the stroke
of a legislative pen, in the category of genuine illness, a brain disease to
boot. Yet, psychiatrists, the families of mental patients, and the general
public regarded, and continue to regard, the use of the political process
to define mental illnesses as brain diseases as signifying momentous
scientific as well as moral progress. Laurie Flynn, then executive director
of the National Alliance for the Mentally Ill (NAMI), declared: "Spurred
on by the aggressive advocacy of NAMI families, the federal government
has finally taken action to place the brain back into the body. Congress
in June [1992] approved legislation to return the National Institute of
Mental Health under the umbrella of the National Institutes of Health....
Moving NIMH to NIH sends an important signal that mental illness is a
disease, like heart and lung and kidney diseases."[78]

Psychiatrists were ecstatic. A jubilant editorial in the *American Journal
of Psychiatry* declared: "The 'remedicalization' of psychiatry ...[and] the
provision of psychiatric care within the mainstream of medical economics
[have generated]...a broad movement toward the privatization of health
care [that] is now a 'megatrend' in mental health economics."[79] Since
few mental patients pay for their "hospitalization," calling this trend
"privatization" is laughable.

10

As the century was drawing to a close, disenchantment with deinstitutionalization—but not yet with antipsychotic drugs—was beginning
to set in. Critics denounced the dumping of the homeless mentally ill on

---

The institution was then called the State University of New York, Upstate Medical
Center, at Syracuse.

the streets and into inadequate "adult homes." In April 2002, the *New York Times* published the results of its yearlong investigation of the fate of thousands of mental patients expelled from state mental hospitals. The report was titled, "For mentally ill, death and misery":

> About 15,000 mentally ill adults...reside in more than 100 adult homes in the state, the majority in the city and its suburbs. Some are now larger than most psychiatric hospitals in the nation. The reality of the homes is far from what was envisioned. In the 1960's, New York, like other states, decided to shutter or sharply scale back its psychiatric wards, where patients often languished for decades. When the profit-making adult homes offered to shelter the discharged patients, the state embraced the idea. Federal disability money was used to pay the homes, which would provide meals, activities and supervision. The homes would bring in outside providers for psychiatric and medical care.... The government spends an average of $40,000 a year on each resident through federal disability and Medicare and Medicaid payments.... In the state's headlong drive to make its psychiatric wards obsolete, officials have publicly maintained for 30 years that the adult homes are a satisfactory substitute. The thinking is this: with psychotropic drugs, residents do not need close supervision. They will see therapists regularly, and when a crisis arises, they will be sent to a psychiatric ward.[80]

New York State Health Commissioner Antonia C. Novello, M.D., promptly issued a whitewash: "Dr. Novello said she will immediately commence a working group of experts to review the care being provided to adult home residents and to offer recommendations on how that care can be improved.... 'The State Health Department is doing more now than ever before to protect and provide a safe environment for residents of adult homes,' Dr. Novello said."[81] Throughout the nation, deinstitutionalized mental patients suffered the same fate. "In 1989, after surveying homes in several states, a Congressional committee called them 'a national tragedy.' ... The homes are typically run by businessmen with no mental-health training.... The homes are staffed largely by $6-an-hour workers who dispense thousands of pills of complex psychotropic drugs each day."[82]

Media exposés of the aftermath of deinstitutionalization abound, but no one in authority has any interest in asking the right questions. To make a career in mental health administration, all that is required is a talent for expressing indignation and laying the blame for the abuse of mental patients on anyone but those responsible for it. The title of a long report in the *Milwaukee Journal Sentinel* in March 2006 summarizes the scandal: "Mentally ill suffer deadly neglect: With a promise of community care, psychiatric wards were unlocked 30 years ago; today, the sickest patients live in squalor":

> The number of long-term psychiatric beds at Milwaukee County's facilities dropped from about 4,000 [in 1976] to roughly 100 today. But when social engineers pushed

the idea of closing mental hospitals and delivering health care in the community, they overlooked a critical element: Where would these people live? Who would take care of those who could not take care of themselves?... Preyed upon by opportunists and neglected by the people we pay to care for them, hundreds of Milwaukee's mentally ill people are fending for themselves. It's killing them—literally.... Tony Hall roasted to death in the stifling heat of an unregulated rooming house. Street thugs murdered David Rutledge. John Collins died after falling from his wheelchair, down the stairs of the unlicensed, mouse-infested group home where his Milwaukee County case-worker placed him. For months after Collins' death, someone kept using his food stamps.... Jim Hill, administrator of Milwaukee County's Behavioral Health Division, who oversees the psychiatric caseworkers, called the living conditions for many of Milwaukee's sickest patients "heartbreaking" but said his case managers often have no choice. "We're not in the housing business," he said. "We're in the mental health treatment business. Did you ask the city building inspectors why they don't go in and close these places down? Honestly, we can't do it all."[83]

Mr. Hill is mistaken. He *thinks* he is in the mental health treatment business, but in fact he *is* in the housing business. How do psychiatrists account for the disastrous consequences of deinstitutionalization? By crediting its alleged successes to neuroleptic drugs, and blaming its failures on me. The review of my book, *Insanity: The Idea and Its Consequences* (1987), in *Contemporary Psychology*, then the official review journal of the American Psychological Association, was entitled: "From the Man Who Brought You Deinstitutionalization." The reviewer, John Monahan, a professor of law, dismissed the book *in toto:* "The crux of Szasz's philosophic position is that psychiatric and psychological practice should be based not on what he derisively refers to as 'coercive paternalism,' but on the more lofty 'principle of free contract.' The problem he seems unable to recognize is that this ideological preference is fundamentally at odds with the social preferences that have shaped our public policy for the past 50 years. Freedom of contract has been in decline."[84]

By disjoining the dubious benefits of new psychiatric treatments from the demonstrable harms they cause, psychiatrists have long managed to enjoy an astonishing lack of blame for their blunders. This is because psychiatry's most harmful practices have been the most helpful for the society it serves. Not surprisingly, social critics have dealt gingerly with the disasters that were the predictable products of psychiatry's vaunted therapeutic triumphs, as if holding psychiatrists responsible for harming their helpless patients would be tantamount to society holding itself responsible for injuring its most helpless members. The snake pits were blamed on public indifference and insufficient funding. Lobotomy was dismissed as a tragic but honest medical mistake. Deinstitutionalization is attributed to my malign influence. "If ever there was anyone who almost single-handedly was responsible for the current mess involving the homeless mentally ill"—declared Mary D. Bublis, M.D.—"Szasz, with his 'urgings' to 'empty the state hospitals' back in the 60's and 70's, could be that person."[85] Rael Jean Isaac and Virginia C. Armat, authors of *Madness in the Streets,* are even more emphatic: "But for all his emphasis on the alleged brutality of psychiatry, it is Szasz's ideology that is truly inhumane."[86] Isaac's premise is that "The mentally ill don't know they're sick.... in mental illness the diseased organ is the brain." She falsely asserts: "Our laws make it impossible to treat the mentally ill against their will."[87] Under the heading, "The Triumph of Thomas Szasz," she and Armat write:

> In making the family impotent to secure treatment, and in making dangerous acts the sine qua non for commitment, the mental health bar has substantially realized the vision of Thomas Szasz. As early as 1963, in *Law, Liberty, and Psychiatry,* Szasz had seen clearly that treatment—involuntary treatment if necessary—was the key to permitting a family to keep close ties with its mentally ill member.... To a large degree, Szasz's dream of turning the mentally ill over to the criminal justice system has also become a reality as dangerousness has replaced the need-for-treatment standard...: "The counterculture denied the very existence of mental illness. ...[as] formulated in the prolific writings of psychiatrist Thomas Szasz."[88]

The claim that I share the views and values of the 1960s counterculture is slanderous; moreover, the "counterculture"—R. D. Laing in particular—*did not deny the existence of mental illness, nor did it repudiate the practice of involuntary mental hospitalization.* Nevertheless, critics regularly bracket my name with Laing's and repeat the canard about my being a spokesperson for the 1960s counterculture.[89] Typically, Dr. Thomas G. Gutheil, professor of psychiatry at Harvard University, opines: "My own view is that he [Szasz] was popular as a sixties kind of guy, an anti-establishment rebel where the facts he distorted were not a problem for the political force of his claims; any smidgin of value he could have had is long eclipsed... "[90]

Myron Magnet, editor of *City Journal,* the Manhattan Institute's[*] quarterly publication, and author of *The Dream and the Nightmare: The Sixties' Legacy to the Underclass,* states: "Of the quartet of writers [Szasz, Goffman, Laing, and Kesey], the most important was Thomas Szasz.... For Szasz mental illness was nothing more than a protest against oppression.... Mental illness is rife today because society is itself sick, as the Kesey-Laing-Szasz refrain would have it."[91] Anthony Daniels,

---

*The Manhattan Institute is a think tank devoted to "fostering economic choice and individual responsibility."

a.k.a Theodore Dalrymple, former British prison-doctor and *City Journal* columnist, agrees: "Then again, perhaps the passersby thought the [homeless, disorderly] man was only exercising his right to live as he chose, as championed by those early advocates for deinstitutionalization of the insane, psychiatrists Thomas Szasz and R. D. Laing. Who are we to judge in a free country how people should live?"[92] Science writer Kenneth Silber states: "He [Magnet] deftly traces the roots of cultural change to Marx, Freud, and the rise of moral relativism. He then presents a thoroughgoing analysis of key intellectual milestones. Among them: Michael Harrington's *The Other America*, Thomas Szasz's The *Myth of Mental Illness*, and Norman Mailer's *The White Negro*.... Szasz argued that there is no such thing as insanity, indeed that madness is a rational response to society's inadequacies. This view soon was adopted by other social thinkers.... Such thinking may have set the stage for the large-scale deinstitutionalization of mental patients."[93]

Conservative columnist Mona Charen agrees: "In 1961 Dr. Thomas Szasz published an influential book called 'The Myth of Mental Illness.' It fit with the nihilistic spirit of the decade. Mental illness came to be seen as a romantic form of social protest.... The march to empty the insane asylums was underway."[94] Charen characterizes me here as a "nihilist." Isaac and Armat regard me as a "do-badder," depriving sick people of the treatment they need. In her book, titled *Do-Gooders* (2004), Charen classifies me as a typical *liberal* do-gooder: "Szacz [sic], author of *The Myth of Mental Illness,* popularized the idea that mental illness did not exist.... Mental illness, said Szacz [sic] to the applause of the academic world, was a social construct, a prejudice, not a diagnosis."[95]

These writers must know that my critiques of the concept of mental illness, involuntary mental hospitalization, and the insanity defense did not endear me to the American Psychiatric Association. This does not stop them from attributing great influence to me in the Association's affairs.[96]

11

As many critics of my writings bracket my name with Ken Kesey's, I want to say a few words about the influence of post-World War II movies on psychiatry. Being closely associated with both sex and violence, psychiatry is a popular subject in the cinema. The most famous psychiatric film of all times, "One Flew Over the Cuckoo's Nest" (1962)—based on Kesey's novel and directed by Milos Forman—was seen by millions and is often credited with stimulating social reform. If by "social reform" we mean advancing the cause of liberating imprisoned "patients" from imprisoning psychiatrists, there is no evidence that it had such an effect. However, a very different film—"The Titicut Follies" (1967), a documentary by the noted filmmaker, Frederick Wiseman (1930-)—might have made a desirable impact, had many people seen it. But it was banned.

In the 1960s, Wiseman received permission to film, for 29 days, inside the Bridgewater State Hospital, an institution for the criminally insane. The movie he made there—his first documentary—was shown to great acclaim at the New York Film Festival in 1967. The Massachusetts Attorney General proceeded to bar public screenings and the state's Supreme Court ruled that the movie constituted an invasion of the privacy of the Bridgewater guards and patients. Today, "The Titicut Follies," if remembered at all, is dismissed as representing the kinds of inhumane psychiatric conditions that, thanks to drugs and deinstitutionalization, we have put behind us.

Wiseman does not interview his subjects, nor does he narrate or comment on what happens. He describes his approach to filmmaking as follows: "[My films are] based on un-staged, un-manipulated actions... I think I have an obligation, to the people who have consented to be in the film, ... to cut it so that it fairly represents what I felt was going on at the time in the original event."[97] In May 1987, "The Titicut Follies" was the subject of a forum at the University of Massachusetts. The anonymous reviewer for the *New York Times* reported:

> It was a rare screening of the film that, under court guidelines, can be shown only to professionals in the legal, human services, mental health and related fields.... A documentary film about brutality at a state hospital for the mentally ill, made 20 years ago and promptly banned, has proved that its power to provoke debate has not diminished.... "Titicut Follies" shows men like Jim, kept naked in solitary confinement for 17 years. Guards who are shown taunting him about his dirty cell later complain that when they control unruly patients with tear gas, the fumes cling to their clothes. The title of the documentary comes from an annual variety show given by inmates and guards; Titicut is an Indian word describing the region south of Boston, where the hospital is located. "Titicut Follies"...is the only American film ever censored for reasons other than obscenity or national security.... The United States Supreme Court has twice refused to hear Mr. Wiseman's appeal. Mr. Wiseman said in an interview this week:... "If the First Amendment of the Constitution protects anything, it's a journalist's right to report on conditions in a prison...." Blaire Perry, a lawyer for Mr. Wiseman who was on the panel, said, "In 20 years, not one patient or his family has ever objected to the showing of the film...." Today, the state hospital is in a modern building. By all accounts, the staff is better trained and there are more legal safeguards protecting the patients, *many of whom have never been convicted of a crime*. But the hospital is still surrounded by barbed wire, staffed by 220 prison guards.... There are 25 nurses and 49 psychiatrists, psychologists and social workers for 436 patients, according to Mary McGeown, a spokeswoman

for the Corrections Department. Bridgewater is still overcrowded, understaffed and underfinanced, according to one panel member, Dr. Robert Fein, assistant commissioner of mental health.[98]

What is the staff better trained *for*? No matter how many psychiatrists, psychologists, nurses, and social workers are in such a "hospital," they are all jailers.

On April 6, 1993—twenty-six years after it was banned—"The Titicut Follies" was shown on the Public Broadcasting System and reviewed by film critic Walter Goodman in the *New York Times* :

> Frederick Wiseman's remarkable first documentary, an unsparing visit to the Bridgewater State Hospital for the Criminally Insane, in Massachusetts, was banned by the state's Supreme Court on the grounds that it violated the privacy of inmates, several of whom were shown naked. The ban was finally overturned in 1991.... As in all his reports, Mr. Wiseman abjures narration. The pictures tell his stories, and he has never presented more powerful pictures. The 90-minute film opens and ends with a chorus line from what was evidently an annual show called "The Titicut Follies." You'll have to guess who among these costumed performers are inmates, who are guards. The stage, where odd behavior reigns, blurs the lines of sanity and confers an hour of equality.... One man outtalks the doctors with a fervent yet coherent plea to be sent back to an ordinary prison.... Many of the encounters have an unsettling ambiguity. A psychiatrist...questions an inmate about his sexual proclivities: "What are you interested in, big breasts or small breasts?" Is he working or just curious? The hardest scene to watch is of a forced feeding. The doctor smokes a cigarette as he inserts a long rubber tube into the patient's nostril and pours a liquid into a funnel; you want to call out to him to flick the lengthening ash onto the floor before it drops into the funnel.... In the years since Mr. Wiseman made "Titicut Follies," most of the nation's big mental institutions have been closed or cut back by court orders. How much this ostensible victory for civil liberties has helped the mentally ill remains in dispute.[99]

"The Titicut Follies," unlike "One Flew Over the Cuckoo's Nest," was a unique film: it humanized madness and depicted the psychiatric invalidation, persecution, and dehumanization of so-called mad persons. For that offense, the American psychiatric establishment, assisted by the American legal establishment, banned the showing of the film. This unique violation of the First Amendment has escaped both legal and psychiatric attention.

Today, the Bridgewater State Hospital is a "health care facility" affiliated with the University of Massachusetts Medical School. In 2003, the National Commission on Correctional Health Care lauded it as its "Facility of the Year." An essay by Jaime Shimkus, publications editor of the organization, presents a brief history of the hospital, but does not mention "The Titicut Follies" or the conditions described in the film.[100]

12

While the media celebrate the supposed discovery of the chemical causes and cures of mental illnesses, psychiatrists and their allies are preoccupied with the politics of housing the chronic mental patient. On the face of it, housing people does not seem to belong in the domain of medicine. Nor would it count as a treatment unless it were tacitly understood that, in a psychiatric context, housing means incarceration. An editorial in the *New York Times*, titled "How to house the mentally ill," explains:

> Across the nation, the mentally ill living on the streets number in the hundreds of thousands. Many of them fear the public shelters now available but are too dysfunctional to take advantage of new cheap housing on their own. Mental health workers know how to get them off the street.... New York City now operates an outreach program empowered to hospitalize the homeless mentally ill, *even against their will*.[101]

Disenchantment with deinstitutionalization has prompted psychiatrists to renew their attack on their old foe, freedom. After criticizing my views, Paul Applebaum, a former president of the APA, states: "That freedom *per se* will not cure mental illness is evident from the abject condition of so many of the deinstitutionalized."[102] Applebaum's assertion that freedom does not cure mental illness illustrates the cynicism with which he treats psychiatry's cardinal claim that mental illness is an illness. Freedom does not cure cancer or heart disease. Why, then, should we expect it to cure mental illness? Because if freedom does not cure mental illness, then psychiatric coercion is justifiable. Declares Applebaum: "[We need] greater authority for the state to detain and treat the severely mentally ill for their own benefit, even if they pose no immediate threat to their lives or those of others.... Our intervention, though depriving them of the right to autonomy in the short term, may enhance that quality in the long run. In such circumstances, benevolence and autonomy are no longer antagonistic principles."[103] Richard Lamb, a prominent advocate for the coercive psychiatric treatment of the homeless, takes this argument a step further. He maintains that certain mental patients have a right to be deprived of their rights:

> Many homeless mentally ill persons will not accept services even with assertive outreach case management. ...if homeless persons with major mental illnesses are incompetent to make decisions with regard to accepting treatment...then outreach teams including psychiatrists should bring all of these patients to hospitals, involuntarily if need be. ... these persons have *a right to involuntary treatment*.[104]

Along with psychiatrists, liberal and conservative social observers alike have rediscovered the charms of the old psychiatric plantations.

James Q. Wilson declares: "Take back the streets. Begin by reinstitu-
tionalizing the mentally ill."[105] Charles Krauthammer agrees: "Getting
the homeless mentally ill off the streets is an exercise in morality, not
aesthetics. ... Most of the homeless mentally ill...are grateful for a safe
and warm hospital bed."[106] If they are grateful, why do they have to be
coerced? Remarking on the plight of the "solitary homeless persons
who live on the streets," George Will opines: "Most are mentally ill."[107]
Marvin Olasky, a professor of journalism, also recommends resurrecting
the state hospital system:

> We need to move from sentimentality to clear thinking about the problem of the
> mentally ill...[who] are on the streets because of the astoundingly sentimental de-
> institutionalization movement that swept through state mental hospitals during the
> mixed-up days of the 1960s, when some had faith that the insane were really sane
> and vice versa.... The solution to this problem [of the homeless mentally ill] only
> seems difficult because of an [sic] *pervasive unwillingness to categorize*. But it is
> clear to anyone who walks the streets that the insane homeless who are unable to
> help themselves desperately need asylum, both in the current meaning of the word
> and in its original meaning of safety.[108]

The original meaning of the term "asylum" and it new meaning in
"insane asylum" are antithetical. Olasky's assertion that the problem
of the homeless mentally ill is due to our "pervasive unwillingness to
categorize" is nothing short of bizarre. The unhappy fate of the former
asylum inmates contrasts sharply, but not unexpectedly, with the happy
fate of the asylums which had been their homes. During the past half a
century, the value of the empty state hospital buildings and the real estate
on which they stood—often in or near large metropolitan centers—has
escalated:

Across the nation, former state hospitals for the mentally ill...are being
converted into homes. Even the ominous Danvers State Hospital, once
described as "the scariest building in the world" and a favorite destina-
tion of ghost-hunting thrill-seekers, soon will be home to laptop-toting
latte drinkers.... Six hundred would-be buyers signed up for the first 60
homes built at the site of the former Dammasch State Hospital, a $500
million project in Wilsonville, Ore., 20 miles south of Portland.... In
Traverse City, Mich., developers of a former asylum overlooking Lake
Michigan have down payments in hand from buyers looking for condos,
and a waiting list should those buyers bow out. Rents at the 500-unit
Octagon, the former New York City Lunatic Asylum on Manhattan's
Roosevelt Island, are 10 percent higher than expected.... Trailblazing
journalist Nellie Bly spent time undercover at the asylum and wrote in
1887 that it was a "human rat trap."[109]

Those particular rat traps have been phased out. The practice of psychiatric coercion has not.

13

Along with drugging-and-deinstitutionalization, lawyers and psychiatrists have greatly expanded the scope of psychiatric coercions, transforming many formerly consensual psychiatric relations into potentially or actually coercive relations. Personal injury lawyers, supported by psychiatric hired guns, are bringing civil suits against psychotherapists for failing to drug patients, failing to protect them from suicide, or failing to protect third parties from patients under their care. Today, any physician practicing psychotherapy, however loosely defined, has three corresponding new professional obligations: (1) to prescribe neuroleptic drugs for his patient and compel him to take the drugs faithfully; (2) to protect him from harming himself, if necessary by preventively incarcerating him; and (3) to protect third parties from being harmed by patients under his care, by warning them of a patient's dangerous propensities and, if necessary, preventively incarcerating the patient. Nonmedical mental health professionals have the same duties. Since they cannot prescribe drugs or commit, they must refer their patients to psychiatrists to carry out these preventive-protective measures.

At the 1980 annual meeting of the American College of Forensic Psychiatry, Melvin Belli, the most prominent tort lawyer at the time, explained: "The trend toward imposing liability on a psychotherapist for failing to inform on his dangerous patients is now firmly established. ... If the therapist unyieldingly clings to his old ethical considerations and refuses to divulge this material, the simple truth is that he will find himself having to pay a jury's verdict of $1 million or more in a wrongful death action."[110]

Invited to respond to Belli's presentation, I observed that the legal requirement that the psychotherapist predict his client's dangerous behavior is not only absurd but also incompatible with the moral and psychological premises undergirding the private, confidential, contractual relationship between patient and therapist. I stated: "The patient does not pay the therapist to have his or her behavior predicted...the issue of predicting patient behavior simply has no relevance to the private psychotherapy situation: the therapist is the patient's hired servant, not his parole officer."[111] Like the confessional, the psychoanalytic situation does not allow for the presence of a third person or party. Because the therapist's participation in insurance coverage negates the privacy of the relationship, and because the law no longer protects the therapist who wants to keep his patient's communications confidential, psychoanalysis as a private and confidential relationship between two competent and responsible adults is now an anachronism.[112]

American psychiatrists saw these legal-political developments as a fresh opportunity to reinforce their image as the protectors of both the patient and the public, expanding the scope of forensic psychiatry, increasing their income by giving expert testimony against colleagues limiting their practices to voluntary clients, and, perhaps most importantly, destroying, once and for all, the distinction between voluntary and involuntary psychiatric relations.

The American Psychiatric Association's 1999 "policy for therapist confidentiality requires mental-health professionals to take actions that might violate confidentiality if a patient explicitly threatens to kill or seriously injure someone."[113] A president of the American Psychiatric Association opined: "In principle, the duty to protect is difficult to reject, especially for members of a profession dedicated to assisting others in need. Indeed, I suspect that ... by seeking to guard potential victims of their patients from harm, clinicians as a group would endorse the trend toward broader duties to rescue."[114] In 1988, the Association formally declared that "breaching confidentiality is acceptable when required to protect third parties."[115] The result is a further expansion of the psychiatrist's powers vis-à-vis the patient and his duties vis-à-vis the state, and the complete abolition of patient autonomy and security for anyone receiving any assistance that may be categorized as a mental health service.

In 1999, commenting on Surgeon General David Satcher's declaration of war on mental illness, Kay Redfield Jamison, professor of psychiatry at John Hopkins Medical School and an enthusiastic advocate of psychiatric coercion in all its forms, joined the chorus: "As someone who studies, treats and suffers from a severe mental illness--manic depression, I commend the surgeon general for his excellent, thoughtful and fair report on mental illness."[116] Jamison celebrates the psychiatric coercions to which she has been subjected, declares the distinction between voluntary and involuntary psychiatric relations to be "misleading and arbitrary," and recommends her personal version of the psychiatric will as a model for such instruments: "I drew up a clear arrangement with my psychiatrist and family that if I again become severely depressed they have the authority to approve, against my will if necessary, both electroconvulsive therapy, an excellent treatment for certain types of severe depression, and hospitalization."[117]

Sally Satel, a Fellow at the American Enterprise Institute who teaches psychiatry at Yale, states: "For addicts, force is the best medicine."[118] The fact that this expert opinion, defining medical violence as "the best medicine," appeared on the editorial page of the *Wall Street Journal* is indicative of how widely Americans approve of the use of psychiatric force and fraud. For addicts, force is needed to stop them from taking the drugs they want to take. For mental patients, force is needed to make them take the drugs they do not want to take. Satel's recommendation for increased psychiatric surveillance and coercion appears on the editorial pages of the *New York Times* as well:

> Society must find a way to handle the thousands of severely mentally ill people who function quite well when on medication but who become violent, homeless or profoundly delusional when not being treated.... Patients know they'll go back to the hospital if they don't participate in treatment.... About half of all schizophrenics have no insight into their own condition and no understanding of why they need medication. As for free will, *the freedom to be psychotic is no freedom at all.*"[119]

14

In our day, coercive psychiatry has entered a new phase. Psychiatrists claim, and the press and the public believe or pretend to believe, that psychiatric coercion is a thing of the past, a practice essentially abandoned. "States had passed well-intentioned laws that allowed people to decide for themselves whether they wanted treatment," explains E. Fuller Torrey, founder and president of the Treatment Advocacy Center. "If you want a definition of insanity, that's it."[120] Yet, at the same time, psychiatrists insist that the medically and morally correct practice of psychiatry requires the judicious use of force and defend the *de facto* expansion of psychiatric coercion.

In previous books, I have documented that, in the course of the last several decades, the use of psychiatric coercion in the United States and the United Kingdom has increased and now affects more people than ever; and that this is not apparent to the public because, aided by the media, contemporary coercive psychiatry wraps itself in the mantle of treatment.[121] Torrey's Treatment Advocacy Center is, in fact, the most prominent and vocal American organization advocating psychiatric coercion:

> The Treatment Advocacy Center (TAC) is a national nonprofit organization dedicated to eliminating legal and clinical barriers to timely and humane treatment for millions of Americans with severe brain disorders who are not receiving appropriate medical care.... The Treatment Advocacy Center is working on the national, state,

and local levels to educate civic, legal, criminal justice, and legislative communities on the benefits of assisted treatment in an effort to decrease homelessness, jailings, suicide, violence and other devastating consequences caused by lack of treatment.... The principle [sic] activities of TAC include: educating policymakers and judges about the true nature of severe brain disorders, advanced treatments available for those illnesses, and the necessity of community ordered treatment in some cases; assisting individuals in states working to promote laws that enable individuals with the most severe brain disorders to receive assisted treatment; promoting innovative approaches to diverting the psychiatrically ill away from the criminal justice system and into appropriate treatment.[122]

"Severe brain disorders" is code for "dangerous mental illnesses"; "assisted treatment" is a euphemism for court-ordered drugging under the threat of involuntary hospitalization; "treatment" is the wrapper inside of which we find involuntary psychiatric diagnosis, forced hospitalization, and the imposition of psychiatric interventions on persons against their will. Torrey's love affair with psychiatric coercion proved to be too much even for the National Alliance for the Mentally Ill (NAMI): "Torrey and TAC departed from NAMI based on NAMI's discomfort with Torrey's extreme pro-forced treatment views."[123]

Torrey claims that the schizophrenic patient's brain disease abolishes his "insight" into being ill and hence his ability to contract: "The physical illness of their brain has affected the part of the brain that governs self-awareness. They are biologically unable to understand that they are sick and need treatment."[124] There is no biological evidence for this claim. Torrey simply cites the patient's rejection of treatment as if it were evidence: "...multiple studies have shown that approximately half of such individuals do not know that they are sick. Many of these individuals will never accept treatment voluntarily, because they are certain that the CIA really did implant electrodes in their brains, which cause their voices."[125] Torrey ignores that, even if his contention were true, it would not, *eo ipso*, make Torrey or any other psychiatrist the patient's guardian.

It should be clear already, and the material presented in this book will make it clearer still, that psychiatric coercion has nothing to do with the bona fide treatment of bona fide disease. The term "psychiatric treatment" is a misnomer: it refers to the incapacitation of the patient by ostensibly therapeutic measures, such as the injection of depot doses of neuroleptic drugs.* In practice, this is how the process works:

Every other week, Jeff Demann drives to a clinic in rural Michigan, drops his pants and gets a shot of an antipsychotic drug that he says makes him sick. "If I don't

---

*For a discussion of coerced psychiatric drugging, see chapter 8.

show up, the cops show up at my door and I wind up in a mental ward," says the unemployed 44-year-old, who lives on disability in Holland, Mich.... "I don't believe in putting this stuff into my body," Mr. Demann says. "It's time for the system to let me go."[126]

The system never lets the Demanns of America go. To escape, they must move to another state. The bottom line is that the avowed aim of psychiatric coercions of all kinds is the *prevention of harm to self and others, not the provision of treatment for an illness.* In 1985, Alan A. Stone, then professor of law and psychiatry at Harvard University and a former president of the APA, observed: "Psychiatry, by calling custodial confinement 'treatment,' gave legitimacy to the practice of locking people up for the rest of their lives whether they were dangerous or not."[127] In 1999, John J. Sandford, a British forensic psychiatrist, observed: "The preventive detention of those with untreatable mental disorders is already widely practiced in England. Under the Mental Health Act (1983) people...[are] detained indefinitely in hospital regardless of response to treatment and on grounds of risk to self as well as others. Secure and open psychiatric hospitals are full of such patients."[128] The history of mental health laws and of standard psychiatric practices illustrates and supports my contention that psychiatric coercion has nothing to do with psychiatric treatment. In 1851, the State of Illinois statute specified that "married women...may be received and detained at the hospital on the request of the husband of the woman...without the evidence of insanity or distraction required in other cases."[129]

Today, the desire to psychiatrically incarcerate persons who are not committable by the lawyers' and the psychiatrists' own criteria looms large in connection with the political need to keep so-called sex offenders confined *after they have served their sentences.* In 1997, the U. S. Supreme Court declared this practice to be constitutional. In *Kansas v. Leroy Hendricks,* the Court declared: "States have a right to use psychiatric hospitals to confine certain sex offenders once they have completed their prison terms, *even if those offenders do not meet mental illness commitment criteria.*"[130]

In November 2005, New York State Governor George Pataki made the headlines when he initiated "an administrative program to commit sexual predators to public psychiatric hospitals indefinitely.... New York became the first state to enact civil commitment for sexual offenders administratively—a move that has triggered strong concerns among psychiatrists."[131] Pataki's order pulls back the curtain. The state's mental health system is like an army. The governor is the general, the psychiatrists are the foot soldiers expected to follow the orders of their superiors. "As citizens, most of us would be comfortable seeing people properly incarcerated if these are considered crimes," said Barry Perlman, M.D., president of the New York State Psychiatric Association (NYSPA). "What we are concerned about is using the mental health system to solve a problem that seems to spill over to it because the criminal justice system cannot adequately handle it." Perlman acts as if he had just discovered that the mental health system and the criminal justice system are twins. Politicians have no illusions about psychiatry; they know that it is an extension of the state's law enforcement apparatus and use it as such:

> The governor directed the Office of Mental Health [OMH] and the Department of Correctional Services to push the envelope of the state's existing involuntary commitment law because he couldn't wait any longer for the Assembly leadership to bring his legislation to the floor for a vote.... The state has begun to identify "appropriate models for treatment" and to hire staff to treat these patients. The state prison system houses more than 5,000 violent sex offenders.... Psychiatrists who have spoken with OMH officials said that state officials estimate commitment costs about $200,000 annually for each patient, which includes facilities and personnel but not potential legal costs from court challenges to the program.... [Richard Rosner, M.D., chair of the NYSPA's Committee on Psychiatry and the Law] said. "On the surface it would appear that state psychiatric services are being used in the service of preventive detention, and that is something that is inconsistent with the American criminal justice system." ...To date, 16 states and the District of Columbia have enacted laws to allow authorities to confine violent sexual offenders in psychiatric hospitals after their prison terms....

It is important to note here that as far back as 1988 the American Psychiatric Association's Council of Psychiatry and Law explicitly approved the use of mental hospitals as prisons. In a document dated November 11-13, 1988, the Council declared: *"Psychiatric patients who no longer require active psychiatric treatment or who are untreatable can still be best managed in a psychiatric setting.... Acquittees who are unable to be discharged to outpatient status should remain under psychiatric care in a hospital environment."*[132] Again, the rank offensiveness of the document-writers' language requires comment. The psychiatric prisoner longing for freedom is treated as if he has power over his own discharge but is "unable" to exercise it: he is termed "unable to be discharged." The writers also duly note that confining a person acquitted of a crime in a building called a "prison" would violate the imprisoned person's fundamental right to liberty, and that confining him in a building called a "hospital" does not violate that right: they know that they can count on the expert medical opinion of psychiatric Jacobins that such confinement protects and insures their right to freedom from the "shackles" of mental illness.

15

Psychiatrists resent being considered jailers. Confronted with the reality that the mental hospital *is* a prison and that the psychiatrist who works there is a jailer, Brandon Krupp, a state-hospital psychiatrist in Rhode Island, quits his post and laments:

> True or false: An American citizen can be committed to a psychiatric unit of a state hospital based on political expediency, without a judicial hearing, without the approval or testimony of any doctors and without any expectation that the forced detention will make the patient better? The answer is true, and though it sounds like it could have happened only in the Gulag, it happened last month right here in Rhode Island with the placement of sex offender Todd McElroy in the state psychiatric hospital. After witnessing first-hand this cynical abuse of the state's mental-health law and practice, I resigned as chief of psychiatric services at the Eleanor Slater Hospital after 12 years of state service. ... The *unprecedented intervention* in the McElroy case now raises some very disturbing questions about *the political use of psychiatry.* ...pretending that a hospital is a prison will not make any of us safer.[133]

Mental hospitals *are* prisons. It is psychiatrists, and mainly psychiatrists, who pretend that they are not. There is nothing "unprecedented" about the McElroy case. On the contrary, reconfining, as mental patients, sex offenders who have served their prison sentences is now a routine procedure in most of the states, and, as I noted earlier, the constitutionality of the procedure has been upheld by the U. S. Supreme Court.

After serving a seventeen-year prison sentence for sexual assault, Todd McElroy was scheduled to be released on October 28, 2005. Media coverage of the case made his release politically inexpedient. Rhode Island Governor Donald L. Carcieri asked "the directors of the Departments of Corrections (DOC) and Mental Health, Retardation and Hospitals (MHRH) to find an 'institutional' way to keep Mr. McElroy off the streets."[134] The officials did their duty.

Krupp was grandstanding. When politicians incarcerate a person in a mental hospital, it is imprisonment. When psychiatrists do it, Krupp implies, it is treatment: "[T]he canons of medical ethics, professional standards, Department of Health regulations and the state mental-health law forbid the use of a psychiatric hospital as a prison." Does Krupp expect any public official—indeed, anyone but a principled psychiatric abolitionist—to admit that a mental hospital is a prison? Krupp continues: "The state mental-health law requires patients to either sign themselves in voluntarily or be civilly committed after a hearing. In Mr. McElroy's case, neither happened. The mental-health law also requires an expectation that patients may benefit from available treatment at the psychiatric facility, but the Eleanor Slater Hospital does not provide any specialty treatment for sex offenders."[135]

Governor Carcieri was not impressed. His spokesman Jeff Neal, "denied that the state's petition to civilly commit McElroy was improper. 'From the governor's point of view, it has never been the state's policy to hospitalize anyone who does not require medical care.' Corrections Director A.T. Wall, who has led the commitment attempt, has said McElroy remains a clear danger to society. And H. Reed Cosper, the state's mental-health advocate—and McElroy's lawyer until the hearing last month—has said McElroy is 'very impaired' and needs some transitional hospitalization after so many years in prison." Krupp, on the other hand, "argued that McElroy wasn't eligible to be committed under the state Mental Health Law 'because he is not dangerous by virtue of his treatable mental illness [schizophrenia], ... and would not benefit from extended inpatient treatment.'"[136] Krupp has no intention of eschewing his power to imprison innocent individuals and refuses to recognize that, because "every confinement of the person is an 'imprisonment,'" it matters not whether the imprisoner is a politician or a psychiatrist. What matters to the modern psychiatrist is his burning ambition to "treat."

Following Krupp's resignation, Steven Sharfstein, president of the APA, defended the "ethics" of the profession in an editorial, titled "Hospital or Prison?", that was at once sanctimonious and self-incriminating. Would the president of the American Medical Association write an editorial with such a title? Noting that "To date 16 states and the District of Columbia have passed civil confinement laws for sexual offenders once their prison terms have ended," Sharfstein emphasized that "civil commitment is based on the premise of forced confinement to a hospital that must offer treatment, not just containment or punishment.... As a medical specialty, we are part of an ethical tradition to put our patients first and to do no harm."[137] These are bare-faced lies. Forced treatment in an environment of forced confinement is coerced, not "offered." It is punishment, not treatment. As for doing no harm, Hippocrates and Galen took for granted, when they used the Latin phrase *primum non nocere,* that anything a doctor did to a patient against the patient's will, *ipso facto*, counted as doing harm.[138]*

16

Psychiatrists now celebrate neuroleptics as miracle drugs that have helped to liberate mental patients from the asylums. Future historians of

---

* If they did use the phrase, which is likely, they would have used it in its Greek form.

psychiatry are likely to have a very different view of this scene. I believe they will see the profession's most notable achievement to have been its ability to convince the public, and perhaps itself as well, that psychiatric imprisonment has been abolished. The creation of this modern Potemkin's Village is the more remarkable inasmuch as psychiatric incarceration is now practiced on a scale never before seen.[139] The facts are sobering.

In 1996, leading authorities in psychiatric epidemiology reported: "Each year in the United States well over one million persons are civilly committed to hospitals for psychiatric treatment. ... It is difficult to completely separate discussions of voluntary and involuntary commitment because voluntary status can be converted efficiently to involuntary status, once the patient has requested release."[140] Indeed so. In 1972, in an article in the *New England Journal of Medicine*, I showed that there is no such thing as voluntary mental hospitalization, that so long as involuntary mental hospitalization remains an option, there can be no such thing. The adjective "voluntary," in the context of mental hospitalization, is a transparent mendacity: *all so-called voluntary mental hospitalizations* are, actually or potentially, involuntary incarcerations, instances of an officially "unacknowledged practice of medical fraud."[141]

Formerly, the fraud was not quite as unacknowledged as it is today. As recently as 1966, Frederick Redlich and Daniel Freedman's popular textbook, *The Theory and Practice of Psychiatry,* seriously considered the problem of psychiatric coercion:

> ... even voluntarily admitted patients are deprived to a degree of some aspects of their ordinary freedom.... Such rules are established in the interest of the patients.... No wonder that mental hospitals have been compared with concentration camps and jails! Szasz actually recommends that all institutions to which patients are sent by compulsion should be called jails. We believe it would be just as erroneous to do this as to call our prisons hospitals.[142]

Fifty years earlier, Karl Jaspers forthrightly acknowledged the obvious, that coercion precludes cooperation and that the relationship between the coercive psychiatrist and the coerced patient cannot be truly therapeutic:

> Rational treatment is not really an attainable goal as regards the large majority of mental patients in the strict sense.... Admission to hospital often takes place against the will of the patient and therefore the psychiatrist finds himself in a different relation to his patient than other doctors. He tries to make this difference as negligible as possible by deliberately emphasizing his purely medical approach to the patient, but the latter in many cases is quite convinced that he is well and resists these medical efforts.[143]

With each new reform, the deceits and ironies of psychiatric history increase. Before deinstitutionalization, mental hospitals were touted as therapeutic institutions. After deinstitutionalization—a "reform" mendaciously attributed to the therapeutic effectiveness of novel psychotropic drugs—the allegedly therapeutic mental hospitals were rediscovered to have also been snake-pits: "With the 'deinstitutionalization' effort that began in the 1960s, hundreds of thousands of mentally ill men and women were released from state institutions. These people escaped *grim conditions and sometimes brutal treatment.*"[144]

Social psychologist M. Brewster Smith, long-time professor of psychology at Harvard, was one of the architects and perpetrators of the sadistic hoax called "deinstitutionalization." Half a century later, Smith regrets the mistake but appears to be none the wiser for the experience. "On the psychosocial side of mental health," he writes, "the case could be made that the rapid and ill-prepared deinstitutionalization of the mentally ill, for which I take some responsibility as an officer of the Joint Commission on Mental Illness and Health of the 1950s, had unexamined consequences that are almost as irreversible as those of psychosurgery."[145]

Psychiatrists, pretending that they have had nothing to do with deinstitutionalization, now complain about "criminalizing the mentally ill" and clamor for new reforms. We have progressed from what Albert Deutsch dubbed "the shame of the States" to the "shame of the Nation"[146]: "It is a national shame that our prisons and jails serve as mental institutions. It reflects a lack of planning, a failure of public commitment, and a single-minded focus on punishment."[147] The solution: more forced psychiatric treatment. This is an especially remarkable proposal inasmuch as mental health experts assert that the number of mentally ill persons in American prisons far surpasses the number of mentally ill in American mental hospitals, and that the two groups are treated similarly. According to Human Rights Watch:

Jails and prisons have become the nation's primary mental health facilities. ...more than 700,000 mentally ill people are processed through prison or jail each year. Chronically underfunded, the country's mental health system does not reach anywhere near the number of people who need it today. Left untreated and unstable, mentally ill people enter the criminal justice system when they break the law. The results, from a therapeutic, humanitarian, and human rights perspective, are appalling. "We are literally drowning in patients," explains one California prison psychiatrist, "running around trying to put our fingers in the bursting dikes, while hundreds of men continue to deteriorate psychiatrically before our eyes."[148]

On May 10, 2005, the Public Broadcasting System's (PBS) Frontline series was devoted to a documentary subtitled "An Image of Prisons as a Warehouse for the Mentally Ill." A PBS review offered this summary of the program: "This documentary, 'The New Asylums,' ... explains that the mentally ill, in the decades after a mass release from mental hospitals, have often wound up in less forgiving confines.... 500,000 mentally ill patients, who in earlier decades would have been treated in hospitals, are now mistreated in prisons. The mental hospitals now house only a tenth of that number."[149] Reginald Wilkinson, director of the Ohio Department of Corrections, explains: "In addition to being the director of the Department of Corrections, I became a de facto director of a major mental health system.... Many of those persons who would have been in state hospitals are now in state prisons. I've actually had a judge mention to me before that, "Hey, we hate to do this, *but we know the person will get treated if we send this person to prison*" (emphasis added).

Psychiatrists and the media lament the results of the last psychiatric reform but do not question the nature of mental illness or the merits of coerced drugging. The reviewer continues: "The bedlam is all too faithfully and nauseatingly depicted.... The show never feels like the problem is being solved nor is its exact origin understood, which is the central frustration in dealing with mental illness. Just by venturing into these Stygian cellblocks, however, 'The New Asylums' is performing a public service." I doubt it. I have viewed the program and I believe that all it accomplished was to reinforce the viewers' beliefs that (most) mental patients are violent subhumans and that it is legitimate to treat them as such. The show's epilogue bemoans "relapse and recidivism... mental-health prison consultant, Fred Cohen, seems as if he's about to suppress his millionth sigh as he describes a penitentiary's in-house tribunal...[that] hands down increased sentences for behavior that is against prison rules but in keeping with an illness's symptoms: cursing, spitting, refusing to give back a food tray." The producers of the program fail to note that imprisoning mental patients in "Stygian cellblocks" and giving them "mental health services" is enormously profitable for the psychiatrists and lawyers who validate the new American *Ward No. 6*s, as well as for the pharmaceutical companies that supply the drugs used to subdue the hordes of involuntary patients.*

"Not only are many, if not most, of the mentally ill people who live in adult homes in New York state in crisis. So is the United States' entire system of mental-health services," concluded a 2002 federal report on the nation's mental health care system. "Mentally ill people today are not

---

* The reference is to Anton Chekhov's short story, *Ward No. 6*

as removed from the 'snake pits' of decades ago that warehoused people with psychiatric disabilities as Americans might like to think."[151]

It is obvious that as long as law, psychiatry, and society define destructive and self-destructive behaviors as mental diseases, assign the duty to control persons who display such behaviors to psychiatrists, who eagerly embrace that responsibility, "seclusion and restraint"—in plain English, psychiatric coercion—will remain a characteristic feature of psychiatric practice. Indeed, recent studies support the impression that the pretense that the "new" mental hospitals are true medical hospitals has rendered them more unsafe for the inmates than were the pre-World War II "snake pits." B. Christopher Frueh and his coworkers examined the experiences of 142 randomly selected adults in "public sector mental hospitals" in South Carolina. The patients reported "physical assault (31 percent), sexual assault (8 percent), witnessing traumatic events (63 percent) ... being around frightening or violent patients (54 percent), ... seclusion (59 percent), restraint (34 percent), takedowns (29 percent), and handcuffed transport (65 percent)."[152] The authors ask, "What kind of message does handcuffed transport send to distressed and vulnerable patients as they begin an episode of psychiatric care?," and answer: "[R]ecent data suggest that the rates of interpersonal violence in psychiatric settings are high.... The complete elimination of seclusion and restraint may eventually prove clinically unrealistic."[153] Robert Paul Lieberman, distinguished professor of psychiatry at the University of California, Los Angeles, coolly concludes: "[T]o press for elimination of seclusion and restraint…is fatuous. ...it would be regrettable if polemics replace sound clinical judgment and empirical evaluation based on the full picture of management of assaultive behavior."[154] Psychiatrists will continue their hopeless struggle to reconcile their putative role as physicians and healers with their actual role as agents of social control and punishment—until they repudiate the combination and actively reject one role or the other.

In the United Kingdom the psychiatric scene is similar to that in the United States. On October 29, 1999, a BBC [British Broadcasting Corporation] report entitled "Forced Treatment of Mentally Ill Doubles," provided the following startling statistics: "The Department of Health says the number of formal admissions to hospital under the [Mental Health] Act rose from 16,000 in 1988-89 to 27,100 in 1998-99. The vast majority of these—some 89%—were people admitted to NHS hospitals under Part II of the Act which deals with emergency admissions and admissions for up to 28 days and up to six months. The number of men sectioned under Part II rose from 6,200 to 12,300 over the 10 years, while the number of women increased by about 48%, from 8,100 to 11,900." A mental-health expert commented: "[W]e are living in a more demanding and violent society.... The increasing focus on protecting the public, following a series of killings by mentally ill people living in the community, could also have contributed to the rise in forced admission to hospital.... The mental health system is in crisis and services are at breaking point."[155]

David Healy, a Reader in Psychological Medicine at the University of Wales, writes: "Compared with 1900,...by 2000 there had been a fifteen-fold increase in rates of admission to psychiatric wards. There had also been a three-fold increase in rates of detention for psychiatric disorders. And psychiatric patients afflicted with schizophrenia and manic-depressive disorder, the disorders at the core of psychiatric business, were likely to spend more time in a service bed during their psychiatric illness than they would have done a century ago."[156] Healy also notes that, in Japan "the asylum population grew dramatically during the chlorpromazine era."[157] "Chlorpromazine era" is still another psychiatric euphemism. The correct term is "the era of chemical lobotomy."[158] One of the most interesting statistics cited by Healy is the increase in the number of forensic psychiatrists: "During the last half of the century, forensic psychiatry was born. Between 1967 and the end of the century, for example, the number of forensic psychiatrists in Britain increased 250-fold."[159] The number of forensic psychiatrists in the United States has also increased exponentially. No private person seeks or pays for "private forensic psychiatric services." Most psychiatrists, most of the time, function as forensic psychiatrists. The number of psychiatrists in the country is an index of the size of the psychiatric-therapeutic state.

17

The American Psychiatric Association's *Diagnostic and Statistical Manual of Mental Disorders* (2000) lists some three hundred fifty discrete mental diseases, a.k.a. "mental disorders."[160] *Kaplan and Sadock's Synopsis of Psychiatry: Behavioral Sciences/Clinical Psychiatry* (2003), the textbook most widely used in American medical schools, lists approximately three hundred "psychotherapeutic drugs" [sic] considered appropriate for the treatment of these diseases.[161] In addition, other products, not included in the list, contain combinations of several psychotropic and so-called depot neuroleptics, a single dose lasting up to six weeks.

This plethora of drugs reflects the psychiatric view, now widely held, that the vexations of life are due to mental diseases caused by chemical imbalances in the brain, and that these can be effectively treated by a rebalancing of the chemicals. Two hundred years ago psychiatrists claimed that mental diseases were due to humoral imbalances in the body, including the brain, which could be rebalanced with appropriate physical treatments. No one has ever demonstrated the existence of diseases affecting the "mind," much less of humoral and chemical imbalances that were causing them.

Unlike the history of medicine, the history of psychiatry consists largely of critiques of its own prevailing practices. The critiques are of two very different kinds. One type, the large majority, is reformist: its targets are defined by and change with psychiatry's prevailing practices—from commitment laws to shock therapies, to the DSM, to psychopharmacology. The other type is radical: its targets are constant and focus on psychiatry's core defects—the nonexistence of mental diseases and the wrongfulness of depriving innocent persons of liberty. Professional psychiatric historians, the press, and the public dwell on the reformist critiques that indirectly validate psychiatry's fables as facts, and valorize its cruelties as compassion. They ignore the radical critiques that confront the professionals, the press, and the public with their complicity in psychiatry's mandates, mistakes, and misdeeds.

Sidestepping vexing questions about the precise nature and definition of the diseases/disorders/maladies/illnesses that psychiatrists diagnose and treat, reformist critiques serially target *the practices that generate the very phenomena that psychiatrists study*. The first psychiatric practice was incarceration. Prior to the existence of madhouses as social institutions, madness was not a medical matter. Madness as medical malady may be said to have been created/invented to rationalize and justify its medical management. In the absence of mental illness, it had to be so. Let me explain.

There have always been sick people, but there have not always been precise medical diagnoses and treatments. Medical diagnoses and medical treatments *were developed alongside the empirical discovery of discrete, new diseases*, for example, measles and mumps, diabetes mellitus and diabetes insipidus. Similarly, there have always been mad people, that is, individuals considered deviant, deranged, feebleminded, senile, and so forth. But there have not always been allegedly precise psychiatric diagnoses and psychiatric treatments. Moreover, psychiatric diagnoses and psychiatric treatments *were not developed alongside the empirical discovery of discrete, new mental diseases*. No one contests this assertion. When I was a young psychiatrist there were but a handful of psychiatric diagnoses/diseases. Now there are more than three hundred. Not one was discovered. All were invented. In the absence of empirically verifiable discoveries, they had to be. What drove the inventions? The inventiveness of psychiatrists needing to prove that they are doctors, that their patients have diseases, and that these maladies require and justify their interventions. From the start, so-called psychiatric treatment was the engine that drove the train of psychiatric diagnostics.

The first "psychiatric treatment" used to "create" mental illness was involuntary mental hospitalization. During most of the nineteenth century, psychiatric dogma decreed that mental illnesses could be effectively treated only in mental hospitals. Subsequently doctors, hospitals, and diagnoses/diseases were needed to justify confinement-as-care, insulin shock, electric shock, and lobotomy. Today, with hospitals serving a subsidiary role in the justificatory rhetoric of psychiatry, psychiatrists need and use drugs to create psychiatric diagnoses/disorders/diseases. *Mirabile dictu,* the use of psychotropic drugs to treat mental illnesses and the number of mental disorders in the DSM expand in tandem. Reformist psychiatric critics note this coincidence, and the media eagerly embrace the new criticism that, like its predecessors, challenges neither psychiatry's alleged scientific basis nor the moral legitimacy of its coercive practices. Lisa Cosgrove, a psychologist, and her coworkers report that "Of the 170 experts in all who contributed to the manual [DSM] that defines disorders from personality problems to drug addiction, more than half had such ties [i.e., financial ties to pharmaceutical companies], including 100 percent of the experts who served on work groups on mood disorders and psychotic disorders.... The process of defining such disorders is far from scientific...You would be dismayed at how political the process can be."[162]

This is reformist psychiatric criticism at its most naive and self-serving. The view that psychiatric classification is political, not scientific, is not a new finding or insight. Psychiatric classification predates psychiatric drug treatment by a century or more. The physicians who classified runaway slaves as suffering from drapetomania, and persons with same-sex interests as suffering from homosexuality, did not do so because of financial ties to drug companies. Would the DSM be more scientific if the psychiatrists who make it up were financially independent of drug companies? The "experts" think it would. The science writer for the *Chicago Tribune* reports that, "100 percent of the experts on DSM-IV panels overseeing mood disorders and schizophrenia/psychotic disorders were financially involved with the drug industry. These are the largest categories of psychiatric drugs in the world—2004 sales of $20.3 billion and \$14.4 billion respectively, " and cites this misguided expert criticism: "'The more lucrative the drug market, the higher the percentage of experts with financial ties—that has to raise serious questions about these panels' objectivity,'" said David Rothman."[163]

The issue is not one of objectivity versus subjectivity. The issue is that of truth versus error, veracity versus deception. The psychiatrist's *raison d'être* is to deal with non-objective phenomena. The important issues psychiatry raises are the questions we dare not ask: Are the phenomena we call "mental illnesses" diseases? Why do psychiatrists, juries, and judges incarcerate innocent persons and excuse persons guilty of crimes? What is a drug? Why does the government prohibit many drugs that used to be available on the open market? Why do we need doctors to prescribe drugs? Why do doctors need diagnoses to prescribe drugs? Where is the evidence that the persons who receive these drugs are sick or that the drugs work? How many people pay out of pocket for these drugs? How many people are forced to take them? And so on, and on.[164]

Notwithstanding much-touted "scientific advances" in psychiatric theories and therapies, the psychiatrist's power and the mental patient's loss of liberty continue to cast a dark shadow over the profession. Two hundred years ago, madness was allocated to the madhouse; the use of force was overt and everyone recognized that mad-doctoring meant coercion. Today, mental illness is located in society; it is everywhere—in the home, the school, the workplace, the prison, the nursing home, as well as the mental hospital; the use of force is, for the most part, covert, and few people realize that psychiatry means coercion. At the same time, the de facto equivalence of mental hospitals and prisons for persons managed as mental patients is now openly recognized, while its significance for psychiatry as a medical specialty is ignored and denied.

In 2001, Andrea Yates was convicted of drowning her five children and sentenced to prison. The appeals court overturned the sentence and ordered a new trial when it was discovered that the psychiatric expert for the prosecution had given false testimony. In February 2006, a judge "freed" Yates on \$200,000 bond, "as long as Yates is *voluntarily committed* to Rusk State Hospital..."[165] Yates's commitment to Rusk State Hospital was no more voluntary than was her commitment to the prison from which she was "released." It is such legal-psychiatric maneuverings that support the myth that psychiatric imprisonment is not imprisonment, but rather a state of freedom.

Despite all this evidence, E. James Lieberman, a distinguished psychiatrist, psychoanalyst, and author, opines, "One rarely hears of someone being committed involuntarily to a mental hospital."[166] Today, conventional wisdom decrees that involuntary mental hospitalization is a thing of the past. It is in bad taste to notice it, much less mention it.

2

Shock and Commotion: Terror Therapy

*Half the harm that is done in this world is due to people who want to feel important.
They don't mean to do harm—but the harm does not interest them. Or they do not
see it, or they justify it because they are absorbed in the endless struggle to think
well of themselves.*

—*T. S. Eliot (1888-1965)[1]*

Life is hazardous. Individuals and communities are destined to live
in fear of disease, crime, famine, war, personal failure, and death. Mad-
doctoring may be said to begin when people stop projecting their amorphous fears onto demonic possession and defending themselves against
witchcraft, and instead start projecting them onto madness as an illness
and defending themselves against "dangerous" madmen.[2] Broadly speaking, we may say that psychiatry begins where religion leaves off.

Historians of psychiatry have lavished a great deal of attention on
witchcraft. Precisely because of that, the role of physicians in the history
of the witch craze remains one of the most misinterpreted aspects of the
history of psychiatry. Gregory Zilboorg did a good job of fabricating an
utterly false but psychiatrically self-flattering interpretation of witches as
mental patients: "He [Johann Weyer] leaves no doubt that but one conclusion is warranted: *the witches are mentally sick people*...[He] stands out
as the true founder of modern psychiatry.... *Unlike surgery and general
medicine, to which the sick man came to ask for help, psychiatry* had to
come out into the open fields of human passions and...*had to liberate the
sick* from the thorns and tentacles of political prejudice, theological tradition, and legal intricacy."[3]* This absurdity has been diligently repeated
by countless subsequent historians of psychiatry.

The recasting of a group of persecuted people from the role of witch
to that of mental patient is a tour de force, the oppressor congratulating

---

*Johann (Johannes) Weyer (1515-1588) was a Dutch physician, "demonologist," and
humanist critic of the persecution of witches.

himself for liberating his victim. Zilboorg correctly notes that the surgical or medical patient seeks help for himself, but the psychiatric patient does not. According to him, the patient has first to be liberated, a task for psychiatrists. This is rubbish, for two important reasons. Who were the witches? In answering this question we must follow Sartre's famous answer to the question of who is a Jew: "The Jew is one whom other men consider a Jew: that is the simple truth from which we must start."[4] There were two quite different kinds of persons whom other people considered to be witches: some were individuals considered socially deviant or frightening, often old women; others were upstanding citizens, men as often as women. In *The Myth of Mental Illness*, I demonstrated the folly of recasting scary, unwanted women—such as the witches in Shakespeare's *Macbeth*—as mentally ill persons.[5] Here I want to offer some brief remarks about the second category of witches.

When Zilboorg asserts, "The witches are mentally sick people," he confuses the reader and perhaps himself. The force of this sentence—and of the image it conjures up and that continues to be portrayed in plays about witch trials—depends on conflating and confusing the "witch" and the "bewitched," accused and accuser. In Salem and elsewhere, the term "witch" referred to the normal person accused of witchcraft-sorcery by "bewitched" girls (and others), whom Zilboorg and others call "hysterical." In fact, the people executed as witches in Salem were upright members of society. It was the bewitched, not the witches, who displayed dramatically abnormal behavior, that is, who faked some sort of malady physicians diagnosed as bewitchment.

The Salem witch trials began with two girls—Betty Parris and Abigail Williams—displaying behaviors that disturbed their parents and community: "These little girls cried out without reason, barked like dogs, and later, with other 'afflicted' young women, accused townspeople of being witches."[6] How was this simple piece of self-dramatized fakery transformed into a vast social drama and the execution of a large number of innocent persons? *It all began with a medical diagnosis.*

Perplexed by what ailed the "afflicted" girls, Betty's father, the Reverend Samuel Parris, took them to be examined by Dr. William Griggs, the only physician in the village. Born in England in 1621, Griggs and his family sailed for Boston in 1635. Not much else is known about Griggs. There was, of course, no medical training or credentialing in the Massachusetts Bay Colony at that time. Anyone could call himself a doctor. "The practice of medicine was often undertaken by ministers and others who could read...ministers often viewed illness as a result of sin."[7] Griggs duly diagnosed the girls as suffering from the "evil hand." The first link in a long chain had been forged. Charles Upham, a scholar of the Salem witch trials, comments: "...so far as the medical profession is concerned, they [physicians] bear a full share of the responsibility for the proceedings. They give countenance and currency to the idea of witchcraft in the public mind and were generally in the habit, when a patient did not do well under their prescription to state that the 'evil hand' was upon him."[8] Ever since, psychiatrist-physicians have certified "popular delusions" as sound judgments, the "madness of crowds" as social realities, and themselves as the proper authorities for authenticating widely shared errors as medical truths. Instances include the pathologizing of masturbation, escape from slavery, homosexuality, sadness, suicide, infanticide, substance abuse, and more—each an illness whose reality the individual doubts at his own peril.[9] Still, the doctors—defenders of social reality—must not be blamed. The good doctor Anthony S. Patton, a retired surgeon, concludes his essay about the good doctor Griggs with this plea: "Whatever Griggs' faults may have been, it was not he alone that caused the problem but the society in which he lived. ...he was only producing a diagnosis accepted by much of society in New England."[10]

One of the witches hanged at Salem was John Proctor, whose servant girl was one of those displaying symptoms of being afflicted with the "evil hand." Proctor seemed to have serious doubts about the existence of witchcraft, believed the "possessed" girls faked their fits, and beat his servant. He paid for it with his life.

> From the start of the outbreak of witchcraft hysteria in Salem, Proctor had denounced the whole proceedings and the afflicted girls as a scam. When his wife was accused and questioned, he stood with her throughout the proceedings and staunchly defended her innocence. It was during her questioning that he, too, was named a witch. Proctor was the first male to be named as a witch in Salem. In addition, all of his children were accused. His wife Elizabeth, and Elizabeth's sister and sister-in-law, also were accused witches. Although tried and condemned, Elizabeth avoided execution because she was pregnant.[11]

Now we know how very right Proctor had been. He saw the method in the accusers' madness. Admittedly, the method is obvious. The powerless were exercising, by means of the widely shared belief in witchcraft, power over their oppressors, real or perceived. In countless cases, this is still the "method in the madness" of persons displaying symptoms of mental illnesses.

2

British psychiatrist William Sargant (1907-1988) approvingly observed: "The history of psychiatric treatment shows, indeed, that from time immemorial attempts have been made to cure mental disorders by the use *of physiological shocks, frights, and various chemical agents; and such means have always yielded brilliant results in certain types of patients.*"[12] He attributed the practice of tormenting-as-treatment to its alleged effectiveness in "curing mental disorders." I attribute it to the human proclivity for sadism. Whatever its ultimate source may be, the torturing of mental patients and rationalizing it as treatment has characterized the practice of psychiatry from its earliest days to the present.*

The notion of madness is inextricably intertwined with the notions of badness and sinfulness. In the Christian worldview, the unrepentant individual guilty of a deadly sin receives his just punishment in hell. Some medieval chroniclers were explicit: for pride, the sinner is broken on the wheel; for envy, he is put in freezing water; for anger, he is dismembered alive; for sloth, he is thrown into snake pits; for greed, he is placed in cauldrons of boiling oil; for gluttony, he is forced to eat rats, toads, and snakes; and for lust, he is smothered in fire and brimstone. Psychiatrists have developed a similar repertoire of torments for "exorcizing" mental illness. The image of the most famous method of torment-as-treatment for madness, placing the sufferer into a pit of snakes, has survived as an eponym-synonym for the mental hospital. Let us begin with a brief glimpse of the origin of the term "snake pit."

The Jewish, Christian, and Islamic faiths require active engagement in the worship of God. In the Age of (Christian) Faith, the person who withdrew from such engagement—who was bored, disengaged, withdrawn—was considered to suffer from *acedia*, a synonym for sloth. Sloth is an obsolete term. *Webster's* defines it as "Indolence; disinclination to action or labor; spiritual apathy and inactivity; the deadly sin of *sloth*." Today we might call such a person depressed or schizophrenic, although we still use "lazy" when not pathologizing. As sins became secularized, many of them became psychiatrized and punished by psychiatric sanctions called "treatments."[13]

In medieval Europe, snake pits had been used as instruments for executing people. Convicts were cast into a pit containing poisonous snakes, where they died from snake-venom poisoning. Subsequently, the term "snake pit" came to be used as a critical name for insane asylums and also for other total institutions, such as schools and prisons, that treated their inmates inhumanely. The image of the modern, mid-twentieth-century

---

* As noted earlier, in this book I use the term "psychiatry" to refer to actually or potentially coercive psychiatric practices, and the term "psychiatrist" to refer to psychiatrists who engage in such practices.

mental hospital as a snake pit was popularized by Mary Jane Ward's best-selling autobiographical novel, *The Snake Pit*, and the popular film based on it.[14] The dust jacket of the original edition explained: "Long ago men tried to shock the insane back into sanity by throwing them into a snake pit—a drastic treatment which by its sudden terror was sometimes successful. Modern methods, though superficially more civilized, often rely on the same brutal shock to achieve their results."

Although Richard Hunter and Ida Macalpine clearly intended their compendium of psychiatric-historical documents as a tribute to their profession, not as a criticism of it, they candidly acknowledge that treatments designed to frighten and injure mental patients played a pivotal role in the history of psychiatry. They try, I think not very convincingly, to put a positive spin on the story: "*Treatment by 'shock and commotion'* came early in the history of psychiatry. It derived and gained support from three different sets of clinical observations...some patients with hydrophobia—long confused with insanity proper—had been reported cured by the shock of 'having been several times cast into Water.'"[15]

In an effort to attribute medical-scientific validity to the psychiatrists' observations-rationalizations, Hunter and Macalpine qualify them as "clinical." This linguistic ennobling conceals a basic truth about psychiatry, namely, that the psychiatrist—unlike other physicians—possesses no special methods of observation or fact gathering. No less an authority than Emil Kraepelin acknowledged this embarrassing fact: "When the alienist confronts his patient and tries to establish that patient's mental condition...*he cannot see more in the patient than could a good, non-psychiatrically trained observer with a little practice and attention.*"[16] Hunter and Macalpine knew this. They recognized that the roots of psychiatric torture lay in the tortures associated with the history of witchcraft, not in "clinical observations": "The method of producing shock *usque ad deliquum*, to the brink of death as the phrase went, [was] similar to the ducking test for witches."[17] Human inventiveness in devising so-called psychiatric treatments by means of "shock and commotion" has proved to be as limitless as is the human capacity for sadism.

3

The policy of punishing witches required distinguishing witches from nonwitches. This was a task for experts, called "inquisitors," who *inquired* into the matter by certain methods and "diagnosed" persons accused of witchcraft as witches (and rarely as nonwitches). One of these methods was the so-called ducking test, which consisted of tying the suspect's right thumb to her left toe and plunging her into a pond. If she floated, she was a witch and was executed. If she sank and drowned, she was innocent and was exonerated. Madness, like witchcraft, is an attribution, presumed to be true until proved false, with the victim deprived of all means of proving its untruth. Madness justifies, indeed requires, that the secular authority imprison and torment the mad person who, by virtue of his alleged condition, poses a threat to the well-being of the community.

The first medical professional to claim ducking as a treatment for insanity was Jean Baptiste Van Helmholt (1577-1644), a celebrated physician in the Netherlands. Helmholt's discovery lay—as did numerous later discoveries in psychiatry—in creating a metaphor that meshed with and captivated the imagination of the public: ducking cured madness by "suffocating the mad Ideas."[18] Van Helmholt's son, Franciscus Mercurius (1618-1699), also a physician, published an account of his father's method:

> The way he took was this, having stript the Parties naked, he bound their hands upon their backs, and ty'd their Feet to a Rope fastned to a Pulley for to let them down more or less deep into the Water; and then setting them upon a Bench with the Backs towards a great Vessel with Water, he pull'd them up by the Rope which was fastned to their Feet, and so let them fall with their Heads downwards to their Waste into the Water, yet so as that their heads did not touch the bottom of the Vessel, and there left them till he judged that their upper Parts were drowned; It may happen indeed that some through fear, or because they are not strong enough to stand out this Method, may miscarry and die; and therefore it is fitting that permission should be procur'd from the Magistrate for the exercising of this practice, as it is usual for the cutting of the Stone [urinary calculus], which is likewise a doubtful Operation and from whence all do not escape with Life. And for as much as *Fools or distracted Persons, by being bereft of their understanding, are of no use in the Commonwealth;* whereas those who are troubled with the Stone may notwithstanding that Disease some way or another contribute to the well-being of it, it is more reasonable that this Method should be used towards the former, than the Operation of Lithotomy practiced upon the latter.[19]

This may be the first reference to the mental patient as a useless member of society, and to killing him as a therapeutic intervention, ostensibly for the patient's good, yet recommended as a method benefiting the community by restoring the madman to social usefulness or terminating his useless life. Franciscus Mercurius Van Helmholt's remarks anticipate by two hundred and fifty years the introduction into psychiatry of such modern methods as destroying the patient's soul by lobotomy rationalized as "psychosurgery," or his body by murder rationalized as "euthanasia."

"Drowning therapy," practiced until the early decades of the nineteenth century, was based on the theory "that if the patient was nearly drowned

then brought to life he would take a fresh start, leaving his disease behind. Most were put in a coffin-like box with holes, lowered with one fell
swoop into water, and kept there until no bubbles surfaced, then taken
out and revived."[20]

4

The pioneer English mad-doctors were educated men. They recognized that the madman was an individual who so conducted himself
that others found it painful or impossible to have social intercourse or
share their homes with him. Trying to bridge the gap between religion,
humoral medicine, and common sense, the doctors concluded that the
insane individual suffered from a *disease of his "corporeal soul,"* and
that healing him required medically punishing him. Explained Thomas
Willis (1621-1675), one of the leading physicians of his age:

> Curatory requires threatenings, bonds, or strokes, as well as Physick.... And indeed
> for the curing of Mad people, *there is nothing more effectual or necessary than their
> reverence or standing in awe of such as they think their Tormentors.* For by this means,
> the Corporeal Soul being in some measure depressed and restrained, is compell'd to
> remit its pride and fierceness; and so afterwards by degrees grows more mild, and
> returns in order: Wherefore, Furious Mad-men are sooner, and more certainly cured
> by punishments, and hard usage, in a strait room, than by Physick or Medicines.[21]

Willis, a pioneer neuroanananatomist and physiologist, coined the terms
"neurologie" and "psycheologie," the latter to denote "the study of the
nature and essence...and powers and affections of the Corporeal Soul or
mind."[22] Willis's choice of words reveals the struggle of a sophisticated
mind trying to reconcile the waning influence of the humoral-religious
concept of disease with the waxing ideas and images of the newly emerging corporeal-secular concept of it.

Although Willis opposed the old idea that madness is related to
"wanderings" of the uterus (hysteria), he clung to treatments based on
the humoral theory of disease: "But yet a course of Physick ought to
be instituted besides, which may suppress or cast down Elation of the
Corporeal Soul. Wherefore in this Disease, Bloodletting, Vomits, or very
strong Purges, and boldly and rashly given, are most often convenient."[23]
Eventually, each fashionable psychiatric treatment-torture is replaced
by another "better," "more humane" method. In the eighteenth century,
the ducking stool for near-drowning the mental patient was replaced by
"rotating" and "tranquilizing" chairs intended to produce adult versions
of what is now called the "shaken baby syndrome." The web site of the
Institute for Neurological Disorders and Stroke defines this syndrome

as "a severe form of head injury that occurs when a baby is shaken forcibly enough to cause the baby's brain to rebound (bounce) against his or her skull. This rebounding may cause bruising, swelling, and bleeding (intracerebral hemorrhage) of the brain, which may lead to permanent, severe brain damage or death."[24]

The idea of treating madness with a machine that would shake up the madman was the brainchild of Erasmus Darwin (1731-1802), the grandfather of Charles Darwin. Trained as a physician in Edinburgh, widely regarded as one of the medical and intellectual luminaries of his age, Darwin practiced medicine in Lichfield in Staffordshire. So great was his reputation that George III invited him to be royal physician, an offer he declined. Darwin had wide-ranging scientific interests, among them the causes and cures of insanity. In 1801, he wrote:

> Another experiment I have frequently wished to try, which cannot be done in private practice, and which I therefore recommend to some hospital physician: and that is, to endeavor to still the violent actions of the heart and arteries, after due evacuations by venesection and cathartics, by gently compressing the brain. This might be done by suspending a bed, so as to whirl the patient round with his head more distant from the center of rotation, as if he lay on a mill-stone.... By this whirling the patient with increasing velocity sleep might be produced, and probably the violence of the actions of the heart and arteries might be diminished in inflammatory fevers.[25]

Darwin shared the medical-scientific fantasies of his time regarding the causes and cures of maladies: they were due to an imbalance of the four humors. He believed insanity to be a disease that affects "the brain and blood vessels," and that these body parts could be restored to health by means of a mechanical device to "compress the brain." Based on Darwin's idea, Joseph Mason Cox (1763-1818), a mad-doctor and the owner of a private asylum, constructed a device that became known as "Cox's chair." In his book *Practical Observations on Insanity* (1804), Cox described his rotating chair and its use.[26] As with the "discoverers" of modern treatments for mental illness—from the shock therapists to the psychopharmacologists—the longer Cox used his instrument, the more convinced he became of its therapeutic powers. In 1813, he wrote: "Since publishing former editions of this work, I have continued the use of the swing, and am not only confirmed in my first opinion of its safety and utility, but convinced of its efficacy in some of the most hopeless maniacal cases."[27] For several decades, Cox's chair enjoyed considerable popularity, especially in German-speaking countries and Scandinavia. In a recent review of the history of Cox's chair, Nicholas J. Wade and his co-workers write:

Spinning in chairs, rotating in swings, prolonged immersion beneath high pressure cold showers, surprise plunges into icy water, or lying in warm baths while cold water was applied to the head, were all methods calculated to debilitate, shock, and soothe sanity back into the system. The rotary treatment was apparently applied more as a *corrective, than a therapeutic treatment.* [In the words of a nineteenth-century Scandinavian asylum doctor:] "After having committed some irrational and spiteful act, the patient is forthwith placed on the rotating chair and revolved at adjusted speed until he becomes quiet, apologizes, and promises improvement, or until he starts to vomit."[28]

5

Benjamin Rush (1746–1813) was a founding father of not only the United States but of American psychiatry. His portrait adorns the seal of the American Psychiatric Association. Here is the crux of Rush's therapeutic credo: "Terror acts powerfully upon the body, through the medium of the mind, and should be employed in the cure of madness."[29]

Rush was a zealous medicalizer of misbehavior as disease and of torture as treatment: "Lying, as a vice, is said to be incurable. The same thing may be said of it as a disease.... Its only remedy is, bodily pain, inflicted by the rod, or confinement, or abstinence from food."[30] He is best remembered as the inventor of a new instrument of terror and torture, which he called the "tranquilizing chair." It was but a small step from the tranquilizing chair to the tranquilizing drug, each administered against the will of the patient.

Rush, too, adhered to the humoral theory of disease and used it to rationalize his interventions. The tranquilizing chair, which, he boasted "binds and confines every part of the body [and] acts as a sedative to the tongue and temper as well as to the blood vessels," was supposed to correct the "disordered blood flow." His regimen of bleeding, purging and blistering "quickly reduced the patient to a weakened and therefore more manageable state."[31] In short, his treatments consisted of inflicting pain on the patient and depriving him of liberty. Despite Rush's unambiguous declarations that he had created the tranquilizing chair to torment the patient, the web site of the University of Pennsylvania Health Systems celebrates Rush and displays a picture of the tranquilizing chair accompanied by this plainly mendacious explanation: "Pictured here is the 'tranquilizing chair' in which patients were confined. ...[It] did neither harm nor good."[32]

In Rush's day, psychiatry was a newborn infant. Many madhouse keepers were clergymen, not physicians. Madness, as the term still implies, was associated with anger, lack of self-control, and suicide ("self-murder")—in short, with behaviors then regarded as sinful. In 1774, when Rush was only twenty-eight years old, he revealingly declared, "Perhaps hereafter it may be as much the business of a physician as it is now of a divine to reclaim mankind from vice."[33]

To distinguish himself from the doctor of divinity, the doctor of medicine could not simply claim that he was protecting people from sin or, as Rush put it, from vice. After all, vice is a moral concept. As a medical scientist, the physician had to reframe badness as madness, and represent madness as a bona fide medical malady. He had to demonstrate, by his language and actions, that his object of study was not the immaterial soul, but a material object, a bodily disease. That is precisely what Rush did. In a letter to his friend John Adams he wrote: "The subjects [mental diseases] have hitherto been enveloped in mystery. I have endeavored to bring them down to the level of all other diseases of the human body, and to show that the mind and the body are moved by the same causes and subject to the same laws."[34] Thus does physical reductionism replace scientific evidence in psychiatry. Today, neuroscientists assert that the mind is the brain and pretend that the claim rests on and is supported by novel discoveries.

Rush did not *discover* that certain behaviors are diseases; he *decreed* that they are: "Lying is a corporeal disease. / Suicide is madness. / Chagrin, shame, fear, terror, anger, unfit for legal acts, are transient madness."[35] The rejection of medicine and of Christianity were also mental illnesses, which he named "derangements in the principle of faith or the believing faculty," describing the "patients" as "persons who deny their belief in the utility of medicine, as practiced by regular bred [trained] physicians, believing implicitly in quacks; [and] persons who refuse to admit human testimony in favor of the truths of the Christian religion."[36]

Everything Rush deplored became an illness. Lamenting the "excess of the passion for liberty inflamed by the successful issue of the [Revolutionary] war," Rush stated: "The extensive influence which these opinions had upon the understandings, passions, and morals of many of the citizens of the United States, constituted a form of insanity, which I shall take the liberty of distinguishing by the name of anarchia."[37] Disappointed with his political efforts, he declared: "Were we to live our lives over again and engage in the same benevolent enterprise, our means should not be reasoning but bleeding, purging, low diet, and the tranquilizing chair."[38] Rush would be proud of the current American psychiatric nosology, which recognizes more than 300 discrete "mental disorders," every one a "brain disease."

Not surprisingly, Rush defined crimes as "derangements of the will" and championed the insanity defense:[39] "I have selected those two symptoms [murder and theft] of this disease (for they are not vices) from its other morbid effects, in order to rescue persons affected with them from the arm of the law, and render them the subjects of the kind and lenient hand of medicine."[40]

6

The language and thought of Van Helmholt, Willis, Cox, and Rush illustrate that psychiatry came into being when the study of the soul was transformed into the study of the mind, the cure of souls became the treatment of madness, the image of the paradigmatic social deviant threatening society changed from that of the heretic to that of the insane, and responsibility for the control of the deviant was transferred from the jurisdiction of church-and-priest to the jurisdiction of medicine-and-psychiatrist. In short, psychiatry is an offspring of religious thought and clerical repression that rested on the alliance of church and state. It is not, and could not have been, an offspring of medical thought and clinical repression resting on an alliance of medicine and the state for the simple reason that there was no such alliance before the advent of mad-doctoring.

For millennia, religion and the church (as well as criminal law) prescribed rules of personal conduct and social behavior and punished transgressions. In Islamic countries, this is still the case. In the West, the vacuum created by the demise of the alliance between church and state in the wake of the Enlightenment was filled partly by criminal and civil law, and partly by a new, ostensibly secular-scientific system of social control, called "mad-doctoring," later renamed "psychiatry." Trying to reconcile religion and science, the pioneer mad-doctors provided a system of explanations for certain socially unwanted behaviors, an ostensibly judicial-medical system of justifications for controlling persons who displayed such behaviors, and a set of institutions for confining certain deviant persons in prisons called "(state) hospitals." The result is the ideology of mental health and an historically novel type of *state security apparatus*, called "psychiatry." This apparatus, which matured toward the end of the nineteenth century, became the servant *par excellence* of the modern therapeutic state in all its seemingly diverse forms—International Socialist (Communist), National Socialist (German), and Democratic Socialist (American and Western European, embraced by the United Nations and the World Health Organization).

The writings of the famous German alienist, Johann Christian Heinroth (1773-1843), exhibit the nakedly political nature of the ideology of early mad-doctoring and the internally contradictory character of its explanations and justifications. Heinroth's *magnum opus*, published in 1818, is tellingly titled, *Textbook of Disturbances of Mental Life, or Disturbances of the Soul and Their Treatment (Lehrbuch der Störungen des Seelenlebens).*[41]

It is unlikely that Heinroth was familiar with Rush's textbook, published six years earlier, which makes the similarities between their views and practices all the more remarkable. Heinroth, however, was more forthright than Rush in acknowledging that the mad-doctor's duty is to serve the interests of the modern secular state, not the interests of the denominated patient. His definition of mental illness is explicitly political: "The complete concept of mental disturbances includes permanent *loss of freedom or loss of reason*, independent and for itself, *even when bodily health is apparently unimpaired*, which manifests itself as a diseased condition, and which comprises the domains of temperament, diseases of the spirit, and will."[42] Prefiguring the rhetoric of contemporary psychiatric dehumanizers supposedly enlightened by modern neuroscience, Heinroth declares:

> All these diseases, however much as their external manifestations may differ, have this one feature in common, namely, that not only is there no freedom but not even the capacity to regain freedom.... Thus, individuals in this condition exist no longer in the human domain, which is the domain of freedom, but follow the coercion of internal and external natural necessity. Rather than resembling animals, which are led by a wholesome instinct, they resemble machines and are maintained by vital laws in bodily life alone.[43]

Psychiatric propagandists and the media tirelessly regale us about recent "breakthroughs" in the understanding and treatment of mental illness. It is all a lie. The truth is that, from a moral and political point of view, nothing has changed. In 1818, Johann Christian Heinroth asserted that mentally ill persons resemble machines. In 1975, Michael S. Moore, a professor of law and philosophy at the University of San Diego, asserted that such patients resemble "infants, wild beasts, plants, and stones—none of which are responsible because of the absence of any assumption of rationality."[44]

Viewing the person who lacks self-control, who is controlled by his passions, as not free is a classic Greco-Roman idea. Shakespeare romanticized it: "The lunatic, the lover, and the poet, are of imagination all compact."[45] Heinroth psychiatrized it: "The man who is fettered by passions deceives himself about external objects and about himself. *This illusion, and the consequent error, is called madness....* In madness the spirit is fettered and man, just as in passion (both being indissolubly linked), is unfree and unhappy."[46] And Edmund Burke warned: "Society cannot exist unless a controlling power upon will and appetite be placed somewhere, and the less there is within, the more there must be without. It is ordained in the eternal constitution of things, that men of intemperate minds cannot be free. Their passions forge their fetters."[47]

The early alienists managed to conflate and confuse the loss of *existential liberty imposed by intemperance and illness with the loss of political liberty imposed by law and enforced by psychiatrists.* Loss of freedom due to physical disease or disability is radically different from deprivation due to the action of a human agent, such as judge, prison guard, or psychiatrist. Muscular dystrophy, multiple sclerosis, stroke, and many other diseases deprive the subject of freedom. But such persons are not, properly speaking, "deprived of political liberty." Nor are they incarcerated by physicians. *As mental illness is a metaphorical illness, so the unfreedom attributed to the mental patient is a metaphorical loss of freedom. It becomes a literal loss of freedom only as a result of the psychiatrist's action.* It must be added, even though obvious, that paraplegic persons do not assault people, because their injury deprives them of the freedom to do so; whereas persons psychiatrists call "paranoids" and "psychopaths" assault people not because they are ill, but because we attribute their lawless behavior to paranoia and psychopathy and, with circular logic, call people who engage in such behavior "paranoids" and "psychopaths." Hence, society and psychiatry need both an insanity defense and buildings in which to imprison and "treat" "insane killers."

Heinroth's assertion that the insane lack freedom—"individuals in this condition exist no longer in the human domain, which is the domain of freedom"—is a *strategic claim.* Because the patient is unfree, the psychiatrist is justified in coercing him: medical control is treatment, psychiatric oppression is liberation.[48] Referring to patients for whom Heinroth believed recovery was possible, he wrote: ""What is needed in such cases is *constraint, which is in no way cruelty or inhumanity, but necessary for the reeducation of such patients to the norm of reason....* For as long as such and similar patients have their will, nothing can be done with them."[49]

Heinroth's aim was to justify not only torture as treatment but also the medical profession's monopolistic control over the study of "mental disturbance" and the treatment of the mental patient: "Since we are speaking of medical art and science, we should think that nobody but a doctor should have a right to make mental disturbance the object of his studies and treatment."[50] Under the revealing heading "Medicina Psychica Politica" [Psycho-Political Medicine], Heinroth declares: "It is the duty of the state to care for mentally disturbed persons whenever they are a burden to the community or present a public danger."[51] Ipso facto, the psychiatrist is an agent of the state.

According to Heinroth, "They [mental disturbances] all have a common starting point, a main principle to which they are subordinated: selfishness."[52] In contrast, "The doctor of the soul (or psyche)...has overcome selfish interests and treats for purely humanitarian reasons."[53] Since the psychiatrist is a physician who nevertheless is not an agent of the so-called patient, his role must be sanctified: "He influences the patient by virtue of his, one may be permitted to say, *holy presence,* by the sheer strength of his being, his glance, and his will."[54] Heinroth asserts that the proper method of curing mental illnesses rests on domination-submission: "First, be master of the situation; second, be master of the patient.... Unless this superiority is established, all treatment will be in vain."[55] He recommends that hospitals devoted specially to the treatment of the insane be built and that they "must also have *a special correction and punishment room* with all the necessary equipment, including a Cox swing (or, better, rotating machine), Reil's fly-wheel,* pulleys, punishment chair, Langermann's cell, etc."[56] This account sounds more like a plan to equip a prison in a totalitarian state with appropriate torture devices than a plan to equip a medical institution with diagnostic and therapeutic instruments.

7

Johann Heinrich Ferdinand von Autenrieth (1772-1835) was born and studied medicine in Stuttgart. In 1797, he was appointed professor of Anatomy, Physiology, Surgery, and Obstetrics at the University of Tübingen, and in 1819, became its chancellor. In his day, Autenrieth was a highly respected physician and medical educator. Because he was not a mad-doctor, his name and work are not mentioned in psychiatric history texts, not even in Hunter and Macalpine's encyclopedic *Three Hundred Years of Psychiatry, 1535-1860.*[57]

Autenrieth invented two devices to control mental patients, both named after him and both widely used in the nineteenth century. The

---

* For more about Reil and Langermann, see chapter 3.

"Authenrieth chamber" was a movable stockade used to confine and move patients who were considered dangerous. The "Authenrieth mask," was a piece of hard wood, with the shape and dimensions of a medium-sized pear with a cross-bar fitted with straps which can be tied at the back of the patient's neck. Heinroth recommended the use of the mask: "Since the oral cavity of the patient is more or less filled by this instrument, the patient can obviously utter no articulate sounds.... *[This instrument] must not be condemned as cruel, since its aim is to produce one of the most healing of restrictions.*"[58] The Autenrieth mask may have inspired the muzzle with which Dr. Hannibal Lecter (Anthony Hopkins) was fitted in the famous 1991 film, *Silence of the Lambs.*[59]

The purpose of the Autenrieth mask is emblematic of the aim of all involuntary psychiatric interventions: the silencing of the patient. The mad person says things people do not want to hear. The psychiatrist responds: "Shut up!" He protects society from the mad person whose speech society considers offensive. "Children should be seen, not heard," declares a popular adage. Psychiatry was created to insure that the insane are neither seen nor heard. Institutionalization, shock treatment, lobotomy, neuroleptic drugs—and, perhaps most simply and most importantly, stigmatizing psychiatric diagnoses—are all *instruments for silencing the subject.* Autenrieth explains: "The doctor can never sufficiently impress upon himself and others the fact that the insane are identical in most respects to stubborn, ill-mannered children and, like them, require stern (not cruel) treatment.... Is not the treatment of mental patients frequently comparable to the education of children? Every finding indicates that the comparison is apt."[60]

Silencing, speaking, listening and refusing to hear—these are the blocks out of which psychiatrists build their theories, therapies, and histories. Silencing the patient is a cure, letting or making the patient speak is also a cure. In either case, it matters not what the patient says or might want to say. The psychiatrist, cloaking himself in the mantle of benevolence and the mystery of being able to "analyze minds," robs the subject of his voice and declares him too crippled in mind to know, much less be able to articulate, his own desires and values. The somatically oriented psychiatrist does not listen to the patient. The psychologically oriented therapist listens, but only to re-interpret the patient's communication.

In addition to his invention of devices for restraining and silencing mental patients, Autenrieth deserves to be remembered for two other contributions: he created what we call "academic medicine," that is, medicine as a discipline studied, taught, and practiced in the setting of a modern university; and he cared, with great humanity, for the mad Johann Christian Friedrich Hölderlin (1770-1843), one of the most celebrated German poets.

Before Autenrieth's time—indeed, until well into the twentieth century—*medical hospital care* was for poor people only. Called charity hospitals, these institutions, financed and operated by municipalities, resembled poorhouses more than hospitals. Prior to World War II, domestic help was plentiful and inexpensive, permitting the upper-class disabled, sick, mad, elderly, and dying to be housed in their own homes (or the homes of relatives). The typical privately practicing physician's practice was conducted mainly in private homes, the impoverished inmates of charity hospitals serving as the "clinical material" for teaching medical students.

Universities, ancient institutions, did not operate hospitals. Autenrieth changed this, establishing a 15-bed "clinic" (hospital) at the University of Tübingen.[61] Regarding his treatment of Hölderlin, a brief summary suffices. Hölderlin had been trained for the clergy, a vocation he quickly abandoned for poetry and music. In 1806, when he was 36 years old, Hölderlin had a "breakdown." His friends took him to Autenrieth's clinic in Tübingen:

> Believing that he is being kidnapped, the poet attempts to jump from the coach.... Arriving at the clinic, Hölderlin is given various sedatives and stimulants, such as digitalis, and the deadly nightshade, Belladonna. During the first part of his stay, he is required to read the Bible, which has a considerably negative effect upon him. Though the clinic is considered to be "humane" in comparison with other clinics, Hölderlin is nonetheless kept under strict observation, and during his outbreaks of madness is presumably forced to wear the facial mask designed by Autenrieth.... Unable to cure the poet, Autenrieth places Hölderlin in the care of the prosperous and intellectual cabinet-maker Ernst Zimmer and his wife. The doctors give Hölderlin "three years at best" to live.[62]

Hölderlin spent the last thirty-six years of his life living with and being cared for by the Zimmer family. It is instructive to compare the course of his "illness" with that of the modern mental patient, living in so-called transitional housing and maintained on neuroleptic drugs under the threat of outpatient commitment orders. In 1835, Ernest Zimmer wrote about his famous guest: "His state of mind was much worse in the clinic.... Since the clinic could do nothing more for him, Autenrieth suggested that I take him into my custody, for he knew of no better place for him. He was and still is a great friend of nature, and his room has a view of the whole Neckar valley, including the Steinlacher valley." Hölderlin often went on strolls with the Zimmers, and spent much of his time playing the piano and flute, making drawings, and creating more poetry.

István Vida, a contemporary Hungarian psychiatrist who was a student at Tübingen, has examined Hölderlin's records and concluded that, for the last thirty-six years of his life, he was well cared for in what was in effect a foster home.[63] The Swiss poet and novelist Robert Walser (1878-1956), who had spent the last forty-three years of his life in an insane asylum and knew of what he spoke, summed up Hölderlin's final years as follows: "I am convinced that Hölderlin was not that unhappy in his last thirty years, as the professors of literature want to make us believe. Being allowed to dream in a modest nook without being obliged to fulfill permanently all the demands of the world is surely not a martyrdom. People only like to see it this way."[64] This is an important observation that requires amplification. Many persons whom psychiatrists call "seriously mentally ill" or "schizophrenic" are withdrawn from the public world. Because they live in their own "private world," which they are unwilling to leave, psychiatrists call them "inaccessible." To better understand how the contemporary psychiatrized mind sees their behavior, we must once again turn to religion.

8

In biblical times, voluntary withdrawal from the world was a recognized and respected option. In the modern secular world, it is not. Our vocabulary still has words, usually used in a religious context, to express such a life choice. The hermit (from the Greek *eremites*, "living in the desert"), or "anchorite" (from the Greek *anachoreo*, "to withdraw"), is a person who retires from worldly life for religious reasons.[65] He seeks solitude to be alone with God, undistracted by the diversions of ordinary social life: he rejects family, sex, work, and socially acceptable standards of dress and cleanliness. "The soul occupied with divine thoughts freed from all distracting cares leads an existence most consonant to man's rational nature, and consequently productive of the highest type of happiness obtainable on this earth."[66] Some anchorites formed groups, became religious orders and founded monasteries. Persons living in such monastic groups—devoted to being "alone with God"—were called "cenobites." Eventually monasteries combining features of the eremitical and cenobitical types of religious life were founded. Anchoritic practices are a part of Christianity as well as Hinduism, Buddhism, and Sufism.

According to Maximos E. Aghiorgoussis, Orthodox Bishop of Pittsburgh, "Since the early years of the Christian era, Christians have been called by Christ Himself to life in the world without being of the world (John 17:13-16). They are distinct from the world, because of their special conduct and their exemplary ethical life.... They practiced chastity, celibacy, poverty, prayer and fasting. These people considered themselves Christians selected to live the life of angels (Matt. 22:30)."[67] The similarities between the solitude-seeking withdrawal of the hermit, the "creative genius," and the "psychotic" are obvious. In the past, people often recognized that "insanity" may be a form of voluntary withdrawal from the world. As a result of "scientific progress in psychiatry," it is now socially impermissible to suggest that a so-called psychotic may choose to act as he does.

In modern societies, populated by masses of atomized individuals living in lonely togetherness, it is virtually impossible for the person who feels tormented by his life to withdraw from it and not be punished. Society treats such a person as the military treats the soldier who withdraws from the front lines by falling ill with battle fatigue/post-traumatic stress disorder. The civilian psychiatrist's job, like that of his military counterpart, is to treat-torment the patient in an effort to make him rejoin his society/battalion. One of the punishments for going "AWOL" is being diagnosed as mentally ill and forcibly cured of it.

Friedrich Nietzsche's (1844-1900) life and breakdown invites such an interpretation. Nietzsche was a "loner." True, he had a mother and sister. However, he felt alienated from them: "I do not like my mother, and listening to my sister's voice makes me miserable, I have always been sick when I was together with them," he wrote to his friend Franz Overbeck in Basel, in 1883.[68]

Nietzsche had a few devoted male friends, but they did not meet his needs. He longed for female companionship, but was incapable of forming a relationship with a woman, or was unwilling to do so. For the better part of his brief, pre-illness life as an adult, Nietzsche was alone in the world. First he lived the life of a hermitic philosopher, then that of psychotic mental patient. Richard Schain calls him first a "homeless philosopher," then an "asylum inmate."[69]

Only ten years, 1879-1889, had elapsed between the time Nietzsche resigned from his professorship in Basel and the time he assumed the role of a madman. *Thus Spake Zarathustra*—written between 1883 and 1885, and published in 1891, two years after the official date of the onset of his insanity—is at once a desperate lament from the depth of Nietzsche's self-imposed solitude and a grandiose, megalomaniacal celebration of himself as "overman" replacing the God that has died. Walter Kaufman, editor and translator of *The Portable Nietzsche*, correctly observes: "the most important single clue to *Zarathustra* is that it is the work of an utterly lonely man."[70]

Nietzsche's prose style is dramatic, moving, and deservedly famous. It is, in a way, one prolonged, anguished *cri de coeur*, an impassioned outcry, entreaty, or protest, or all of them together. In the foreword to *Ecce Homo* (1888/1908), Nietzsche says, "*Hear me! For I am such and such a person! Above all, do not mistake me for someone else!*" [71] Who, at that time, wanted to know who Nietzsche was? No one!

In *Thus Spake Zarathustra*, Nietzsche *is* both Zarathustra and "the saint/hermit." At the age of thirty, Zarathustra abandons his home for a retreat in the mountains. After living and meditating in solitude for ten years, he leaves his retreat to share his wisdom with humanity. A saint/hermit tries to persuade Zarathustra to reconsider: "It will be a waste of time, don't trouble yourself. Men are ungrateful. Men are distracted.... It's much better to be a hermit like me, it's much better to live in the forest with the birds and the beasts...simply worshiping God." Zarathustra tells him that "God is dead" and proceeds with his mission. Humanity, more interested in comfort than in "heroic living," rejects Zarathustra.[72] The monastic Zarathustra in his mountain retreat makes one think of Nietzsche in his mountain retreat in Sils Maria (near St. Moritz). The view that "God is dead" was no longer news at the end of the nineteenth century. In "Zarathustra's Prologue," Nietzsche protests, speaking through Zarathustra: "I love man."[73] Nietzsche may have loved man, whatever such an all-encompassing yet vacuous phrase might mean, but he loved solitude more, and withdrew into it.

Nietzsche recognized that he was trying to escape from the world. He struggled with the option of killing himself, but decided not to do so. In 1880, he wrote to Otto Eiser, his physician: "My existence is a fearful burden. I would have long ago thrown it over if I had not been making the most instructive tests and experiments in the spiritual-moral area in exactly this condition of suffering and enduring almost total deprivation."[74] Of what was Nietzsche "deprived"? Of intimacy, of which he was incapable, and he knew it: "The energy for absolute solitude and release from customary relationships, my insistence on not allowing myself to be cared for, to be served, to be doctored—that revealed an absolute certainty of instinct about what was necessary at that time."[75] A year later, Nietzsche began his eleven-year career as a mental patient—cared for, served, and doctored around the clock.

Everyone needs both intimacy and solitude. Some people need solitude more than others. Cynthia Ozick uses the metaphor of the anchorite to characterize the writer: "He is in the private cave of his freedom, an eremite, a solitary; he orders his mind as he pleases."[76]

Virginia Woolf also loved solitude, which she found in her marriage to Leonard Woolf and her periodic bouts of madness. She offered this moving description of her longing for secular isolation:

> We do not know our own souls, let alone the souls of others. Human beings do not go hand in hand the whole stretch of the way. There is a virgin forest in each; a snow field where even the birds' feet is unknown. Here we go alone, and like it better so. Always to have sympathy, always to be accompanied, always to be understood would be intolerable. But in health the genial pretense must be kept up and the effort renewed—to communicate, to civilize, to share, to cultivate the desert, educate the native, to work together by day and by night to sport.

And she added this cogent comment about the moral condemnation we place on such withdrawal: "In illness this make-believe ceases...we cease to be soldiers in the army of the upright; we become deserters."[77] Deserters, indeed. And society does not let deserters go unpunished, lest too many of its members be tempted to take that course.

3

Moral Treatment: Renaming Coercion

[T]he medical treatment of [mental] patients began with the infringement of their personal freedom.

—*Karl Wernicke (1848-1905)*[1]*

1

Through much of the nineteenth century, "moral treatment"—a term first used by William Tuke in 1796, and by Philippe Pinel in 1801 (*traitment moral*)—was considered correct psychiatric practice. This concept of treatment meshed with the concept of mental illness as "moral insanity." Like most concepts framed in the specialized idiom of psychiatry, "moral treatment" does not lend itself to clear definition. Historians of psychiatry characterize the method as "optimistic," even though it rests on a theoretical commitment to "*a physiological basis for mental disorder*: insanity was caused by brain damage.... The notion that mental illness resulted from physical impairment was rarely challenged."[2]

In practice, the only clear and constant element in the practice of moral treatment was the legally authorized coercion of the patient by the doctor. The matching concept of "moral insanity" is also vague. Primarily, it was used to convey the idea that *the essential nature of mental disorder was psychological*, concerned with man's spiritual life, personal habits, and interpersonal relations. The terminology points to the beginning of the medicalization—indeed, the neuroanatomical localization—of eccentric and illegal behavior and, at the same time, the recognition that mental diseases, unlike bodily diseases, manifest themselves in ways that are inherently "moral." Definitions of these obsolete terms in modern medical dictionaries are consistent with these interpretations. *Dorland's Illustrated Medical Dictionary* defines "moral insanity" as "a 19th cen-

---

* The full quotation reads: "Remarking on the purpose and goals of psychiatric clinics, Carl [sic] Wernicke noted that the medical treatment of patients began with the infringement of their personal freedom."

tury concept corresponding roughly to antisocial personality disorder; a disorder of emotions and habits without impairment of the intellectual faculties in which the moral sense (concern for the rights and feelings of others) is stunted (moral imbecility) or absent (moral idiocy)"; and "insanity" as "mental derangement or disorder, *a legal rather than a medical term* denoting a condition due to which a person lacks criminal responsibility for a crime and therefore cannot be convicted of it."[3]

The assertion that insanity is a "legal rather than a medical term" is only partly true. "Insanity" is a term that psychiatrists have claimed and disclaimed as it has suited their needs. Between 1844 and 1921, the official journal of the profession, now called the *American Journal of Psychiatry,* was published under the title *American Journal of Insanity.*[4] Aggressively interrogated in court by a district attorney, psychiatrists are wont to assert that "insanity has no medical meaning." The fact remains that the law speaks of insane persons; that individuals are incarcerated in accordance with "mental health laws," not "brain health laws"; and that the medical jailers in charge of insane persons are psychiatrists, not neurologists.

In short, the semantics of early psychiatry contains unmistakable signs of the view that insane behavior is immoral behavior; that insane conduct is often illegal conduct; that if insane conduct is illegal, the individual committing the prohibited act is not legally responsible for it; and that the concept of insanity is susceptible to both juridical and medical definitions.

The practice of what was called "moral treatment" developed along different lines in different countries. I will present brief sketches of the English, French, German, and American versions of the story.

2

In England, the history of moral treatment is closely associated with the Quaker family Tuke, in York. In 1796, William Tuke (1732-1822), a tea and coffee merchant, not a physician, opened the doors to his private asylum, which he called "The Retreat." For Tuke, this was a humanitarian-philanthropic enterprise. His aim, he said, was to provide "a place in which the unhappy might obtain a refuge—a quiet haven in which the shattered bark might find the means of reparation and of safety."[5] Tuke viewed the founding of the Retreat in political rather than medical terms: He desired, he said, to "carry[ing] out the noble experiment, as to how far the insane might be influenced through the medium of the understanding and the affections, and how far they may be beneficially admitted to the liberty, comfort, and general habits of the sane."[6] The Retreat quickly acquired the reputation of being the best asylum in Europe.

William Tuke's work was continued by his eldest son Henry Tuke (1755-1814), his grandson Samuel Tuke (1784-1857), and his great grandson, Daniel Hack Tuke (1827-1895). Henry and Samuel Tuke were businessmen and philanthropists. Daniel Tuke was a physician and a famous expert on mental diseases. In 1813, Samuel Tuke published a small book titled, *Description of the Retreat, an Institution Near York, for Insane Persons of the Society of Friends.* He wrote:

> Neither chains nor corporal punishments are tolerated, on any pretext, in this establishment. The patients, therefore, cannot be threatened with these severities.... To the mild system of treatment adopted at the Retreat, I have no doubt we may partly attribute, the happy recovery of so large a proportion of melancholy patients.... If it be true, that oppression makes a wise man mad, is it to be supposed that stripes and insults, and injuries, for which the receiver knows no cause, are calculated to make a madman wise? or would they not exasperate his disease and make excite his resentment?... The superintendent...is fully of the opinion that a state of furious mania, is very often excited by the mode of management.[7]

Tuke was well aware that psychiatric slavery generates problems that only its abolition can solve, but he was not ready to act on the basis of that conclusion. Yet, Hunter and Macalpine, who cannot be accused of naiveté regarding the history of psychiatry, are so carried away by their enthusiasm for the Quaker psychiatric reformers that they baldly, but erroneously, state that the success of the Retreat "led a quarter of a century later to the completion of the work started by Pinel and the Tukes when *John Conolly abolished all restraint in a large public asylum and banished the principle of fear from moral treatment.*"[8] This is a startlingly false claim, contradicted by material cited by Hunter and Macalpine themselves. In an essay on "Moral Treatment at the Retreat, 1796-1846," Anne Digby, a historian, states: "The 'external' control of the patient, either through physical restraint or through medication, was practiced on a lesser scale at the Retreat than had been usual in some earlier asylums, although *neither means of treatment were entirely eschewed.*"[9] Clearly, confining a person in an asylum, or anywhere else, constitutes restraint, and everything done to a person so restrained is, by definition, an act of coercion. This is not to gainsay the importance of Conolly's criticism of psychiatric coercion.

In 1839, John Conolly (1794-1866), professor of the practice of medicine at London University, became the superintendent of the Middlesex County Lunatic Asylum at Hanwell. His interest in psychiatry having begun long before, Conolly made his reputation nine years earlier with the publication of his *Inquiry Concerning the Indications of Insanity, With Suggestions for the Better Protection and Care of the Insane* (1830). Therein precisely lay Conolly's problem and therein lies the problem for all psychiatric "reformers": How can an adult citizen in a free society be "protected" from harming himself or others without being coerced? The answer is that he cannot. In a modern secular society, the freedom to harm oneself is a human right, and so, too, is the liberty that may lead to harming another, in the sense that preventive detention is incompatible with the rule of law. Conolly knew and acknowledged this. "What is required," he wrote, "is, that no person, who is not insane, should be treated as an insane person. That all who are insane, should be properly taken care of.... That all persons of unsound mind should be *the property of the State, and be controlled by public officers*."[10] Surely, this does not sound as if Conolly had "abolished all restraint in a large public asylum."[11] Of course, Conolly does not ask whether a person ought to have a right to be insane, and not be molested because of it by doctors and the state, just as he has a right to be ill with, say, gout, and not be molested because of it by doctors and the state. Nor does he say how to distinguish sane persons from insane persons.

Precisely because Conolly recognized that insane asylums were carceral institutions, he accepted that the entire psychiatric enterprise rested on the powers of a benevolent state. This view was widely shared by the leading opinion makers of his day, and is illustrated by the mushrooming growth during Conolly's life time of state lunatic asylums in both Europe and the United States. Everywhere, the new psychiatry rested on the same statist-socialist, medical-paternalistic psychiatric premises.

Notwithstanding the Quaker influence, in England, too, moral treatment came down to coercion, however "mild." Medical advances, especially during the latter half of the nineteenth century, made psychiatrists feel more secure in their conviction that "insanity" was a serious, usually incurable, brain disease, that "the insane" were biological degenerates, and that it was the neuropsychiatrist's job to protect society from the insane. General William Booth (1829-1912), founder of the Salvation Army, expressed this view in no uncertain terms. Recommending an "Asylum for Moral Lunatics," he stated: "There are men so incorrigibly lazy that no inducement that you can offer will tempt them to work.... Sorrowfully, but remorselessly, it must be recognized that he has become lunatic, morally demented...and that upon him, therefore, must be passed the sentence of permanent seclusion from a world in which he is not fit to be at large."[12]

3

In France, the history of moral treatment (*traitment moral*) is associated with Philippe Pinel (1745-1826) and his followers. Psychiatric historians celebrate Pinel as a pioneering humanitarian physician and attribute the discovery of moral treatment to him. The crux of Pinel's alleged achievement lies in the transformation of undisguised psychiatric brutality into torture disguised as treatment.[13] Perhaps nothing illustrates the centrality of coercion to the practice of psychiatry more dramatically than the sanctifying of Pinel as the "liberator" of the madman. However inadvertently, the legend of Saint Pinel also points to the recognition-cum-denial of the fact that efforts to reform psychiatric imprisonment are doomed to failure. Repeatedly, the mental patient is liberated. Yet he continues to be enslaved.

Pinel, the son of a barber surgeon born in the south of France, received an excellent education for his time and was greatly influenced by the encyclopaedists, particularly Jean-Jacques Rousseau (1712-1778). Planning to become a priest, Pinel enrolled in the Faculty of Theology at Toulouse in 1767 but left three years later for the Faculty of Medicine, from which he graduated in 1773. In 1778, Pinel moved to Paris carrying with him letters of recommendation to several prominent Parisian intellectuals. At the salon of Mme. Helvétius, widow of the celebrated Encyclopedist Claude-Adrien Helvétius (1715-1771), he became acquainted with Pierre Jean Georges Cabanis (1757-1808), the leading French physician of his day.

In 1783, four years into the French Revolution, the government appointed Pinel "physician of the infirmeries" at the Bicêtre, a dungeon that "housed about four thousand imprisoned men—criminals, petty offenders, syphilitics, pensioners, and about two hundred mental patients."[14] He received this appointment not because of professional merit but because of friendship with leading Jacobin physicians, among them Cabanis and Michel-Augustin Thouret (1748-1810).[15] In 1804, Pinel was made Chevalier of the *Légion d'Honneur*. Today, his statue stands outside the Salpêtrière in Paris.

The Pinel legend masks the fact that his ceremonial unchaining of the mental patient, reprised in book after book and rememorialized in painting after painting, is a medical re-enactment of Exodus and/or of Jesus's healing of the epileptic and the leper. It is the founding miracle of the new Jacobin religion of psychiatry.[16] The legend has proved amazingly successful in distracting the attention of both the public and the medical profession from the most obvious and important feature of the origin of psychiatry, namely, that it is a creature of the modern centralizing state, an auxiliary to the prison system, with the psychiatrist's role defined as that of an officer charged with the correction of the inmates' incorrect behavior. Pinel created modern psychiatry as a medical specialty not by demonstrating that mental diseases are diseases, but by defining coercion as treatment. *The adjective "moral" in "moral treatment" refers to the fatal self-contradiction at the heart of psychiatry: the psychiatrist claims to be a physician and diagnoses the subject as ill, yet confines and punishes him as if he were a criminal, and calls the punishment "moral treatment."* By arranging and rearranging, in various patterns, the two basic elements of psychiatry—the fiction of mental illness and the fact of coercion-therapy—psychiatrists erect ever more impressive and costly pyramids of bogus diseases and brutal treatments.

In 1795, Pinel was appointed chief physician of the *Hospice de la Salpêtrière*, a post that he retained for the rest of his life. His *magnum opus, Traité médico-philosophique sur l'aliénation mentale, ou la manie (Medical-Philosophical Treatise on Mental Alienation, or Mania)*, was published in 1801 and quickly became enormously influential in both Europe and the United States. The English translation, published in 1806, is entitled, *A Treatise on Insanity, in which are Contained the Principles of a New and More Practical Nosology of Maniacal Disorders than has yet been Offered to the Public, etc.*[17] In Section II, under the subtitle, "The Moral Treatment of Insanity," Pinel states:

> If met, however, by a force evidently and convincingly superior, he submits without opposition or violence. This is a great and invaluable secret in the management of well regulated hospitals.[18] ...The estimable effects of coercion illustrated in the case of a soldier.... All fair means to appease him being exhausted, coercive measures became indispensable.[19] ...In the preceding cases of insanity, we trace the happy effects of intimidation, without severity; of oppression, without violence.[20] ...For this purpose the strait-waistcoat will generally be found amply sufficient.... Improper application for personal liberty, or any other favor, must be received with acquiescence, taken graciously into consideration, and withheld under some plausible pretext.[21] ...To effect and expedite a permanent cure, unlimited power in the choice and adoption of curative measure were given to his medical attendant.[22]

As these excerpts show, Pinel regarded the madman as a headstrong, ill-behaved child, and himself as his father whose duty is to break the child's will and domesticate him. He ended the *Traité* with a flattering plea addressed to government authorities: "For the accomplishment of these our earnest wishes, we look up to the councils of a firm government, which overlooks not any of the great objects of public utility."[23] Pinel, let us not forget, was a Jacobin. He was among the spectators witnessing the beheading of Louis XVI. The guillotine, too, was the creation of a Jacobin, Dr. Joseph Ignace Guillotin (1738-1814), a member of the Revolutionary Assembly, who developed his machine at the Bicêtre and tried it on cadavers of the inmates.

I share Edmund Burke's view of the French Revolution as a human catastrophe of unparalleled historical significance. Jacobinism presaged the chaos and cruelty that were the trademarks of International Socialism and National Socialism in the twentieth century. One of the Jacobins' principal aims was to dechristianize society: they converted the clergy from priests into patriots, from servants of God into agents of *la patrie*. The result was the *sacralizing of the state,* a curse that the French and many other Westerners celebrate as a blessing. After World War II, the new Jacobins set out to demedicalize medicine: they converted physicians from servants of their patients into agents of *public health.*[24] The result is the *therapeutizing of the state,* an oppression most people in the West, especially liberals, regard as a "liberation," ensuring health care for all.[25]

The transformation of the physician from servant-healer of the patient into employee-agent of the state occurred first and remains most obvious and troubling in psychiatry. Pinel was, literally, an employee and agent of the Jacobin state and is an appropriate exemplar of the torturer as treater. C. S. Lewis painted this portrait of Pinel's modern successor:

> We know that one school of psychology already regards religion as a neurosis. When this particular neurosis becomes inconvenient to the government, what is to hinder the government from proceeding to "cure" it? Such "cure" will, of course, be compulsory; but under the humanitarian theory it will not be called by the shocking name of Persecution. No one will blame us for being Christians, no one will hate us, no one revile us. The new Nero will approach us with the silky manners of a doctor, and though all will be in fact as compulsory as *tunica molesta* or Smithfield or Tyburn, all will go on within the unemotional therapeutic sphere where words like "right" and "wrong," or "freedom" and "slavery" are never heard.... But it will not be persecution. Even if the treatment is painful, even if it is life-long, even if it is fatal, that will be only a regrettable accident, the intention was purely therapeutic.... But because they are "treatment," not punishment, they can be criticized only by fellow experts and on technical grounds, never by men as men and on grounds of justice.*

4

The term "moral therapy" did not become a part of the German psychiatric vocabulary. In their psychiatric practice, German-speaking

* The tunica molesta or "flaming shirt"—a garment impregnated with flammable substance and set ablaze—was a commonly used instrument of execution in ancient Greece and Rome. Nero sentenced scores of Christians to be killed by this means.

physicians, like their English and French counterparts, relied on coercion. Respecting psychiatric theory, they became the founders and leaders of modern organic psychiatry, that is, the doctrine that mental illnesses are diseases of the brain.

During the first several decades of the nineteenth century, the English and the French ruled psychiatry. By mid-century, German-speaking psychiatry had conquered the field; it retained its leadership until past World War I. The very term psychiatry (*Psychiatrie*) is of German origin, having been coined in 1808 by Johann Christian Reil (1759-1813), one of the outstanding medical scientists and physicians of his age.[27] Such was his reputation that in 1810 Wilhelm von Humboldt invited him to participate in the organization of the medical school at the newly founded University of Berlin. He was a friend and physician of Johann Wolfgang von Goethe. Reil was not a psychiatrist. However, he was a man of broad interests and knowledge who played an important role in the early history of psychiatry. In addition to coining the term "psychiatry," he also coined the term "noninjurious torture." He believed that frightening mental patients was an effective and legitimate method of treating them.[28]

The French system of insane asylums was, as we have seen, a product of the Jacobin state and was considered "humanitarian." The German system was also a product of an autocratic state, albeit one considered "reactionary." According to Emil Kraepelin, the German (Prussian) state insane asylum system was created in 1805 by Karl August von Hardenberg (1759-1822), a Prussian statesman. "The state," Hardenberg declared, "must concern itself with all institutions *for those with damaged minds*, both for the betterment of the unfortunates and the advancement of science. In this important and difficult *field of medicine* only unrelenting efforts will enable us to carve out advances for the good of suffering mankind. Perfection can be achieved only in such institutions."[29] Writing in 1917, at the height of World War I, Kraepelin repeated Hardenberg's words and added these revealing remarks: "The great war in which we are now engaged has compelled us to recognize the fact that science could forge for us a host of effective weapons for use against a hostile world. Should it be otherwise if we are fighting an internal enemy seeking to destroy the very fabric of our existence?"[30]

Kraepelin's remarks make clear that he regarded psychiatry as an arm of the state, similar to the military forces, whose duty is to protect the fatherland from "an internal enemy" that, like a hostile army, seeks to destroy it. The evil genius of psychiatry lay, and continues to lie, in its ability to convince itself, the legal system, and the public that, in matters defined as psychiatric, there is no conflict between the legitimate interests of the individual and the legitimate interests of the ruling class.

In 1804, Johann Gottfried Langermann (1768-1832)—the director of an asylum in Bavaria whom Zilboorg characterizes as a "psychiatric humanist"—advocated "that doctors should when necessary resort to imprisonment, punishment, and flogging."[31] Although all nineteenth-century psychiatrists believed in insanity and coercion, some entertained doubts about the medical nature of mental illness and the possibility of a truly medical therapy for it. Heinrich Neumann (1814-1884) insisted, "we shall never be able to believe that psychiatry will make a step forward until we decide to throw overboard the whole business of classification.... There is but one type of mental disturbance and we call it insanity."[32] This cuts to the core. Insanity is a type of "crime" against society: it is that "mental disturbance" which justifies the imprisonment of the "disturbed/disturber." The psychiatrist's only tool, Neumann asserted, is coercion: "The mental patient must be handled like an ill-behaved child, and the measures used to correct the child can also be used to advantage with the lunatic."[33]

Outside the sphere of psychiatry, coercion is crime, if committed by the individual, or punishment, if authorized by law and imposed by the criminal justice system. In psychiatry, coercion is therapy. Why? Because *the psychiatrist's avowal of therapeutic intent, endorsed by the law, transforms the victim's imprisonment into his care and protection. Mutatis mutandis, the criminal's disavowal of criminal intent, endorsed by the psychiatrist and the law, transforms crime into mental illness.* These two formulas continue to be dear to the hearts of psychiatrists, politicians, and other people looking to psychiatry as the guardian of the social order.

One of the most important psychiatrists—or, more precisely, neuropsychiatrists—of the modern era was Wilhelm Griesinger (1817-1868). Griesinger had extensive medical experience and made important contributions to neurology before devoting himself to the study and treatment of mental patients. In 1859, he became head of an institution for mentally retarded children in Mariaberg, a small town in southern Germany. In 1860, he left for Zürich, became a member of the *Medizinalkommission*, and participated in the founding of *Burghölzli*, the new Cantonal (state) mental hospital. In 1865, Griesinger settled in Berlin to assume leadership of the psychiatric clinic, and also of the department of nervous diseases established on his initiative at the *Charité*. He founded the *Archiv für Psychiatrie und Nervenkrankheiten* (*Archive for Psychiatry and Nervous*

Diseases) that quickly became one of the leading journals in its field. Insanity had long been associated with brain disease. However, it was Griesinger who insisted on viewing mental diseases in the same way modern scientific physicians viewed bodily diseases, through the lens of pathology.* The first edition of Griesinger's epoch-making work *Pathologie und Therapie der Psychischen Krankheiten* had been published in 1845, thirteen years before Rudolf Virchow (1821-1902) published his revolutionary *Cellular Pathology as Based upon Physiological and Pathological Histology*. Griesinger's work became the foundation of modern "scientific psychiatry." It was translated into English, as *Mental Pathology and Therapeutics*, in 1867. Griesinger began this work with a plea for the localization of mental diseases and their symptoms: "There was no doubt in his mind that the brain is the seat of mental diseases. He is known for writing: 'Psychological diseases are diseases of the brain,' and 'Insanity is merely a symptom complex of various anomalous states of the brain.'"[34] Griesinger argued not only that madness was a disease of the brain, but that it was the consequence of a single disease of the brain:

> According to this concept of the "unitary psychosis" (*Einheitspsychose*), the manifold symptoms of madness were not the result of different diseases but different stages of a single disease process. For Griesinger the soul became a function of the brain.... By the time of the English translation Griesinger's views on the nature of insanity were "well nigh universally admitted to be correct." During the late nineteenth century it was the most widely used text in psychiatry. This popularity was no doubt due to the combination of Griesinger's astute clinical observations and his strict adherence to the principle that mental diseases were not inherently different from other diseases of the nervous system.[35]

Griesinger's psychiatric legacy was solidified by Theodor Hermann Meynert (1833-1892), a German-born Viennese neuropsychiatrist and one of Freud's teachers. He began his textbook, *Psychiatrie* (*Psychiatry,* 1884), with this statement: "The reader will find no other definition of 'Psychiatry' in this book but the one given on the title page: *Clinical Treatise on Diseases of the Forebrain.* The historical term for psychiatry, i.e., 'treatment of the soul,' implies more than we can accomplish, and transcends the bounds of accurate scientific investigation."[36]

In a review of nineteenth-century Swedish psychiatry, historian of science Roger Qvarsell states: "In the 1860s, the debate among psychiatrists about the real nature of mental disease was over.... Almost all

---

* That is to say, through the lens of somatic pathology. The invention of the literalized metaphor of psychopathology lay in the not very distant future.

medical scientists and medical authorities were at this time convinced that mental diseases were of the same nature as somatic disorders."[37] *Plus ça change...*

5

The history of moral treatment in the United States reprises the rationalizations of coercion as care already popular in England and France. Albert Deutsch begins his account with the familiar legend of Saint Pinel: "Almost his first act at the Bicêtre was to strike off the chains from fifty-three lunatics, many of whom had been weighed down with fetters for years in the belief that they were dangerous.... Their violent behavior had resulted quite naturally from the oppressive tortures inflicted on them."[38] If the inmates were harmless, as Deutsch would have it, why hadn't Pinel set them free? Deutsch does not ask the question. Instead he presents the obligatory canard of Pinel as a humane psychiatric reformer whose coercions, unlike those of his inhumane colleagues, are kind and therapeutic.

"What was the essence of this 'moral treatment'?" Deutsch asks. He answers by quoting T. Romeyn Beck, a prominent early nineteenth-century New York physician, who defined "moral management" as "consist[ing] in removing patients from their residence to some proper asylum. ... [and] convinc[ing] the lunatics that *the power of the physician and keeper is absolute; ... punish disobedience peremptorily...use the strait waistcoat, confine them in a dark and quiet room, order spare diet.*"[39] Zilboorg, too, connects moral treatment with the mirage of nonrestraint: "The French were skeptical of its efficacy. The Americans were almost violently opposed to it."[40] The terms "psychiatry" and "nonrestraint" denote antithetical practices.

The Jacobin philosophy of psychiatric humanism, in which the madman is viewed as a wayward human being rather than an irreparably damaged object, had far-reaching consequences whose ripple effects are still being felt. The medicalization of misbehavior meant that the "condition" was curable and, further, that since madness was such a calamitous illness, the effort to cure it amply justified the use of force. Soon, the ever-optimistic American practitioners of moral treatment reported spectacular successes in curing insanity. Thus began a period in psychiatry Deutsch aptly dubs the era of "the cult of the curability of insanity."[41] Today we are in the midst of another such era, "the cult of the treatability of insanity with drugs."

In 1820, George Man Burrows, an English mad-doctor, had declared that the notion that insanity was incurable was erroneous. Thanks to the principles and practices of moral treatment, he was able to cure 81 percent of all his mental patients. The Americans quickly overtook him. Dr. Eli Todd, head of the Hartford Retreat in Connecticut, then recognized as the foremost American superintendent of a mental hospital, reported a cure rate of 91.8 percent.

Reform now followed reform. The result was a triumph for the mad-doctor, and a tragedy for the madman. In principle, the mental patient was restored to full citizenship. In practice, he became a non-person: a "ward of the state," in the words of Horace Mann (1796-1859), social reformer and "father of American education."[42] The prevailing Zeitgeist and social changes, combined with the agitations of do-gooders such as Mann and Dorothea Lynde Dix (1802-1887), led to the sprouting of lunatic asylums all over the nation, each claiming greater success in the curing of insanity than the last. By 1843, perfection was at hand. Dr. William M. Awl, superintendent of the Ohio State Lunatic Hospital in Columbus, recorded in his annual report: "Per cent of recoveries on all recent cases discharged the present year, 100."[43] Other superintendents of lunatic asylums claimed to have achieved similar results. "The records of this Asylum, " reported Dr. Luther V. Bell, head of the McLean Asylum in Boston, "justify the declaration that all cases, certainly recent...recover under a fair trial. This is the general law." Dr. Thomas S. Kirkbride, superintendent of the Pennsylvania Hospital for the Insane, asserted: "The general proposition that truly recent cases of insanity are commonly very curable...may be considered as fully established."[44] The peddlers of today's psychiatric drugs make similar claims.

Although Deutsch was a pious psychiatric apologist, many of his observations are valid and some of his remarks are relevant to the present psychiatric scene. On the exaggerated therapeutic claims of mid-nineteenth-century American psychiatrists, he comments as follows: "The belief, based on the reports of cures of recent cases, that insanity was easily curable if treated early enough, rapidly impressed itself on the public and professional mind and soon reached the plane of established dogma. But what of the psychiatric profession as a whole? Did it raise any objections to the spread of this fallacy? On the contrary: except for a very few instances, it not only subscribed wholeheartedly to the current misconceptions but stimulated and strengthened them as best it could."[45] Did these pioneer psychiatrists engage in systematic deception and self-deception? Do modern neuroscientific psychiatrists engage in lying to the public and themselves?

"The myth of easy curability lasted long and died hard," concludes Deutsch. It was still alive in 1875 but then quickly expired. "Disillusioned, the public cast off the cloak of false optimism that had been woven with the warp of error and woof of short-sighted opportunism." The older psychiatric attitude revived: "Once insane, always insane!"[46] A version of this belief characterizes present psychiatric opinion as well, with this difference: Court-ordered, life-long ingestion of psychiatric drugs is likely to keep the insane person "in remission."

6

The alienist's claim that insanity was an easily curable disease laid the ground for the division of modern secular societies into two classes of citizens, sane and insane, unmolested by psychiatrists and permanently enslaved by them. Dorothea Lynde Dix, an unhappy but energetic woman, found this to be the ideal arena in which to vent her blind reformist zeal. She dedicated herself to establishing psychiatric plantations all over the United States.

Dix was born in 1802 in a small town in Maine. Her father was an itinerant Methodist preacher, alcoholic and abusive. Her mother was said to have been "mentally unwell." Later in life Dix commented, "I never knew childhood."[47] Spurning marriage, she first chose to work as a schoolteacher for girls and later, when she was almost forty, found her calling in institutions housing society's unwanted members, prisons and insane asylums. A biographer states, "In her life her goals were not defined, she simply did whatever would best help people." Like so many reformers, she wrought great harm whose effects are still with us.

Dix's second career began in 1841, when she entered the East Cambridge Jail to teach a Sunday School class for women inmates. The experience of coming to know drunks, criminals, prostitutes, retarded individuals, and the mentally ill—all housed together in unheated, unfurnished, and foul-smelling quarters—changed her life. She proceeded to visit jails and almshouses, where the mentally ill were housed, and drew up a document for the Massachusetts legislature that first led to expansion of Worcester State Hospital and then sparked a nationwide movement for the creation of state insane asylums. Although Dix was in poor health, she managed to cover every state east of the Mississippi River, playing a major role in founding thirty-two mental hospitals and fifteen schools for the feebleminded.

Dix's reformist zeal meshed with the temper of her times. Growing in numbers and becoming more urbanized, American families and communities wanted to get their troublesome members out of sight and out of mind. Dix offered to satisfy their need and to soothe them with the fiction that her proposed psychiatric plantations would make the slaves healthy and happy.

In the late 1840s, Congress was making generous donations of public land to states for use to the advancement of public education and public works. By 1848, more than 100 million acres of land had already been apportioned to various states for educational purposes. Dix conceived the idea of petitioning the federal government, urging it "to grant to the states, on the basis of population, 5 million acres of land, the proceeds of the sales of which were to be used exclusively for bettering the condition of the indigent insane."[48] Although this petition proved unsuccessful, it marked the beginning of the allocation of vast sums of public funds ostensibly for the benefit of mental patients, but actually for the benefit of their oppressors. It also marked, as Deutsch correctly notes, the beginning of the idea that caring for the insane is a responsibility of the *national government,* an idea the socialist Deutsch warmly endorses. In her *Memorial to Congress,* Dorothea Dix declared:

> I confide to you the cause and the claims of the destitute and of the desolate, without fear or distrust. I ask, for the thirty states of the Union, 5,000,000 acres of land, of the many hundreds of millions of public lands, appropriated in such manner as shall assure the greatest benefit to all those who are in circumstances of extreme necessity, and who, through the providence of God, are wards of the nation, claimants on the sympathy and care of the public, through the miseries and disqualifications brought upon them by the sorest afflictions with which humanity can be visited.[49]

Note that Dix used the term "sorest affliction," rather than the term "insane," to identify the objects of her benevolence. Explains Deutsch: "Wards of the nation! Here was a brand-new concept of governmental responsibility for mentally ill dependents."[50] The first bill, inspired by Dix's *Memorial,* failed in Congress. Dix persevered and raised her request to 10 million acres, adding to it 2,250,000 acres for deaf mutes, for a total of 12,250,000 acres. Astonishingly, in 1854 the bill passed both houses! All it needed to become law was for the President Franklin Pierce to sign it. However, the proposal was blatantly unconstitutional and Pierce refused to sign it. His veto is of the utmost interest both historically and for its relevance to our present medical-economic predicaments.

One need not be a constitutional scholar to understand that the Founders' "original intent" was to create a carefully limited federal government, with laws governing most of the day-to-day affairs of the people entrusted to the states. Were the federal government to fund and oversee the management of human misery, categorized with grab-bag terms like "destitution" and "insanity," it would inexorably exercise the kind of power over people against which the Founders had fought. This, in part, is how Pierce justified his veto:

> The bill entitled "An act making a grant of public lands to the several States for the benefit of indigent insane persons," which was presented to me on the 27th ultimo, has been maturely considered, and is returned to the Senate, the House in which it originated, with a statement of the objections which have required me to withhold from it my approval. ... It cannot be questioned that if Congress has the power to make provision for the indigent insane without the limits of this District it has the same power to provide for the indigent who are not insane, and thus to transfer to the Federal Government the charge of all the poor in all the States. It has the same power to provide hospitals and other local establishments for the care and cure of every species of human infirmity, and thus to assume all that duty of either public philanthropy or public necessity to the dependent, the orphan, the sick, or the needy which is now discharged by the States themselves or by corporate institutions or private endowments existing under the legislation of the States. *The whole field of public beneficence is thrown open to the care and culture of the Federal Government. Generous impulses no longer encounter the limitations and control of our imperious fundamental law*; for however worthy may be the present object in itself, it is only one of a class. It is not exclusively worthy of benevolent regard. Whatever considerations dictate sympathy for this particular object apply in like manner, if not in the same degree, to idiocy, to physical disease, to extreme destitution. If Congress may and ought to provide for any one of these objects, it may and ought to provide for them all. And if it be done in this case, what answer shall be given when Congress shall be called upon, as it doubtless will be, to pursue a similar course of legislation in the others? *It will obviously be vain to reply that the object is worthy, but that the application has taken a wrong direction. The power will have been deliberately assumed, the general obligation will by this act have been acknowledged, and the question of means and expediency will alone be left for consideration.* The decision upon the principle in any one case determines it for the whole class. The question presented, therefore, clearly is upon the constitutionality and propriety of the Federal Government assuming to enter into a novel and vast field of legislation, namely, that of providing for the care and support of all those among the people of the United States who by any form become fit objects of public philanthropy. I readily and, I trust, feelingly acknowledge the duty incumbent on us all as men and citizens, and as among the highest and holiest of our duties, to provide for those who, in the mysterious order of Providence, are subject to want and to disease of body or mind; but I can not find any authority in the Constitution for making the Federal Government the great almoner of public charity throughout the United States. To do so would, in my judgement, be contrary to the letter and spirit of the Constitution and subversive of the whole theory upon which the Union of these States is founded.[51]

Equating humanism with statism and attributing the neglect of the destitute insane to individualism, Deutsch was appalled by Pierce's veto: "So was the great 12,250,000 Acre Bill finally defeated by the penstroke of one man."[52] One hundred fifty years ago Pierce saw that which, ironically, we can no longer see because we take it for granted—namely, that if the federal government assumed responsibility for relieving the people of illness and poverty, the result would be the pervasive loss of liberty that is the fruit of the Therapeutic-Welfare State.

Although Dix failed to federalize the care of the mentally ill in America—it remained for Lyndon Johnson to complete that job—she succeeded in creating a building boom in public mental hospitals supported by the states, hence the name "state hospital" for mental hospital. "In all," writes Deutsch, "she [Dix] was directly responsible for the founding or enlarging of thirty-two mental hospitals in the United States and abroad."[53]

It should have been obvious from the start that the grand nineteenth-century state hospitals would become psychiatric plantations, providing secure employment and comfortable living quarters for the staff, and snake pits for the inmates. Revealingly, when the Trenton (New Jersey) State Hospital opened its doors in 1881, the aging Dorothea Dix made her home there. For her it was an asylum: she was cared for and could come and go as she pleased. She died there in 1887, at the age of 85.

7

Although the notion of moral treatment is associated most closely with Pinel and his followers in France, the problem of coercion—intrinsic to the social mandate of the madhouse keeper—was confronted most clearly and courageously by British mad-doctors who tried to resolve the contradictions inherent in their dual roles as carers and coercers. Their efforts were destined to fail. By contrast, the contemporary psychiatrist glories in his role as coercer and contemplates banning contractual psychiatry because it fails to protect the subject from his freedom to kill himself and is therefore "medically negligent." The problem of suicide, as I shall now show, played a central role in nineteenth-century English debates about the limits of moral treatment and continues to play a major role in legitimating the psychiatrist's mandate to exercise "benevolent coercion."

It is not possible to understand psychiatry or the history of psychiatry without understanding and appreciating the connections among religion, suicide, madness, and the insanity defense.[54] In the Christian worldview, human life is God's gift and property. Hence, suicide is self-murder, *felo de se* (felony against oneself). Inasmuch as the legitimacy of the Christian sovereign's rule rested on his special relationship to God, self-murder was also an offense against him and was accordingly punished by both canon and criminal law.

With suicide defined as a species of murder, the persons sitting in judgment of self-killers had the duty to punish them. Since punishing suicide required doing injustice to innocent parties—in particular the wives and minor children of the deceased—eventually the task proved to be an intolerable burden. In the seventeenth century, men sitting on coroners' juries began to recoil against desecrating the corpse and dispossessing the suicide's dependents of their means of support. However, their religious beliefs precluded repeal of the laws punishing the crime. Their only recourse was to evade the laws: The doctrine that the self-slayer is *non compos mentis* and hence not responsible for his act accomplished this task.

The transformation of *self-killing from a deliberate act* into the *unintended consequence of a disease (of the brain)* is an integral part of the pseudo-science of psychiatry and the vastly influential institutions of social control that rest on its claims called "theories" and coercions called "treatments." The "insanitizing of suicide" antecedes the birth of psychiatry. Psychiatry is a result, not the cause, of the transformation of self-murder from sin-and-crime into illness-as-excuse.

The impetus for excusing self-murder did not come from its beneficiaries, the victims of the law against suicide. Indeed, it could not come from them: The suicide was dead; his family, bereft of means and reputation, was powerless. Instead, the impetus came from those who needed the reform and had the political clout to bring it about: the coroners and coroners' juries who sought to evade the burden of having to impose harsh penalties on the corpses of suicides and the widows and orphans they left behind.

The practice of routinely excusing self-killers as insane led inevitably to practices and policies ostensibly directed at preventing suicide, principally incarceration of the potential self-killer in an insane asylum. That practice, in turn, reinforced the belief that persons who kill themselves are insane, that the insane are likely to kill themselves, and that persons deemed dangerous to themselves or others are justifiably deprived of liberty under psychiatric auspices. For three hundred years, the legal and medical justification for psychiatric preventive detention—civil commitment—has rested comfortably and securely on that set of beliefs.

Why did the insanity defense against self-murder develop when it did and where it did? The answer lies in the rapid economic development of England in the seventeenth century and the accompanying spread of culture and social sensibility. For the first time in history, people at large, not just a few philosophers, began to take seriously the twin ideas of personal liberty and right to property. One result, as noted already, was that men sitting on coroners' juries found it increasingly more difficult to deprive innocent wives and children of their dead husbands' and fathers' possessions. But they were in a bind. Repeal of the laws against self-murder was politically unthinkable, yet the penalty for the offense was morally unacceptable.

There is an important similarity between the former dilemma involving the prohibition of suicide (self-murder) and the need to punish it, and the contemporary prohibition of feticide (abortion or murder of the fetus) and the need to punish it. Both acts entail the deliberate taking of human life (homicide). Both may be treated as crimes. In the climate of modern popular opinion, both acts are practically unpunishable. Rational criminal sanction against abortion would require that the agent, the pregnant woman, be punished more severely than her deputy, the abortionist. Absent an alliance between church and state or medicine and state, there can be no *rational* criminal sanctions against either abortion or suicide.[55]

In eighteenth-century England, the solution to the dilemma of punishing self-murder as prescribed by law was to treat the person guilty of the crime as if he were a lunatic. This maneuver allowed society to condemn self-killing as a moral and legal offense, maintain the religious and legal sanctions against it, and provided a seemingly enlightened mechanism for not punishing the act as required by law. Faced with tough choices about delicate matters, people often prefer evasion to confrontation. The evasions we call the "insanity defense," "diminished capacity," "psychiatric disability," and so forth pose a deadly and widely unappreciated threat to political liberty.

Life is full of dangers, mainly of two types, natural and human. Earthquakes and floods are instances of dangers from the physical environment; theft, assault, and murder are instances of dangers from the human environment. From Hobbes and Locke to the Framers of the Constitution, political philosophers have agreed that the principal (or only) moral justification for the state, as a political entity with a monopoly over the rightful use of force, is the protection of people from injury at the hands of other people, criminals at home and enemies abroad. In other words, the legitimacy of the state rests on a tacit understanding or "compact": in exchange for our renouncing, as private persons, the use of force in relation to our fellow man, the state protects us from theft, assault, and murder.

The proposition that the self-killer, as a lunatic, is a danger to himself from which he needs the coercive protection of the state violates this core principle. Evading the penalty for self-murder by insanitizing the deed legitimizes the fiction of a self divided against itself and, derivatively, legitimizes the idea of insanity that, in turn, entails the assumption of dangerousness to self and others, as well as the vast psychiatric edifice built on these ideas. Thus has arisen and developed the belief and social practice that it is the duty of the state to protect, by force, insane persons from themselves and others from insane persons. *The end result is a radical expansion of the authority, legitimacy, and power of the state—from its use of force to protect people from others to its use to protect people from themselves.*[56]

The idea of excusing the self-killer by attributing to him the fictitious malady called "insanity" was invented as a tactic for the merciful treatment of his survivors. It was too good a gambit to be limited to suicide. In the United States today, there is virtually no situation in which the notion of mental illness may not be brought into play to diminish or annul the actor's responsibility for his action; to deny his role as moral agent and redefine him as a victim; and to hold others responsible for the deleterious consequences of his behavior. By the same token, virtually no behavior deemed undesirable by authorities is immune from being subjected to "therapeutic" social controls.

The more society relies on therapeutic controls, the more their use reinforces belief in the reality of mental illness and, generally, in the rationale of treating bad habits as if they were diseases. In the process, the public loses sight of the fact that bad habits are not diseases; that the diagnosis of (mis)behaviors does not make them diseases; and that psychiatrists have nothing to do with treating diseases, but everything to do with regulating behavior.

The insanity defense is not merciful. Involuntary mental hospitalization is not a treatment. Both are coercive methods of social control. Both rest on the attribution of an absence of *mens rea* to the actor. Both result in the "protected" person's being deprived of liberty. Both function as tactical weapons in society's and psychiatry's war on dignity, liberty, and responsibility.

4

Dauerschlaf: Requiescat in Pace

To die, to sleep; / To sleep: perchance to dream: aye, there's the rub; / For in that sleep of death what dreams may come, / When we have shuffled off this mortal coil, / Must give us pause: ...

—William Shakespeare, Hamlet *(3, 1, 66-68)*

1

Folk wisdom views life as perpetual tumult and turmoil, with the grave as the sole and final place of rest. A person dies and people say, "May he rest in peace," though everyone knows that cadavers need neither rest nor peace. Henry Ward Beecher observed, "There is but one easy place in this world, and that is the grave."[1] Similar remarks abound. The metaphor of death as rest and sleep is alive and well.

In the popular view, insanity greatly magnifies the ordinary turbulence of life, turning it into a state of perpetual torment, a veritable hell on earth. Terms associated with mental illnesses—such as agitation, anger, anxiety, obsession, compulsion, hallucination, delusion, furor, and rage—suggest a state of uncommon unrest. It is reasonable, then, to view rest as a remedy for such disorders.

Sleep is to the mind what rest is to the body: it lets us suspend our need to be alert and responsive to our environment, human and physical. We need sleep more than food: we can go without eating much longer than we can without sleeping. Sleep deprivation is a familiar form of torture and the cause of the loss of higher mental functions, often resulting in symptoms mimicking those of "mental illnesses." Such common-sense observations have no doubt contributed to the notion of sleep as therapy. Hypnotics, that is, chemicals that help us to sleep—such as alcohol and opium—are among the oldest discoveries of man and have long been a mainstay of self-medication, medical therapeutics, and mad-doctoring.

Given the importance of rest and sleep for our health and well-being, it is not surprising that chemicals that make us relax and sleep have been among the most sought-after substances of mankind. We call such drugs "sedatives," "hypnotics," and "narcotics." These drugs must be distinguished from chemicals that make us feel more alert and energetic—such as caffeine, nicotine, amphetamines, and cocaine—called "stimulants." Until after the end of World War II, the distinction between sedatives and stimulants was clear.[2] With the beginning of America's prolonged war on drugs the distinction between these two classes of drugs, exhibiting diametrically opposite pharmacological actions, became conflated: sedatives and stimulants alike were classified as "narcotics." The pharmacological distinction between them was replaced by the criminological distinction—legal and illegal drugs. All illegal stimulants became "narcotics"; cocaine traffickers became "narcoterrorists." The classification of cocaine as a narcotic signifies the thoroughgoing politicization of the pharmacology of psychoactive drugs, just as the classification of psychiatric prisons as hospitals and coerced poisoning as treatment signify the thoroughgoing medicalization of a large part of the criminal law.

One of the casualties of this process is the cessation of rational discourse about the true pharmacological properties of controlled substances in general, and psychiatric and psychedelic drugs in particular.[3] The advertising, both on television and in the print media, of the currently fashionable sleeping pill, Ambien, is an example: "Ambien CR (zolpidem tartrate extended-release tablets)...FDA approved for the treatment of insomnia. ...is *non-narcotic*..."[4] The *Merriam-Webster Dictionary* defines "narcotic" as "a drug (as opium) that in moderate doses dulls the senses, relieves pain, and induces profound sleep..."; and it defines the term "narcosis" as "a state of stupor, unconsciousness, or arrested activity produced by the influence of narcotics or other chemicals." A "non-narcotic sleeping pill," like a "living corpse," is an oxymoron with powerful rhetorical possibilities.

Therapeutic agents used to remedy real diseases—such as drugs, x-radiation, anesthesia, and surgery—are potentially damaging to the body. Hence, in medicine, the general rule is that the proper dose of a remedy is the smallest dose needed to do the job. More is worse, not better. In psychiatry, this rule tends to be reversed. The principle governing much of psychiatric therapeutics has been and still is that if a particular dose of a remedy seems beneficial, more of it is likely to be even more beneficial. We have seen this principle played out with respect to the use of mental hospitalization, rest, sleep, electric shock treatment, psychosurgery, psychotherapy and psychoanalysis, and, today, drugs.

This phenomenon has not escaped the attention of thoughtful psychiatrists. D. G. Cunningham Owens, Reader in Psychiatry at the University of Edinburgh and the author of an authoritative text on the extrapyramidal effects of antipsychotic drugs, emphasizes: "The recommended dose [of chlorpromazine] from the manufacturer was up to 100 mg per day orally or a maximum of 25 mg for the first intramuscular (i.m.) injection. Delay and Deniker opted for a 'very high' dose of 75 -100 mg i.m. daily.... As would be repeated many times with many drugs, it was when chlorpromazine crossed the Atlantic that 'megadoses' entered practice. By the mid-1950s, doses of 1000 - 2000 mg per day were being used in the USA."[5]

David Healy adds this important comment: "[I]t is far from true that older (somatic) treatments were abusive because they were unscientific; once antipsychotic therapy became theory driven, when it was linked to the dopamine hypothesis of schizophrenia, the theory probably helped legitimate therapeutic abuse. It was theory that drove crippling megadose regimens of antipsychotics, just as theories from the best scientific centers in the world had previously driven psychosurgery."[6] Terms such as "therapeutic abuse" and "megadose"—which imply "overdosing" and "overtreating"—divert attention from the simple fact that the drugs in question are introduced into the denominated patients against their will. In psychiatry, so-called somatic treatments have been and are virtually synonymous with involuntary treatments. Healy's explanation is an excuse. "Psychiatric abuses"—epitomized first by forced hospitalization and now by forced drugging—are driven by a combination of sadism, grandiosity, naiveté, venality, and corruption. Today, pharmaceutical companies in effect bribe psychiatrists to administer psychoactive drugs to as many people as possible and write glowing reports about the drug's therapeutic effectiveness and lack of side effects.

2

The idea that insanity is due to "nervous exhaustion," a fatigue of the brain or nervous system, best treated by rest, has a long history. In the nineteenth century, the American neurologist, Silas Weir Mitchell (1829-1914) raised the notion to the status of medical dogma. His so-called "rest cure" exercised a profound influence on psychiatric thinking and therapeutics from the 1880s until well after World War I. In the early decades of the twentieth century, the work of the famous Russian physiologist-physician Ivan Petrovich Pavlov (1849-1936) lent support to the idea that overstimulation of the central nervous system causes disease and that mental rest is a treatment for it. Because prolonged rest qua prolonged sleep requires intensive medical and nursing support in a hospital setting, sleep treatment has never achieved the popularity of other methods, such as ECT or drug therapy. At the same time, it has never disappeared from the psychiatric scene and stands as an important reminder of how the most elementary restorative functions of the human organism may be abused by turning them into coerced medical procedures.

Silas Weir Mitchell was born into a wealthy family in Philadelphia, the seventh physician in three generations. After graduating from Jefferson Medical College in 1851, he traveled in Europe and studied medicine in Paris for a year. He then engaged in a busy medical practice and did experimental work on snake venoms. During the Civil War, Mitchell was placed in charge of Turner's Lane Hospital in Philadelphia, a 400-bed army hospital for nervous diseases. This work gave him extensive experience in dealing with persons who malingered, a phenomenon that had by that time been thoroughly neurologized. Mitchell recognized that the person who assumes the sick role is not really sick and that malingering—even if it is called "nervous fatigue," "hysteria," or some other disease-sounding name—is not a bona fide disease. Nevertheless, like nearly everyone then and today, he used medical-diagnostic terms—principally "hysteria" and "neurasthenia"—to identify it. Also, he reasoned that if a little rest is good, more is better, and thus developed the "rest cure," consisting of prolonged bed-rest combined with supervised nutrition and massage. This treatment, named after him, made him world famous. Had Mitchell been German, he might have called his method *Dauerruhe.**

Mitchell was a prominent physician, writer, poet, and founder of the American Neurological Association as well as a "proper gentleman," which made his dramatic bedside interventions all the more remarkable. Attending a woman so sick she was thought to be dying, Mitchell dismissed all present in the room and soon left himself. "Asked of her chances of survival he remarked: 'Yes she will run out of the door in two minutes; I set her sheets on fire.'"[7] Confronted with another hysterical woman who claimed to be unable to get out of bed, he "threatened her with rape and commenced to undress. He got to his undergarments when the woman fled the room screaming."[8] That sort of persiflage has passed, and still passes, for medical treatment and illustrates our enduring hypocrisy about distinguishing between disease and nondisease; more precisely, it illustrates our collective passion for a *dual understanding and misunderstanding* of that distinction. In his

---

* *Dauer* is duration, *Ruhe* is rest, and *Schlaf* is sleep.

magnum opus, titled *Fat and Blood* (1878), Mitchell describes his "rest therapy" as follows:

> In carrying out my general plan of treatment it is my habit to ask the patient to remain in bed from six weeks to two months. At first, and in some cases for four or five weeks, I do not permit the patient to sit up or to sew or write or read. The only action allowed is that needed to clean the teeth. In some instances I have not permitted the patient to turn over without aid, and this I have done because sometimes I think no motion desirable, and because sometimes the moral influence of absolute repose is of use. In such cases I arrange to have the bowels and water passed while lying down...I insist on the patient being fed by the nurse, and, when well enough to sit up in bed, I insist that the meats shall be cut up, so as to make it easier for the patient to feed herself.... Usually, after a fortnight I permit the patient to be read to—one to three hours a day—but I am daily amazed to see how kindly nervous and anaemic women take to this absolute rest, and how little they complain of its monotony.... All the moral uses of rest and isolation and change of habits are not obtained by merely insisting on the physical conditions needed to effect these ends. If the physician has the force of character required to secure the confidence and respect of his patients he has also much more in his power, and should have the tact to seize the proper occasions to direct the thoughts of his patients to the lapse from duties to others, and to the selfishness which a life of invalidism is apt to bring about. *Such moral medication belongs to the higher sphere of the doctor's duties,* and if he means to cure his patient permanently, he cannot afford to neglect them.[9]

Did Mitchell and his legions of followers believe that coerced passivity and fattening were curative agents? Or did they recognize that these measures were merely the props of the doctor's "moral medication"? The question is rhetorical and may be asked about all psychiatric hocuspocus. I raise it here to illustrate the thoroughgoing medicalization of morals that has characterized psychiatric practices from their early days to the present.

Mitchell knew that rest and weight gain were medical props, "moral medications," as he put it. "What is so large a part of success in treatment," he emphasizes, "[are] the moral methods of obtaining confidence and *insuring a childlike acquiescence in every needed measure."*[10] In other words, the real therapeutic agent is male medical authority, reinforced by the family and society. Mitchell knew what he was doing, and many of his patients knew it as well. He was teaching self-assertive, "rebellious" women a lesson, and many of his patients never forgave him for it.[11] The roster of Mitchell's female patients represented a veritable Who's Who of prominent late nineteenth-century American women, including Jane Addams, Rebecca Harding Davis, Charlotte Perkins Gilman, and Edith Wharton. One of Mitchell's famous male patients was Clarence Hemingway, the writer's father and a physician, who subsequently committed suicide by shooting himself. Ernest Hemingway, too, received psychiatric treatment at a famous clinic and then shot himself to death.[12]

As the "wage slavery" of modern industrialism became the epitome of the enemy for Marxism, so the "rest cure" of modern psychiatry became the epitome of the enemy for feminism. Ironically, but predictably, "liberated" female psychiatrists have eagerly joined the ranks of the most destructive male psychiatrists. Many of them have specialized in child psychiatry, coercing and exploiting the most helpless members of society.

Despite all the evidence to the contrary, Zilboorg characterizes Mitchell as a "pure somatologist."[13] It is clear that Mitchell knew his hysterical patients were not sick but merely playing the sick role: "I see every week—almost every day—women who when asked 'what's the matter' reply, 'Oh, I have nervous exhaustion.' ...A hysterical girl is, as Wendell Holmes has said in his decisive phrase, a vampire who sucks the blood of the healthy people about her."[14] The contemporary reader may be inclined to dismiss Mitchell's rest cure as just another silly quack remedy. That would be a big mistake. As late as the 1930s, many intelligent and well-informed persons—among them Leonard and Virginia Woolf—regarded Mitchell's rest cure as the best treatment for a nervous breakdown. Leonard Woolf was a fanatic believer in the efficacy of the rest-and-fattening therapy for Virginia's madness, and Virginia willingly submitted to this therapeutic degradation ceremony.[15]

In the final analysis, the rest cure, like hypnosis, required the subject's cooperation and was therefore a feeble means of rendering her helpless. It also did not provide much rest, inasmuch as the patient remained conscious and often actively resisted the restrictions imposed on her. However, Mitchell's rest cure helped pave the way to new, radical forms of rest treatments, such as *Dauerschlaf* or "prolonged sleep," the invention of a Swiss psychiatrist, and sleep as "annihilation," the invention of D. Ewen Cameron, a Scotch-Canadian psychiatrist.[16]

3

While Mitchell is credited with inventing prolonged rest as a treatment for mental diseases, the Swiss psychiatrist Jakob Klaesi (1883-1980) is credited with inventing so-called "sleep treatment" or *Dauerschlaf*. Klaesi's first report on sleep therapy was published in 1920. In fact, such treatments had at that time been in use for half a century: "Ether, chloroform, alcohol, opium and its derivatives were employed as long ago as 1870 to produce long periods of unconsciousness in attempts to break up psychotic mechanisms."[17] Klaesi used Somnifene, a mixture of diethylamine salts and diethyl and allyl isopropyl barbituric acid, and kept his patients sedated for ten days. Subsequently, a host of drugs were used to induce prolonged narcosis in mental patients, among them Avertin, Chloral, Luminal, Sodium Luminal, Pantopon, paraldehyde, Trional, mysoline, soneryl, Adalin, and Amytal—and, in our day, Thorazine.[18]

The most important thing to keep in mind about sleep therapy is that it has nothing to do with sleep. When physicians use chemicals to render unconscious a person undergoing a major operation, they call it "anesthesia." When they do the same thing to a person on a ventilator, they call it a "medically induced coma." When psychiatrists do the same thing to a mental patient, they call it "sleep therapy"; the term instantiates the mendacity intrinsic to coerced psychiatric practices. Critics of this piece of fraud soon complained: "We have no right to speak about fatigue when no work has been done."[19] Nor do we have a right to speak about sleep when we ought to talk about chemical narcosis. Once again we see here the rhetorical abuse of analogies at work. Although sleep therapy is no longer used, at least in the United States, it is an important part of relatively recent psychiatric history.

In 1959, Silvano Arieti's authoritative *American Handbook of Psychiatry* reported the use of various drugs in "continuous, or prolonged, sleep treatment." He added that, after the advent of chlorpromazine it was included among the sleep-producing drugs favored by psychiatrists. In the chapter on sleep therapy, he concludes: "The procedure is not without risk, the mortality averaging 1 to 3 per cent. Possible major complications include cardiovascular collapse, bronchopneumonia, acute renal insufficiency with anuria, respiratory depression, dehydration fever, toxic confusional states, occasional brief delirious episodes, and withdrawal type convulsions at the termination of the treatment."[20] Mental illness, let us keep in mind, is not and cannot be a cause of death. Psychiatric treatment can be and is a remarkably frequent cause of death, not to mention being a cause of loss of liberty, property, dignity, and the right to trial for crime. Freedman, Kaplan, and Sadock's *Modern Synopsis of Comprehensive Textbook of Psychiatry/II* (1976) states:

> [Klaesi] used injections of a barbiturate mixture to keep patients in a state of continuous narcosis for about 10 days, with brief daily dose reductions to permit the patient to take nourishment and use the bathroom. Complications were frequent, with seizures and delirious states...and there was a substantial mortality rate. Today, chlorpromazine (Thorazine) is given in daily doses of 400 to 1,600 mg. in combination with various adjuvant hypnotics to keep the patient asleep for about 20 hours daily. Reports of overall results of 70 percent recovered...are difficult to interpret in light of the fact that almost all patients received concomitant ECT and antidepressant drug therapy.... Four out of 500 patients died during treatment (two from aspirated vomitus).[21]

That's a nearly 1 percent mortality. Nevertheless, David Healy believes there was therapeutic value in sleep therapy: "The barbiturates were such effective sedatives that their use gave rise to sleep therapy, which involved putting people into continuous sleep for several days or even weeks to give their nervous system a chance to stabilize.... *In hospital settings*, this approach *clearly cured* a number of acute illnesses, even fairly severe ones.... Finally, in addition to the *effective sleep therapy in treating schizophrenia, clinicians saw that barbiturates actually cured one form of schizophrenia, catatonic schizophrenia.*"[22] Healy's qualifying of sleep therapy as being administered in "hospital settings" is odd. Where else could this procedure have been performed? Also, if sleep therapy is effective, why has it been abandoned?

There is controversy not only about the value of sleep therapy but also about Klaesi's basic perspective on psychiatry. Roland Kuhn, a Swiss psychiatrist and psychopharmacologist, interviewed by Healy, casually mentions, "When I came into psychiatry in Berne [in the late 1930s] we were already doing sleep therapy with Klaesi and also cardiazol [metrazol] shock treatment and insulin therapy."[23] In contrast, Henri F. Ellenberger, a Swiss psychiatrist and psychiatric historian and author of the much-praised tome, *The Discovery of the Unconscious: The History and Evolution of Dynamic Psychiatry*, compares Klaesi with Nietzsche, Vaihinger, Adler, Freud, Fromm, and Sartre: "Those who were taught psychiatry by Professor Klaesi in Berne could not help but notice the striking analogy of many of his ideas with those of Adler (though he never referred to him).... Klaesi contended that neurosis resulted from a conflict between cratophorous instincts, that is from egoistic domination instincts and aristophorous instincts, that is, social instincts."[24] Then, contradicting himself, Ellenberger compares the medical treatment of syphilis, a disease, with the psychiatric treatment of mental illness, a nondisease: "New trends were manifested in psychiatry. Wagner-Jauregg's treatment of general paresis by malaria became generally known and applied.... Klaesi in Switzerland worked out a new kind of prolonged sleep therapy using Somnifene.... *Psychiatrists gradually came to admit that severe mental illness could be treated by physiological methods.*"[25]

Ellenberger claims to be a devotee of the existential-psychotherapeutic approach to psychiatric problems. In fact, he is a neurological reductionist, a perspective he equates with "scientific psychiatry": "In spite of the dark clouds steadily gathering over the world and the spreading of obscurantism over Europe, scientific psychiatry pursued its progress.

Two Italians, Cerletti and Bini, announced their discovery of a powerful therapeutic agent: electroshock therapy. The method, which had been devised to treat schizophrenia, later proved to be more successful in the treatment of severe depression."[26]

Ellenberger ignores coercion, compulsory hospitalization, the insanity defense, and every other aspect of psychiatric force and fraud, and applauds every somatic treatment: "Manfred Sakel in Vienna published the results of research he had been conducting over several years on a new physiological treatment of schizophrenia with insulin shock therapy. It was the first time that schizophrenia could be treated successfully with purely physiological methods, and it appeared as a vindication of the old organicist psychiatry against the newer dynamic trends."[27] And again: "Another new physiological treatment of mental illness was introduced by von Meduna. By means of metrazol injections he produced epileptic attacks in schizophrenic patients, and many successes were recorded."[28] Ellenberger's writings illustrate what most historians of psychiatry see as their proper task: putting a positive spin on the profession.

4

In France, sleep treatment for mental illness traces its roots to the great psychiatrist-psychologist Pierre Marie Felix Janet (1859-1947), best known for his work on hypnotism and hysteria. Janet acknowledged Mitchell's work and wrote:

> Just as the tendency which leads to the taking of food is first manifested under the form of hunger, so the tendency which leads to repose, in its initial stage of activation, manifests itself as fatigue, and this fatigue is speedily dispelled by absolute rest. Now, seeing that a great many pathological disorders resemble those induced by fatigue, would it not be proper to apply in their case a treatment akin to that we instinctively use for the relief of fatigue, to apply the method of repose?[29]

Eschewing drugs, Janet used hypnosis to produce "prolonged somnambulism," putting patients into a trance for three to four days, waking them periodically to eat and pass urine and feces. "But the great defect of the method," he noted, "is that it is only applicable to suggestible and hypnotizable hysterics."[30] Little did people realize that Mitchell's and Janet's relatively harmless antics would grow into one of the deadliest "treatments" for nondiseases.[31]

After chlorpromazine was introduced into psychiatry, French psychiatrists first used it for producing sedation for sleep treatment. In 1956, Jean Delay, Pierre Deniker, and R. Pauwels described their experience using chlorpromazine alone and in combination with barbiturates, keeping patients "narcotized" for 5 to 10 days. They credited the work of "certain Swiss authors" and of "Pavlovians," but did not say who the patients were or what ailed them. They concluded by enthusiastically recommending chlorpromazine as neuroleptic therapy of great flexibility (*"la cure neuroleptique se présente comme une méthode thérapeutique d'une grande souplesse"*).[32]

Recalling the early 1950s at Saint Anne hospital in Paris, French psychiatrist Thérèse Lempérière tells Healy: "You must remember that at this time we used to do a great number of sleep cures for the most agitated patients. Delay and Deniker had difficulty in persuading people that chlorpromazine had some antipsychotic specificity."[33] In 1957, three psychiatrists at the University of Liège in Belgium published their study of the use of chlorpromazine for sleep therapy. Their paper was summarized in English:

> The authors draw the conclusions of a study of three hundred-fifty-three cases covering a large field of psychiatric pathology...treated either by a potentialized sleep-cure (barbiturates associated with chlorpromazine, [or] by a neuroleptic cure (chlorpromazine, reserpine, etc.). The plain sleep-cure (barbiturates alone) was given up.... In many cases, it proved necessary to associate electroshock or insulin shocks with the [neuroleptic] therapy.... The potentialized sleep-cure is most indicated with non-psychotic patients; especially in neurosis and anxious psycho-neurosis, in severe psychastheny (of the phobic type); in the detoxification cure with alcoholics.... Striking results were obtained in cases of true schizopfrenia [sic].[34]

It is clear from the tenor of both articles that the patients had no say about what kind of treatment they were receiving. The authors were enthusiastic about the success of their treatments. They did not say whether the patients agreed or not. In the war on mental illness, the psychiatrists are the soldiers of fortune, the patients the prisoners of misfortune.

5

In the Soviet Union, the Russian physiologist-physician Ivan Petrovich Pavlov (1849-1936) developed a version of sleep therapy. Pavlov's fame rests on his work on gastric physiology, specifically his discovery of a type of learning he called the "conditional reflex," for which he was awarded the Nobel Prize in Physiology and Medicine in 1904. In the 1890s and 1900s, Pavlov began to investigate gastric function in dogs by externalizing a salivary gland to collect, measure, and analyze the saliva produced in response to food under different conditions. He noticed that the dogs tended to salivate before food was actually delivered to their mouths, and set out to investigate this "psychic secretion," as he called it. After carrying out a long series of experiments, manipulating the stimuli before presenting the food, he formulated the "basic laws" for what he called the establishment and extinction of "conditional reflexes." Although it is popularly believed that Pavlov signaled the impending presentation of food to his dogs by ringing a bell, this proves to be a legend. His writings record the use of a wide variety of auditory and visual stimuli, but ringing bells was not one of them.

It is important to note that Pavlov's phrase "conditional reflex" was mistranslated from the Russian as "conditioned reflex": "scientists reading his work concluded that since such reflexes were conditioned, they must be produced by a process called conditioning."[35] This concept of learning became the basis of John B. Watson's and B. F. Skinner's "behaviorism." Conditioned reflexes are learned, through "positive or negative stimuli," or, in plain English, rewards and punishments, pleasure and pain. The expectation of pleasure may lead a person to smoke a cigarette, and the expectation of pain to avoid a fire. In contrast, innate reflexes—for example, sneezing—are instinctive, unlearned reactions to stimuli.

Gradually, Pavlov became interested in applying his theories to the explanation and treatment of mental diseases. According to Joseph Wortis (1906-1995), an eclectic American psychiatrist and student of Soviet psychiatry, "Pavlov was convinced that sleep, hypnosis, and hysteria represented different types and degrees of inhibition, and came to regard certain morbid conditions in both animal and man as reflections of partial inhibitory states. He also concluded that inhibition often develops in response to stress to spare the organism further stimulation and strain."[36] The Pavlovians, as this excerpt shows, had their own neurologistic jargon, preferring terms that referred to the central nervous system to terms that referred to an individual qua choice-making person or moral agent. Wortis continued: "As a result, Pavlov not only recommended an especially quiet sheltered routine for such [nervous] patients but encouraged the reinforcement of this protective inhibition by the use of sleep. In 1935 he reported a case of catatonic schizophrenia successfully treated by this method."[37]

There is scant information in English about Pavlovian sleep therapy. The best source I could find is *Sleep Therapy in the Neuroses* (1959/1960), by the Soviet psychiatrist B. V. Andreev: "Modern sleep therapy is based on Pavlov's concept of protective or restorative inhibition and on the findings of corticovisceral physiology and pathology. ...neurosis is a functional disorder of the higher nervous activity...presenting the nervous system with tasks beyond its powers.... Sleep treatments induced by hypnosis without the use of any form of sedative drug can be regarded as ideal in neurotic states of various kinds."[38]

Although Pavlov was not a psychiatrist, there was in Leningrad a "Pavlov Clinic for Nervous Diseases." In the Pavlovian view, according to Andreev, "Patients must be told that ... Pavlov's method of sleep therapy...[is] the most humane and rational form of treatment.... During the treatment, the patient must as far as possible be shielded from external stimuli. In order to avoid excitement the patients should not be allowed to keep in touch with their relatives. For sleep therapy, a separate, isolated ward is essential, and an isolated department is even better."[39] It is not clear precisely what methods the Russians used to put patients to sleep. Behind the Pavlovian rhetoric stood, of course, the by now familiar reality of Soviet psychiatry as an integral part of the Gulag—the persecution, torture, and murder of unwanted persons by medical personnel using psychiatric drugs.

A brief comment about Wortis is called for here. Born into an American-communist family, he himself was an idealistic communist, supportive of the Soviet political system and Soviet psychiatry. Although remarkably blind to "benevolent" coercion, political as well as psychiatric, he was nevertheless an acute observer of the twentieth-century psychiatric scene. For Wortis, and for many American twentieth-century psychiatrists, only capitalism was coercive and evil. A year before he died, in an interview with the psychoanalytic historian Todd Dufresne, Wortis explained that "he tried to practice what he preached. After 'about ten years or more' in private practice as a self-styled psychotherapist, he 'decided to make an honest living by working for a salary in a hospital. *I always thought it was bad enough to have to see a doctor, and that you shouldn't have to pay more on top of that. So I never liked private practice.*' As he remarked, he was always a proponent of universal health care."[40] The italicized sentences illustrate the mindset of the coercive psychiatrist. The patient is like an infant utterly dependent for survival on being suckled by his mother. The doctor is like the mother, free to feed or not feed the baby. What is utterly lacking in this image is reciprocity—between infant and parent, patient and doctor. Wortis ignores that normal mothers—and fathers, too—have a "need" to nurture their infants. Moreover, mental patients are not infants, and psychiatrists are not their parents.

The psychiatrist-patient relationship as modeled on the parent-child relationship suits the personal needs of the psychiatrist who likes to dominate and control his patients (and others). It does not suit the needs of the mental patient whom the arrangement deprives of autonomy.

6

Although only peripherally related to the theme of the present work, it is necessary here to mention an important consequence of Pavlovian ideas, namely, behaviorism and behavior therapy. The school known as behaviorism was founded by the American psychologist John Broadus Watson (1878-1958). Its central tenets are "that scientific psychology must focus on the relationship between environmental contingencies and behavior, rather than on the presumed contents of consciousness, and that the principles governing the behavior of humans and other animals are essentially identical."[41]

Watson was a colorful person with a colorful career. He became a star professor at Johns Hopkins University, only to be forced from his chair because of a "sexual scandal," that is, dalliance with a woman who was not his wife. After leaving academic psychology, he became highly successful in the advertising business. Watson's most important book, *Psychology from the Standpoint of a Behaviorist*, was published in 1919. Acknowledging his indebtedness to Pavlov's work on conditioned reflexes, he adapted the "reflexological" terminology to human behavior. In 1920 he published his most famous conditioning experiment, producing, in a young child, a "conditioned fear" of a white rabbit by repeatedly pairing it with the loud "clang" of a metal bar. This conditioned fear was then shown to generalize to other white furry objects, including a Santa mask and Watson's own white hair.

Behaviorism's next star was B. F. (Burrhus Frederic) Skinner (1904-1990). From 1948 until the end of his life, he was a professor of psychology at Harvard, famous as the author of *Walden II*, a utopian/dystopian account of a community run according to his behaviorist principles. Like the fame of all great psychologists and psychiatrists, Skinner's depended in part on his own idiosyncratic terminology, with its flagship term "operant conditioning." In Skinnerian jargon, the organism (not person) "operates" on the environment. During this "operating," the organism encounters a special kind of stimulus, called a "reinforcing stimulus," or simply a "reinforcer." This stimulus has the effect of increasing the "operant," that is, the behavior occurring just before the reinforcer. This is operant conditioning: "the behavior is followed by a consequence, and the nature of the consequence modifies the organism's tendency to repeat the behavior in the future."[42] Thus do trivia become—with the aid of pretentious rhetoric, professional authority, and shameless hucksterism—grand psychological theories and the bases of psychiatric treatments, such as "behavior (modification) therapy," exemplified by the so-called "token economy."

Skinner passionately believed in the practical usefulness of his views, particularly in the imposition of "operant conditioning" on the inmates of state mental hospitals. One of his followers explains:

> Behavior modification is the therapy technique based on Skinner's work. It is very straight-forward: Extinguish an undesirable behavior (by removing the reinforcer) and replace it with a desirable behavior by reinforcement. It has been used on all sorts of psychological problems—addictions, neuroses, shyness, autism, even schizophrenia—and works particularly well with children. There are examples of back-ward psychotics who haven't communicated with others for years who have been conditioned to behave themselves in fairly normal ways, such as eating with a knife and fork, taking care of their own hygiene needs, dressing themselves, and so on. There is an offshoot of b-mod called the token economy. *This is used primarily in institutions such as psychiatric hospitals, juvenile halls, and prisons.* Certain rules are made explicit in the institution, and behaving yourself appropriately is rewarded with tokens—poker chips, tickets, funny money, recorded notes, etc. Certain poor behavior is also often followed by a withdrawal of these tokens. The tokens can be traded in for desirable things such as candy, cigarettes, games, movies, time out of the institution, and so on. *This has been found to be very effective in maintaining order in these often difficult institutions.*[43]

The term "behavior therapy" is another misnomer: in practice it refers to a human relationship consisting of a dominant person endeavoring to change the behavior of a person who is forced or chooses to submit to him. It is similar to hypnotherapy minus the theatrics of sleep or trance.

5

Iatrogenic Epilepsy: And Other Electrical-Therapeutic Miracles

Our concern as medical men is with the body. If there be such a thing as disease of the mind, we can do nothing for it.

—John Hughlings Jackson (1835-1911)[1]*

1

Grand mal epilepsy, manifested by convulsions and loss of consciousness, is a serious neurological illness. Although Hippocrates (b. 460 B. C.) attributed the disease to natural causes, for millennia people preferred to believe that seizures were caused by deities or demons and regarded the disease as either sacred or accursed.

The demonic origin of epilepsy, accepted by the Gospel writers, meant that its cause was possession, and hence its proper treatment was exorcism by holy men skilled in the practice of casting out devils. Jesus regularly engaged in this practice. When the religious explanation of epilepsy was replaced by the medical explanation of it, the belief that the disease is due to possession was replaced by the belief that it is due to madness. But madness was not so easily cast out. Indeed, the first tangible result of the medicalization of epilepsy was that suffering from the disease became a major social handicap. Only after the World War II did physicians change their attitude toward the epileptic, from demeaning him as a defective dependent, to respecting him as an individual with the same rights and responsibilities as anyone else.

The first modern physicians to observe patients suffering from epilepsy were general practitioners who knew their patients as persons, not "cases." They concluded that most epileptics were not seriously disabled. Sir John Russell Reynolds (1828-1896), the most prominent nineteenth-century English physician writing on epilepsy, recognized that the

---

*Jackson is the generally acknowledged "father of English neurology."

disease was due to the abnormal excitability of the cerebral cortex and recommended *Cannabis indica* (marijuana) for its treatment.[2] He stated: "Epilepsy does not necessarily involve any mental change...considerable intellectual impairment exists in some cases; but that is the exception, not the rule...ulterior mental changes are rare."[3] When psychiatrists looked at the epileptic, they saw what they were predisposed to see wherever they turned their gaze—namely, insanity and dangerousness. Although this alleged connection bore no relation to reality, that fact did not diminish the psychiatrists' influence on legislators, as the history of epileptic colonies and the sterilization of epileptics illustrates. It was enough that the psychiatrists were useful. It was not necessary that they also be right.

The psychiatric stigmatization and persecution of the epileptic may be dated from 1873, when Sir Henry Maudsley, the acknowledged founder of British psychiatry, renamed epilepsy "epileptic neurosis" and cast the epileptic in the role of a Frankensteinian monster. He wrote: "The epileptic neurosis is certainly most closely allied to the insane neurosis.... A character which the insane neurosis has in common with the epileptic neurosis is that it is apt to burst out into a convulsive explosion of violence."[4] Maudsley maintained that insane persons are biologically disposed to engage in destructive behavior, for which they are not morally or legally responsible; and that they must, therefore, be permanently incarcerated under the watchful eye of the psychiatrist. His approach to epilepsy, based on commingling it with insanity, reflects this bias: "The two diseases most closely related in this way [that is, being hereditary], are insanity and epilepsy; the descendant of an epileptic parent being almost if not quite as likely to become insane as to become epileptic, and one or other of the descendants of an insane parent not infrequently suffering from epilepsy."[5]

Maudsley had not a shred of evidence to support the claim that epilepsy and insanity are closely related diseases. But he had the power of his authority as a great physician and expert on diseases of the mind—unmatched and uncontested at that time, not only in the English-speaking world but in all advanced countries—and he used it to incriminate the epileptic, along with the insane, as a crazed killer:

> I shall now, then, proceed to point out what I conceive to be the most important conditions which are precedent of an outbreak of insane homicidal impulse. These are the *insane neurosis* and the *epileptic neurosis* in both of which the tendency is to convulsive action.... It is a remarkable and instructive fact that the convulsive energy of the homicidal impulse is sometimes preceded by a strange morbid sensation,

beginning in some part of the body and mounting to the brain, very like that which, when preceding an attack of epilepsy, is known in medicine as the *aura epileptica*.[6]

Note Maudsley's treacherous use of the oxymoron, "convulsive action." Properly speaking, action is the name we attach to the deliberate, voluntary movement of a person; in contrast, we call an involuntary movement of a muscle a reflex, convulsion, or seizure. We hold persons accountable for actions, but not for reflex movements.

Maudsley's epileptic killer is a science-fiction creature. He is a machine, not a man; an innocent bystander, as it were, who happened to inhabit a body filled with "the convulsive energy of the homicidal impulse." In the New Testament view, the epileptic is possessed by demons. In Maudsley's view, he is possessed by "homicidal impulses." This was not medical progress, replacing superstition with science. It was medical propaganda, replacing clerical with clinical superstition, theological therapy with therapeutic incarceration. From the patient's point of view, Maudsley's management of the disease by life-long imprisonment rather than exorcism was hardly an improvement.

By the end of the nineteenth century, the view that epileptics are likely to be dangerous because they are afflicted with an irresistible urge to commit violent acts was psychiatric dogma. Hungry for the spooky and the sensational, journalists and the public embraced this view, which still lingers in the popular mind.

2

Placed in the same category as the insane, epileptics became subject to incarceration.[7] This was a new development in the history of epilepsy. Prior to the 1890s, epileptics lived like other people—with their families and relatives. Epileptics who were considered insane were confined in madhouses, like other insane persons, because they were considered insane, not because they had epilepsy. Toward the end of the nineteenth century, psychiatrists began to agitate for the construction of institutions specifically for the treatment of epileptics. By the time the century ended, epileptics were slaves, and psychiatrists masters, in state facilities popularly called "epileptic colonies." The institutions were so called because they were run largely by the inmates themselves, who received little or no pay. Most of the inmates were poor. They received room, board, and medical care, gratis. Like grateful children, the least they could do was help their "parents."

The advocates of epileptic colonies directed their sales pitch to the families of epileptics, offering them a legitimate, indeed laudable, means of getting rid of their unwanted relatives. The doctors promised that the inmates would receive better care in the institutions than they could receive at home. Since the colonies were state facilities, the inmates were housed and fed at taxpayers' expense. Institutionalizing the epileptic under therapeutic auspices relieved non-epileptics not only of their obligation to care for their afflicted dependents, but also of their feelings of guilt for rejecting them.

The epileptic colonizers recognized that with every increase in the number of persons housed in their institutions, their power and profit would increase as well. Even before the first epileptic colony in America opened its doors, the New York State Lunacy Commissioners declared: "There can be no question as to the desirability of the State making special provisions for epileptics of the *dependent and semi-dependent class, apart from the insane.*"[8] A century earlier, physicians had gained control over lunatics. It was time to go after the non-lunatics. Epileptics were the perfect target. "The entire question [of how best to care for epileptics] can be solved," declared the clinicians bent on colonial conquest, "by the creation of colonies, the admission to which is *not to be regulated by the mental condition of the patient.*"[9] If the mental condition of the patient was irrelevant to the business at hand, why was their care delegated to specialists in mental diseases? No respectable physician or jurist asked that question, then or later.

Even before physicians understood that the proximate cause of an epileptic seizure was an abnormally heightened excitability of the cerebral cortex, they knew from experience that sedatives, such as opium, were useful for controlling convulsions. In 1835, potassium bromide was discovered and was soon employed in the treatment of insomnia. Some twenty years later, Sir Charles Locock learned of a person who, after medicating himself with bromides, complained that the drug virtually eliminated his sexual desire. Locock believed that masturbation caused epilepsy and reasoned that potassium bromide was an "anaphrodisiac" that might be an effective treatment for the disease. That proved to be the case.[10] The drug treatment of epilepsy had arrived.

For the next half-century, bromide was the standard treatment for epilepsy. However, its use left much to be desired, as adequate suppression of seizures often required doses large enough to cause sedation, interfering with normal existence. The next advance in the treatment of epilepsy occurred in 1903, with the discovery of barbiturates. The long-acting barbiturate, phenobarbital, proved to be especially helpful, enabling many epileptics to take enough of the drug to reduce the frequency of seizures without making them too sleepy in the bargain. Phenobarbital remained the drug of choice for treating seizure disorders until 1938, when it was displaced by Dilantin, the first in a class of drugs with specifically anti-convulsant properties. Today, several anti-convulsant drugs are available for treating seizure disorders.

Partly as a result of the development of Dilantin, the policy of seg-regating epileptics began to lose its appeal. By 1950, only one epileptic colony remained, the Indiana Village for Epileptics. In 1955, it became the New Castle State Hospital.[11] Most of the buildings formerly used to store epileptics were renamed and are now used for storing developmentally disabled persons.

The practice of confining epileptics in colonies lasted about half a century, from 1890 to 1940. As long as it was in vogue, people believed that epileptic colonies were progressive, therapeutic institutions, and that incarcerating epileptics in them was the best and most humane treatment for the patients. As late as 1949, Albert Deutsch stated: "The model colony provides the patient with an environment from which many of the dangers he faces in normal community life, as well as stresses injurious to his mental health, are eliminated.... It relieves society in some measure of a source of potential danger to public safety, since certain types of epileptic seizures are often accompanied by *homicidal impulses.*"[12]

Similar falsehoods appeared in medical textbooks as well. The 1942 edition of *Cecil's Textbook of Medicine,* the standard text when I was a medical student, explained:

> Between attacks, the frank epileptic is usually a constitutional psychopath of the most disagreeable sort...[Epileptics] are self-centered, unable to grasp the viewpoint of others, and childishly uncomprehending when forced to accept the opposite view.... Like manic-depressives and other psychotics, they are apt to adjust their depressions through this means [alcoholism], and are likewise easy victims of delirium tremens.... Institutional treatment properly directed along strictly modern lines affords the best possible means of handling [epileptics].... In properly conducted institutions the epileptic...[is] taught to view his malady in its proper light, and learn to enjoy the inestimable advantages of outdoor life.[13]

Thirty years later, when one of my daughters was a medical student, gone were the "constitutional psychopathy" of the epileptic and the advantages of "institutional treatment." Passing over the long history of the medical persecution of epileptics in discreet silence, physicians were now advised: "It is important to emphasize that the patient should be allowed to live as normal a life as possible.... Every effort should be made to keep children in school, and adults should be encouraged to work."[14] Since then, neurologists have gone even further, enjoining the physician to treat the person afflicted with epilepsy as an autonomous moral agent. A current textbook of neurology counsels: "It is important to remember that the goal of treatment is to assist patients in their efforts to overcome or at least adapt to the consequences of epilepsy. This means that treatment consists of things done in collaboration with patients rather than to or for them."[15]

The differences between neurological and psychiatric attitudes towards patients could hardly be more dramatic. The neurologist deals with persons suffering from *demonstrable brain diseases and eschews coercing them.* The psychiatrist deals with persons allegedly suffering from *hypothetical (*nondemonstrable*) brain diseases and clings to his power to impose unwanted interventions on them.*

The modern history of epilepsy is full of ironies. When epilepsy belonged to psychiatry, psychiatrists emphasized the similarities *between epilepsy and insanity.* Today, when epilepsy no longer belongs to psychiatry, neurologists emphasize the *differences between epilepsy and mental illness.* The Epilepsy Foundation of America states: "Not many years ago, people with epilepsy ... were sometimes treated as if they were insane.... No state allows commitment based solely on a person's epilepsy.... The EFA does not believe that epilepsy is a reason to take an individual's freedom away."[16] Will there ever come a day when the American Psychiatric Association makes the same statement about mental illness?

Believing is indeed seeing. The disease we call epilepsy is the same today as it was in 1893. But the beliefs of physicians about epilepsy and our social policies toward epileptics are very different indeed. Michael Trimble, an English authority on the relationship between epilepsy and psychiatry, comments: "By the 1950s, the view was that patients with epilepsy were exactly like anybody else and did not have any special susceptibility to psychopathology."[17]

A recent historical-political event merits notice here. In 1964, in the aftermath of the assassination of President Kennedy, there was a momentary revival of the psychiatric myth that epilepsy may cause murder. Not long after Lee Harvey Oswald, Kennedy's alleged assassin, was taken into custody, he was assassinated by Jack Ruby. Celebrity lawyer Melvin Belli came to Ruby's defense, claiming that his client was not guilty because he had suffered from an epileptic fugue when he shot Oswald. The defense failed, not because it was ridiculous—it was no more ridiculous than other insanity defenses that have succeeded—but largely because the American neurological profession united in refuting the claim. Belli was unable to find a single neurologist willing to testify for the defense. In an editorial in the *Journal of the American Medical Association*, Samuel Livingston, a prominent neurologist, warned: "The 'average reader' who has recently been exposed to the many newspaper articles relative to the Jack Ruby murder trial can understandably get the impression that epilepsy, murder, and crimes of passion are related.... I find no evidence of a higher rate of criminal activity among epileptics than among nonepileptics.... I certainly would not question the fact that an epileptic might kill, not because he has epilepsy, but because he is a human being."[18]

There is a lesson for psychiatry in the recent history of epilepsy. A hundred years ago, people found it intolerable to witness a person having a seizure, falling down, perhaps injuring himself. The public wanted to be spared this spectacle. To accommodate it, psychiatrists declared that epileptics needed to be confined in institutions. Today, people find it intolerable to witness a person talking to himself, contemplating suicide, perhaps killing himself. The public wants to be spared this spectacle. To accommodate it, psychiatrists declare that (seriously ill) mental patients need to be confined in institutions.

That is not the official version of the story. It is considered unprofessional to acknowledge that doctors dispose of Unwanted Persons at the behest of society. The professionally correct perspective on the incarceration of epileptics and mental patients is that such policies serve the purpose of caring for sick and dependent persons. As recently as 1944, Samuel W. Hamilton, psychiatric advisor to the Mental Hygiene Division of the United States Public Health Service, stated: "Still another group that *needs* special institutional accommodation is the convulsive disorders.... The idea of the separation of buildings into many different groups was thoroughly carried out at the Craig Colony in western New York, to create for *appreciative patients* homes where they could be comfortable and have suitable occupation for life."[19]

The rhetoric of the therapeutic segregationist who creates "homes" for "appreciative patients" sounds eerily similar to that of the racial segregationist's creating ghettos for "appreciative Negroes." Hamilton was not satisfied with institutionalizing only epileptics and mental defectives, and, of course, the mentally ill. He added, "Since many alcoholic persons are unable to control themselves, the necessity of institutional control is obvious."* The hypocrisy intrinsic to this rhetoric makes the

---

*The same tactic has been used to justify the segregation and coercive treatment of "sex offenders" (a category that used to include homosexuals) and "drug abusers" (including alcoholics).

predicament of the person caught in the web of therapeutic segregation even worse than that of the person caught in the web of punitive segregation. When we imprison a murderer, we do not say he *needs* to be deprived of liberty; we say he *deserves* to be punished. But when we imprison the epileptic or the mentally ill, we say he *needs* to be treated; we do not say that we don't like his behavior and want to be rid of him.

In the history of epileptic colonies there is, finally, an important medical-political lesson that we are eager to ignore. When treatment for epilepsy was nonexistent or rudimentary, psychiatrists used the epileptic's alleged need for treatment as a pretext for confining him. Subsequently, as the physician's *pharmacological* power to treat epilepsy increased, his *political* power to deprive him of liberty, in the name of therapy, diminished and quickly disappeared. Let us apply this formula to psychiatry. If the psychiatrist has no effective remedies for mental illness, then he cannot appeal to treatment as a justification for depriving the patient of liberty. And if the psychiatrist does possess effective treatments for mental illness, then the patient's alleged need for treatment ceases to be a legitimate reason for depriving him of liberty. This is the argument that has been advanced to justify psychiatric deinstitutionalization. The deinstitutionalization of mental patients, however, led to the creation of a new set of coercions, once more justified by psychiatric-therapeutic rationalizations—such as outpatient commitment and forced drugging; whereas the deinstitutionalization of epileptic patients led to no comparable new forms of neurological-therapeutic coercions.

3

Once physicians understood the neurophysiological mechanism of epilepsy, it became clear that seizures, accompanied by cerebral anoxia, cause brain damage. The more seizures, the more brain damage. The goal of treating the epileptic patient, in the words of the Epilepsy Foundation USA, is to prevent "a person from having seizures..."[21] The goal of treating the mental patient, according to the advocates of electroconvulsive therapy (ECT, also called "electric shock treatment"), is to give the patient seizures, the more severe the illness, the more seizures. I shall summarize how this bizarre and barbarous procedure came into being, gained popularity, and continues to have ardent advocates not only among psychiatrists but also among patients.

Faced with the nondiseases called "mental illnesses" and animated by *furor therapeuticus,* psychiatrists pounce on any chance observation, or pseudo-observation, to create interventions justified as treatments for mental diseases. The urge to treat the mental patient and the need to provide a medical rationale for the particular method of treatment generate the theory of therapeutic action, as the histories of the three types of convulsive therapies—insulin, metrazol, and electrical—illustrate.

The first so-called shock treatment was insulin coma therapy. In 1921 insulin was discovered. A year later it was tried on human beings, and diabetes became a treatable disease. The early preparations of insulin were crude and made the regulation of the diabetic patient's blood-sugar level difficult. Some patients received too little insulin, others received too much. If a person with insulin-dependent diabetes receives too little insulin, the consequences are hyperglycemia (too much glucose in the blood), diabetic coma, and death. If he receives too much insulin, the consequences are hypoglycemia (too little glucose in the blood); lightheadedness, loss of consciousness and involuntary, epileptic-like movements, called "insulin shock," brain damage, and death.

Diabetes is a common disease. Some mental hospital patients treated with insulin for their diabetes developed episodes of hypoglycemia, after which they appeared to be improved. In 1927, while working as a young doctor at a mental hospital in Berlin, Manfred Joshua Sakel (1900-1957), a neuropsychiatrist born in the Ukraine (then a part of Austria-Hungary), allegedly successfully treated a woman addicted to morphine with injections of insulin, and, presto, a cure for mental illness was at hand. Sakel had an instant explanation for how it worked: "My supposition was that some noxious agent weakened the resilience and the metabolism of the nerve cells.... A reduction in the energy spending of the cell, that is in invoking a minor or greater hibernation in it, by blocking the cell off with insulin will force it to conserve functional energy and store it to be available for the reinforcement of the cell."[22] Sakel dubbed his method "insulin shock treatment." The era of "modern somatic treatment in psychiatry" had arrived. Did insulin therapy "work"? David Healy says it did.

Healy affects to be skeptical about the effectiveness of current somatic treatments, but tends to see value in somatic treatments that have been abandoned as worthless. His views about insulin shock treatment are illustrative. "Recent research," he claims, "suggests that ICT [insulin coma therapy] might have been doing a lot more good than we now think.... Insulin stimulates appetite, and this property almost immediately led many psychiatrists to use it to treat agitated states. Following this rationale, Sakel used it on opiate addicts."[23] According to Sakel, this was not his rationale. Healy adds: "Clearly, it [ICT] must somehow have changed glucose levels..."[24] Really? "ICT clearly worked...in the sense that it had neurological effects. It worked in terms of generating enthusiasm in the staff. And it probably also worked for some 'psychotic' conditions..."[25] In short, ICT *clearly* benefited the psychiatrists, but only *probably* the patients. Even more absurdly, Healy asserts that ICT worked because "A therapy that did not produce some good would surely have faded away, given the intense amounts of labor involved and the risk of fatalities.... [Max] Fink showed that chlorpromazine and ICT were equally effective."[26] They are equally effective in legitimating psychiatry as a form of medical practice by means of chemical assaults called "treatments" forcibly imposed on patients.

In 1930, Sakel began to treat persons diagnosed as psychotic and soon reported to have achieved spectacular results with schizophrenics. In 1933, he claimed that "more than 70% of his patients improved after insulin shock therapy." Two large studies carried out in the USA in 1939 and 1942 gave him fame and helped his technique to spread rapidly around the world.[27] Insulin shock became the "standard of care" (a concept and term not yet invented) for the treatment of schizophrenia. Insulin wards, with hundreds of people subjected to hypoglycemia, became a standard fixture of progressive mental hospitals. In his interview with Heinz Lehmann (1911-1999), the first psychiatrist in Canada to use chlorpromazine, Healy asked him, "What was Sakel like?" Lehmann, an old-fashioned psychiatric autocrat, replied: "I had the impression then [in 1938 or 1939] that he was a bit flaky...I thought that he liked the good life and to feel important."[28]

Insulin shock therapy had, however, two major drawbacks: It was dangerous for the patient and troublesome for the staff. The unconscious patient had to be given glucose by nasal tube to bring him out of his coma. The patient could suffer permanent brain damage or die of hypoglycemia. The search was on for a simpler and safer method of inducing convulsions.

In 1933, the same year that Sakel announced his results with the insulin-coma therapy, the Hungarian psychiatrist Meduna László (Ladislaus von Meduna, 1896-1964) began his search for a chemical agent to produce "physiological seizures." Unaware of Sakel's work, Meduna seized on the spurious observation that epilepsy and schizophrenia are antagonistic conditions. I say spurious because Bleuler and other psychiatrists in the pre-shock era saw epilepsy and schizophrenia as related conditions. The new view was a complete reversal. No longer did epilepsy cause insanity; instead, it cured it. It was Meduna rather than Sakel who sold this fantasy to both the psychiatric profession and the public:

He [Meduna] found that 16.5% of epileptic patients who developed psychotic symptoms had a remission of epilepsy.... There were anecdotal reports of cures of schizophrenia in patients who developed epileptic seizures. Meduna had then the idea that seizures could be used to treat schizophrenia.... Finally, he discovered that camphor dissolved in oil was effective in animals as well as in humans.... On January 23, 1934, he tried the injection of camphor oil in a severe 33-year-old catatonic patient. After just 5 treatments, catatonia and psychotic symptoms were abolished.... Soon, Meduna discovered pentylenetetrazol, or metrazol (brand name Cardiazol), a powerful convulsant agent, as being more effective and quick-acting than camphor, and started using it in intramuscular and intravenous injections. He published his results in 1935 and his results quickly provoked a commotion in psychiatry around the world, because schizophrenia was then considered a hereditary and incurable condition.[29]

In his 1939 monograph, *Die Konvulsionstherapie der Schizophrenie* (*Convulsive Therapy in Schizophrenia*), "Meduna claimed an astounding 95% remission rate in acute schizophrenic patients, his results were said to have been reproduced in other centers around the world, and metrazol shock treatment became commonplace."[30] Despite all the evidence to the contrary, most historians of psychiatry accept Meduna's rationalizations and repeat the mendacious legend of his "discovery" of iatrogenic epilepsy as a cure for schizophrenia. In their frequently quoted *History of Psychiatry*, Franz Alexander and Sheldon Selesnick write: "In the late 1920's Ladislaus Joseph von Meduna...observed that the glial tissue [in the brain] had thickened in epileptic patients. When he compared their brains with those of deceased schizophrenic patients he noted that the latter showed a deficiency of glial structure. On the basis of these findings...Meduna became convinced that schizophrenia and epilepsy were incompatible diseases and that a convulsive agent administered to schizophrenics would therefore cure them."[31]

Alexander and Selesnick are guilty of misrepresentation: They fail to mention that in his classic 1911 text on schizophrenia, Eugen Bleuler, like Henry Maudsley before him, observed a direct, rather than an inverse, relationship between epilepsy and schizophrenia. "Many of our [schizophrenic] patients," he wrote, "were first sent to us with the diagnosis of epilepsy, and were so labeled in the clinics."[32]

The American Psychiatric Association's centennial celebratory volume, *One Hundred Years of Psychiatry* (1944), summarizes the official psychiatric version of the story of the origin of shock treatment as follows: "Somewhat as the treatment of general paralysis with tryparsamide paralleled malaria therapy...so was the treatment of schizophrenia by means of insulin shock paralleled by the use for the same purpose of pentamethylenetetrazol (metrazol), as a convulsive agent."[33]

The comparison is absurd. General paralysis is a clearly defined, objectively diagnosable neurological disease, due to infection with the treponema pallidum. Schizophrenia is merely a diagnosis, a disease name. Schizophrenics are not paralyzed and do not die two or three years after falling ill. Nevertheless, having defined schizophrenia as a disease, psychiatrists wanted to be able to treat it. But they had not the foggiest notion of what it was, much less what to do about it. At this point, coincidental advances in medicine once again determined the course of psychiatric quack-therapeutics. Neuroscientist Renato M. E. Sabbatini explains: "The early decades of the 20th century witnessed a major revolution in the understanding and treatment of mental diseases. Until then, people with psychoses were usually locked away in insane asylums, receiving only limited custodial care and sometimes social support, with practically no effective therapeutic options left to the alienist, as psychiatrists were called then."[34] The truth is less rosy. "Eventually," Sabbatini concludes, "psychiatry recognized that his theory of biological incompatibility between epilepsy and schizophrenia was unfounded, but that artificially-induced convulsions were useful to reduce schizophrenia."[35] Contemporary psychiatrists still correlate epilepsy with mental illnesses and even with suicide. Researchers at Columbia University in New York and the University of Reykjavik, Iceland, "believe...that epilepsy is linked to both depression and suicide.... Surprisingly, however, they found no statistically significant link between suicide and depression. ...the results [of their studies] suggest common underlying brain mechanisms for suicidal behavior and epilepsy."[36] Note the appearance here of the specter of suicide, the veritable incubus of the psychiatrist's nightmare. Suicide is the act of an actor, not the disease of an organism. Transformed into a "mental health problem," suicide haunts contemporary psychiatry perhaps even more than the communism of *The Communist Manifesto* (1848) haunted modern Europe.[37]

We must keep in mind the basic problem, conceptual as well as practical, underlying so-called treatments for schizophrenia: psychiatrists have no objective criteria or tests for diagnosing the disease; there is no way physicians can be certain that a person has schizophrenia, or whether the alleged disease is or is not being ameliorated. Furthermore, most persons subjected to treatment for schizophrenia, especially prior to the 1960s, were de facto prisoners, individuals confined in mental hospitals against their will. This is still largely the case, even if the patients are not physically confined. In view of these circumstances, it is not surprising that every new treatment for schizophrenia—from insulin shock, to metrazol shock, to electric shock, to lobotomy, to neuroleptic drugs—was initially claimed to be a magical cure and later declared to be worthless or harmful.

4

Sakel and Meduna succeeded in fabricating a rationale and establishing a professional justification for giving mental patients epileptic convulsions against their will. By the time the Italian psychiatrists Ugo Cerletti (1877-1963) and Lucio Bini (1904-1964) started to experiment with electrically induced seizures, the therapeutic value of iatrogenic convulsions was taken for granted in medicine and the media. All that remained was to describe the "discovery." Cerletti provided two detailed accounts of it. To convey the tone as well as the content of these accounts, I offer extensive extracts from both. The first was published in the *American Journal of Psychiatry* in 1950:

Convulsions were to be induced with a therapeutic aim since the good clinical results obtained by Meduna's method were ascribed to them. For this the old transcranial method followed by physiologists was sufficient. But this idea then, and for a long time to come, appeared Utopian, because of the terror with which the notion of subjecting a man to high-tension currents was regarded. The spectre of the electric chair was in the minds of all and an imposing mass of medical literature enumerated the casualties, often fatal, ensuing upon electric discharges across the human body. Nowadays, after twelve years of experience with electroshock, that terror may seem to have been exaggerated; but cases of death caused by low tensions (forty volts) had been described.... The fact is that no one at the clinic seriously thought of applying electric convulsions to man.... Nevertheless I, who had gone to such lengths in striving to preserve dogs from death when given electrically induced convulsions, had now come to the conviction that a discharge of electricity must prove equally harmless to a man if the duration of the current's passage were reduced to a minimum interval.... This inactivity in the face of so momentous a question greatly depressed me, so that I immediately jumped at the information, given me by my colleague, Professor Vanni, that "at the Rome slaughterhouse pigs are killed by electricity." As though to justify my passiveness and to settle my hopes by facing a real fact, I decided to see this electric slaughtering with my own eyes, and immediately went to the slaughterhouse.

There I was told that the application of a current across the pigs' heads had been in use for some years. The butchers took hold of the pigs near their ears with a large scissor-shaped pair of pincers. The pincers were connected to the lighting plant with wires, and terminated in two teethed disc-electrodes enclosing a sponge wet with water. As they were seized, the pigs fell on their sides and were soon taken by fits (convulsed). Then the butcher, taking advantage of the unconscious state of the animal, gave its neck a deep slash, thus bleeding it to death. I at once saw that the fits were the same as those I had been producing in dogs, and that these pigs were not being "killed by electricity," but were bled to death during the epileptic coma.

Since a great number of pigs was available at the slaughterhouse for killing, I now set myself the exact opposite of my former experiments' aims; namely, no longer to make efforts to keep the convulsed animals alive, but rather to determine what the conditions must be for obtaining their death by an electric current. Having obtained authorization for experimenting from the director of the slaughterhouse, Professor Torti, I carried out tests, not only subjecting the pigs to the current for ever-increasing periods of time, but also applying the current in various ways: across the head, across the neck, and across the chest. Various durations (twenty, thirty, sixty or more seconds) were tried. It turned out that the more serious results (prolonged apnea sometimes lasting many minutes and, exceptionally, death) appeared when the current crossed the chest; that this application was not mortal for durations of some tenths of a second; and, finally, *that passage of the current across the head, even for long durations, did not have serious consequences....* These clear proofs, certain and oft repeated, caused all my doubts to vanish, and without more ado I gave instructions in the clinic to undertake, next day, the experiment upon man. Very likely, except for this fortuitous and fortunate circumstance of pigs' pseudo-electrical butchery, electroshock would not yet have been born.

A schizophrenic of about forty, whose condition was organically sound, was chosen for the first test. He expressed himself exclusively in an incomprehensible gibberish made up of odd neologisms, and since his arrival from Milan by train without a ticket, not a thing had been ascertainable about his identity. Preparations for the experiment were carried out in an atmosphere of fearful silence bordering on disapproval in the presence of various assistants belonging to the clinic and some outside doctors.

As was our custom with dogs, Bini and I fixed the two electrodes, well wetted in salt solution, by an elastic band to the patient's temples. As a precaution, for our first test, we used a reduced tension (seventy volts) with a duration of 0.2 second. Upon closing the circuit, there was a sudden jump of the patient on his bed with a very short tensing of all his muscles; then he immediately collapsed onto the bed without loss of consciousness. The patient presently started to sing at the top of his voice, then fell silent. It was evident from our long experience with dogs that the voltage had been held too low. I, bearing in mind the observations with repeated applications of the day before upon pigs, made arrangements for a repetition of the test. Someone got nervous and suggested whisperingly that the subject be allowed to rest; others advised a new application to be put off to the morrow. Our patient sat quietly in bed, looking about him. Then, of a sudden, hearing the low toned conversation around him, he exclaimed—*no longer in his incomprehensible jargon*, but in so many clear words and in a solemn tone—"'Not a second. Deadly!"

The situation was such, weighted as it was with responsibility, that *this warning, explicit and unequivocal*, shook the persons present to the extent that some began to insist upon suspension of the proceedings. Anxiety lest something that amounted to superstition should interfere with my decision urged me on to action. I had the electrodes reapplied, and a 110-volt discharge was sent through for 0.5 second. The immediate, very brief cramping of all the muscles was again seen; after a slight pause, the most typical epileptic fit began to take place. True it is that all had their hearts in their mouths and were truly oppressed during the tonic phase with apnea, ashy paleness, and cadaverous facial cyanosis—an apnea which, if it be awe-inspiring in a spontaneous epileptic fit, now seemed painfully never-ending—until at the first deep, stertorous inhalation, and first clonic shudders, the blood ran more freely in the bystanders' veins as well; and, lastly, to the immense relief of all concerned, was witnessed a characteristic, gradual awakening "by steps." The patient sat up of his own accord, looked about him calmly with a vague smile, as though asking what was expected of him. I asked him: "What has been happening to you?" He answered, with no more gibberish: "I don't know; perhaps I have been asleep."

That is how the first epileptic fit experimentally induced in man through the electric stimulus took place. So electroshock was born; for such was the name I forthwith gave it.[38]

In the same article, Cerletti relates the rapid intensification and extension of the use of ECT in the treatment of various conditions:

Bini in 1942 suggested the repetition of ECT many times a day for certain patients, *naming the method "annihilation."* * This results in severe amnesic reactions that appear to have a good influence in obsessive states, psychogenic depressions and even in some paranoid cases. "Clustering" of treatments, shocking daily for three or four days followed by a three-day rest, is less intense but sometimes effectual. The method of annihilation has made possible studies of amnesia and of hallucinations, delirium, and moria occurring during the treatment.... Depressed and aged patients show disturbances earlier than young or excited patients. The "annihilation syndrome" has been compared by Cerquetelli and Catalano with the psychopathology following prefrontal leukotomy.... Electroshock has also been applied in certain general physical illnesses though all have a constitutional "nervous" background. Recovery has been frequently reported in asthma,...in psoriasis, prurigo, and alopecia areata. .... It is worth noting that any of our therapeutic methods such as prolonged sleep, narcoanalysis, insulin coma, epileptic coma, electronarcosis, etc., have in common the factor of the induction of a state of unconsciousness. The second idea has to do with the patient's fear of therapy, which leads some to want to stop it. On being asked the reason, they reply: "I don't know, I am afraid." "Afraid of what?" "I don't know, I have fear...." There must be a vague recollection—organic memory—of the first "terror-defense" reaction....[39]

In a report published six years later, Cerletti repeated much the same story but added a few fresh details:

During this period of unconsciousness (epileptic coma), the butcher stabbed and bled the animals without difficulty. Therefore, it was not true that the animals were killed by the electric current: the latter was used, at the suggestion of the Society for the Prevention of Cruelty to Animals, so that the hogs might be killed painlessly.... At this point I felt we could venture to experiment on man, and I instructed my assistants to be on the alert for the selection of a suitable subject. On April 15, 1938, the Police Commissioner of Rome sent a man to our Institute with the following note: "S.E., 39 years old, engineer, resident of Milan, was *arrested at the railroad station while wandering about without a ticket on trains ready for departure. He does not appear to be in full possession of his mental faculties, and I am sending him to your hospital to be kept there under observation....*" The condition of the patient on April 18 was as follows: *lucid, well-oriented.* He describes with neologisms deliriant ideas of being telepathically influenced with related sensorial disturbances; his mimicry is correlated to the meaning of his words; mood indifferent to environment, low affective reserves; physical and neurologic examination negative; presents conspicuous hypacusic and cataract in left eye. A diagnosis of schizophrenic syndrome was made based on his passive behavior, incoherence, low affective reserves, hallucinations, deliriant ideas of being influenced, neologisms. This subject was chosen for the first experiment of induced electric convulsions in man.... Naturally, we, who were conducting the

---

*The aptly named "method of annihilation" was later adopted by the Scottish-Canadian psychiatrist, D. Ewen Cameron. See chapter 6.

experiment were under great emotional strain and felt that we had already taken quite a risk. Nevertheless, it was quite evident to all of us that we have been using a too low voltage. It was proposed that we should allow the patient to have some rest and repeat the experiment the next day. All at once, the patient, who evidently had been following our conversation, said clearly and solemnly, without his usual gibberish: "Not another one! It's deadly!"[40]

Cerletti's accounts allow us to draw some inferences from them:

- The first person given ECT was a vagrant who was shocked against his explicit protest.
- S.E., the denominated patient, did not seek psychiatric help. In fact, he was a prisoner, having been arrested by the police, for "wandering about." Instead of being tried for his offense, he was sent to Cerletti "for observation." Cerletti disobeyed the instructions of the Rome Police Commissioner. Instead of observing S.E., Cerletti used him as an experimental subject for ECT.
- Cerletti makes no reference to obtaining permission for his experiment from the police or any other authority. Having received the prisoner from the police, Cerletti regarded him as his patient and himself as the sole judge of the treatment he should have. Throughout the experiment, S.E. was treated as an animal or thing. After the first shock, when he announced "clearly and solemnly: 'Not another one! It's deadly!,'" his seemingly rational communication did not deter the physicians experimenting on him. On the contrary, it seemed to intensify Cerletti's desire to continue his experiment.[41]

Cerletti, like all psychiatrists inventing a new psychiatric "treatment," created a theory about the mode of its action. His student, Ferrucio di Cori, explained: "He [Cerletti] formulated a theory that the humoral and hormonal changes provoked in the brain by the epileptic attack lead to the formation of substances which he called 'acroagonines'—substances of extreme defense. These substances, when injected into the patient, would have therapeutic effects similar to those resulting from electroshock."[42] When mental patients exhibit such reasoning, psychiatrists say they have "delusions." When psychiatrists exhibit such reasoning, they say that they are formulating "theories."

Frank J. Ayd, a leading post-World War II advocate of ECT, recalled Cerletti's reminiscing about the electroshocking of his first patient: "When I saw the patient's reaction, I thought to myself: This ought to be abolished! Ever since I have looked forward to the time when another treatment would replace electroshock."[43] David Shutts, author of *Lobotomy: Resort to the Knife,* confirms the story: "Cerletti later regretted his decision: 'It was not long after I had first witnessed electrically produced convulsions in man...that I came to the conclusion that we must get away from the use of electroshock. When subjecting unconscious patients to such an extremely violent reaction as these convulsions, I had a sense of illicitness and felt as though I had somehow betrayed these patients.'"[44]

The development of electroconvulsive treatment is an example of modern therapeutic totalitarianism in *statu nascendi:* handed over to the psychiatrist by the police, the mental patient is treated as a non-person, without his or anyone else's consent. In a society that permits this type of human relationship because the psychiatrist claims it is "therapeutic," the so-called patient cannot expect the law to protect him. The "abuse" of ECT by D. Ewen Cameron, which I discuss in the next chapter, dramatically illustrates this contention.

5

Since its introduction into psychiatry in 1938, the popularity of ECT has waxed and waned and waxed again. In the early 1960s, in the wake of my writings and those of Erving Goffman, and especially of Ken Kesey's novel *One Flew Over the Cukoo's Nest* and the film based on it, the image of ECT became temporarily tarnished. I may note in this connection that while Kesey was working on the screenplay of *One Flew Over the Cuckoo's Nest*, he wrote to the magazine *Madness Network News:* "I'm into the first rewrite of the Cuckoo's Nest screenplay. But I haven't been in a nuthouse for more than ten years. Your paper came at a perfect time to remind me of something unrememberable. Thanks. / Also, we are bringing out a magazine in the Fall called *Spit in the Ocean.* The theme of the first issue is Old in the Streets. Have you got a piece telling what it's like to be an old looney and observations therein? / Long live Thomas S. Szasz!"[45]

Soon, ECT was rehabilitated and "reemerged in the 1980s and 1990s as 'the gold standard antidepressant treatment modality.'"[46] "In my case," declared actor and TV host Dick Cavett, "ECT was miraculous." Producer Joshua Logan stated, "All I wanted to do was lie there and enjoy this cool peace flowing through me." Norman Endler, a professor of psychology at York University in Canada; Martha Manning, a clinical psychologist and former professor at George Mason University; novelist William Styron; and actress Patty Duke Astin are among the vocal advocates of ECT. One grateful ex-patient described receiving ECT as similar to "receiving a blessing in a sanctuary."[47] Both the American Psychiatric Association and the National Alliance for the Mentally Ill (NAMI) strongly support

ECT, and so do many ECT patients, celebrities as well as mental-health professionals. The most active and prominent supporter of the procedure today is Max Fink, often called "the grandfather of American ECT." Born in 1923, Fink is certified in neurology, psychiatry, and psychoanalysis, and is currently professor emeritus of psychiatry at the State University of New York at Stony Brook. He is the author of several standard works on ECT, founding editor of *Convulsive Therapy*, now *The Journal of ECT*, consultant to the FDA, and consultant to the U.S. Army on the Feasibility of Using Incapacitating Agents Against Terrorists.[48] In 2004, Fink assembled the pro-ECT testimonials of scores of professionals, among them those of Sherwin Nuland, M.D., professor of surgery at Yale University Medical School, author, and medical and psychiatric historian, and Leon Rosenberg, M.D., former dean of Yale University Medical School.[49] Nuland wrote:

> From my late thirties until my early forties, I underwent a period of depression that gradually deepened into an intensity that I finally required admission to a mental hospital, where I stayed for more than a year. Neither medication, psychotherapy, the determined efforts of friends nor the devotion of the few people whose love never deserted me had even the most minimal beneficial effect on my worsening state of mind. Finally, faced with my resistance to all forms of treatment till then attempted, the senior psychiatrists at the institution in which I was confined recommended the draconian measure of lobotomy. I was, in fact, completely disabled by pathological preoccupations and fears. Obsessions with coincidences; fixations on recurrent numbers; feelings of worthlessness and physical or sexual inadequacy; religious anxieties of guilt and concerns about God's will.... I was saved from the drastic intervention of lobotomy by the refusal of a twenty-seven-year-old resident psychiatrist assigned to my case to agree with his teachers. At his insistence, a course of electroshock therapy was reluctantly embarked upon. At first, the newly instituted treatment made not a whit of difference. The number of electroshock treatments mounted, but still no improvement took place. The total would eventually reach twenty. Somewhere around the middle of the course, a glimmer of change made itself evident, which encouraged the skeptical staff to continue a series of treatments they had begun only to mollify a promising young man in training. I recovered so well, in fact, that in the four remaining months of hospitalization, I lost all but the dimmest memory of the obsessions and saw my depression disappear entirely.[50]

About Rosenberg we learn only that "in 1998, around the time of Rosenberg's 65th birthday, he awakened in an agitated state after restless nights of insomnia [and] attempted suicide by drug overdose. He was admitted to the closed ward of a psychiatric hospital. Electroconvulsive therapy was prescribed." Fink quotes Rosenberg:

> After the fourth ECT, I was noticeably less depressed. My appetite returned, as did my ability to sleep. After eight treatments, my mood was fully restored. I experienced no confusion, memory loss, headache, or any other symptom sometimes attributed to ECT. I felt so well that, with some trepidation, I prepared to go back to work.... I now

understand that I was brainsick ("diseased of the brain and mind") when I tried to kill myself. I view my suicide attempt as the end result of mental illness in the same way I view a heart attack as the end result of coronary artery disease. Both are potentially lethal, both have known risk factors, both are major public health problems, both are treatable and preventable....[51]

Meaning is something we attribute to our experiences, good and bad, virtuous and wicked. If we look for meaning—for our roles in our joys and sorrows alike—we "find" it, or believe we do. If we do not look for meaning in them, we find our tragedies "meaningless"—the impersonal results of events outside our control, the consequences of pathophysiological processes in bodies, or the results of influences exerted by celestial bodies. "The fault, dear Brutus, is not in our stars, / But in ourselves...," wrote Shakespeare four hundred years ago.[52] Thanks to psychiatric progress, we now know better.

There is a vast literature on ECT, the majority of writers endorsing the procedure as therapeutic and life-saving, a minority condemning it as brain-damaging. Supporters of ECT have their own official organization, the Association for Convulsive Therapy, and their journal, *The Journal of ECT*, covering "all aspects of contemporary electroconvulsive therapy, reporting on major clinical and research developments worldwide. Leading clinicians and researchers examine the effects of induced seizures on behavior and on organ systems; review important research results on the mode of induction, occurrence, and propagation of seizures; and explore the difficult sociological, ethical, and legal issues concerning the use of ECT."[53]

Opponents of ECT also abound. A web site devoted to criticizing Max Fink states: "[Fink] argued for years that the therapeutic effect from ECT is produced by brain dysfunction and damage. ... In 1956, he stated that the basis for improvement from ECT is 'cranio-cerebral trauma.' In 1966, Fink cited his own research indicating that 'there is a relation between clinical improvement and the production of brain damage or an altered state of brain function.'"[54] Most neurologists regard it as self-evident that epileptic seizures cause brain damage and that all injury to an intact brain is harmful. Berkeley, California neurologist John Friedberg, author of *Shock Treatment Is Not Good For Your Brain,* states:

From a neurological point of view ECT is a method of producing amnesia by selectively damaging the temporal lobes and the structures within them.... ECT produces a form of brain disease, with an estimated incidence of new cases in the range of 100,000 per year. Many psychiatrists are unaware that ECT causes brain damage and memory loss because numerous authorities and a leading psychiatric textbook deny these facts.... Assuming free and fully informed consent, it is well to reaffirm the individual's right to pursue happiness through brain damage if he or she so chooses.

But we might ask ourselves whether we, as doctors sworn to the Hippocratic Oath, should be offering it.[55]

Dr. Sidney Samant, a neurologist and electroencephalographer, agrees: "I have seen many patients after ECT, and I have no doubt that ECT produces effects identical to those of a head injury. After multiple sessions of ECT, a patient has symptoms identical to a retired, punch-drunk boxer. ... Electroconvulsive therapy in effect may be defined as a controlled type of brain damage produced by electrical means."[56]

Nevertheless, today ECT is widely practiced. In December 1999, David Satcher, Surgeon General of the United States Public Health Service, issued his first-ever report on mental health in the United States and gave electroshock the coveted stamp of approval, "safe and effective."[57]

6

D. Ewen Cameron (1901-1967), Scottish-born physician, founding chairman of the department of psychiatry at McGill University Medical School in Montreal, first head of the World Psychiatric Association, president of both the American and Canadian Psychiatric Associations, and a celebrated pioneer in the somatic treatment of mental illness, was widely regarded as a humane and "progressive" psychiatrist. In 1944, when he became the head of the Allan Memorial Institute, the headquarters of the McGill psychiatry department, he declared that "no doors in the Allan would be locked.... patients could not be locked up if they were to realize that they still belonged to society."[58] In fact, Cameron's patients were not only locked up, they were abused as few patients have been in the barbarous history of psychiatry. His fame, or infamy, resides in his having adopted Lucio Bini's "method annihilation"—that is, giving patients ECT several times a day to produce severe amnesia—and in having participated in clandestine, CIA-sponsored "experiments" on mental patients.

On January 6, 1998, thirty-one years after Cameron's death, the Canadian Broadcasting Corporation (CBC) aired a radio documentary titled, "MKULTRA, 'Dr.' Ewen Cameron, Psychiatrist and Torturer." An announcer introduced the program:

Behind closed doors, human guinea pigs in shocking mind control experiments conducted by our government and the CIA.... The horrors of "the sleep room...." In the 1960s, Dr. Ewen Cameron conducted CIA-funded experiments on troubled Canadian patients he was meant to help. A Fifth Estate investigation revealed how one Canadian government secretly supported these horrific experiments, and then another blocked the victims' fight for justice. It's the classic story of good turning to evil in its most simplistic terms.... Inspired by the exuberant post-war optimism and technology, Cameron thought he'd achieved a major scientific breakthrough—how to repair a damaged human mind. The media rejoiced—even coined a phrase which would become a tragically silly oxymoron: "beneficial brainwashing."[59]

A woman patient who had felt "tired and depressed" then related her story. A family member told her: "Why don't you go to Montreal and visit this Dr. Ewen Cameron, this famous man, who has all of these accolades, and have an assessment. So we went. ...and that was the end of my life. Within three weeks Dr. Cameron decided to call me an acute schizophrenic, and shipped me up to the 'sleep room....' I was in a coma for 86 days." She and eight other of Cameron's victims sued the CIA. After a litigation lasting ten years, the plaintiffs settled out-of-court, for 750,000 Canadian dollars. According to the CBC, it was "an ambiguous victory. Ottawa refused to acknowledge any wrongdoing at the Allan, a conclusion backed up by a legal review of what happened there."

What happened was that the Canadian government had retained its own expert and relied on his report. The expert was "Dr. Frederick Grunberg, one of Quebec's leading psychiatrists, who made two controversial assertions: that the patients hadn't suffered irreparable harm, and that they had consented to the treatment." At the end of the program, the listeners were left with this conclusion: "It's been more than 33 years since the Allan put an end to the practices initiated by its most notorious doctor. It has recovered its world-class reputation as a leader in the treatment of mental illness." Thus was an ostensible media exposé of massive psychiatric fraud and force by the McGill Department of Psychiatry transformed into one more psychiatric whitewash. Cameron and the famed Allan Memorial Institute were exonerated of medical wrongdoing. The blame for what went wrong was laid on the CIA, the Canadian Government, and the exceptional horrors of mental illness that justified exceptional treatments. Cameron wasn't a bad guy, after all; he was only trying to cure patients with a terrible illness, with their consent.

7

While Cameron was alive, psychiatrists and psychologists never criticized his psychiatric practices. After he died, most of them lamented his practices. For example, Donald Olding Hebb (1904-1985)—head of McGill's psychology department during Cameron's tenure and himself a prestigious physiological psychologist who had nothing to fear from Cameron—had remained silent for years. With Cameron dead, he expressed only scorn for him. Hebb told John Marks, author of *The*

Search for the "Manchurian Candidate," an indispensable volume for understanding the history of modern psychiatry: "That was an awful set of ideas Cameron was working with.... If I had a graduate student who talked like that, I'd throw him out.... He was eminent because of politics." Marks adds: "Nobody said such things at the time...D. Ewen Cameron read papers about 'depatterning' with electroshock before meetings of his fellow psychiatrists and they elected him their president."[60]

An anonymous McGill psychiatrist was even more critical: "I probably shouldn't talk about this but Cameron—for him to do what he did—*he was a very schizophrenic guy*, who totally detached himself from the human implications of his work.... God, we talk about concentration camps. I don't want to make this comparison. But God, you talk about what 'we didn't know it was happening' and it was—right in our own back yard."[61]

But Cameron still has defenders. One is Thomas A. Ban, a Hungarian-born psychiatrist and psychopharmacologist. Ban received his medical degree in Budapest, subsequently fled to Canada, did his psychiatric residency in Montreal, and then joined Cameron's team. In an interview with David Healy in 1994, Ban spoke about Cameron at length. He begins with this stage-setting comment: "Cameron had been critical of psychoanalytic theory, rejected what psychoanalysis stood for.* Now I am not saying that the Cameron affair was created by the psychoanalysts."[62] Of course, that is exactly what Ban is saying; and because he, too, closes his eyes to the carceral character of psychiatry, his defense of Cameron unwittingly becomes an indictment:

> What is somewhat surprising is that no one ever pointed out that while Cameron's team was depatterning a patient on one bed, another team on another bed of the sleep room was busy doing anaclitic therapy—one of those therapies based on psychoanalytic therapy in which adults are treated as babies. After all, Cameron's idea to erase everything one had learned, get rid of the pathogenic patterns, create a *tabula rasa*, and try to rebuild things from scratch, program in new behavior, was not as way out as some people have perceived it. And even if many people had forgotten it conveniently, Cameron had only introduced the term depatterning for a treatment which was in use, but referred to as regressive ECT by others. As you know, there were all kinds of treatments in those days—apomorphine-induced vomiting and atropine-induced toxic psychosis were considered to be therapeutic.[63]

Healy comments: "It was all very strange because around 1960/62, Cameron was one of the three or four big names in the world." Ban

---

*Psychoanalysis may be said to stand for many deplorable practices but coercion is not one of them. Psychoanalysis rests on a consensual relationship between doctor and patient. "Coerced psychoanalysis" is a contradiction in terms.

continues: "He was one of the Nuremberg psychiatrists and one of the psychiatrists who examined Rudolph Hess...it was actually [Robert] Cleghorn's [Cameron's successor at the Allan Memorial Institute] team which commissioned the work which found *no memory impairment in the depatterned patients...*"[64] Note that Ban gives Cameron credit for creating a *tabula rasa* by erasing his patients' memories *and* for creating no memory impairment in them. Healy then asks, "Why is getting funds from the CIA such a potent stick to beat people with?" Ban replies:

> Because it can be implied that CIA-funded studies were used for the development of brainwashing techniques....* There were many distinguished scientists who got funds from the CIA.... Harris Isbell, who was director of the addiction research center in Lexington; Jolyon West, who was chairman of the department of psychiatry in Los Angeles, and Leo Hollister, one of the most prominent clinical psychopharmacologists of the United States. But there were many well-known psychologists too. I read that Hans Eysenck, Carl Rogers and Fred Skinner...[65]

In 1963, four years before his death, Cameron retired abruptly, "for unexplained reasons."[66] More than thirty years after Cameron's exposure, Joel Paris, the current chairman of the McGill Department of Psychiatry, continues to paint a glowing picture of this Mengele of modern psychiatry. I cite this from a web site titled "History of the McGill Department of Psychiatry":

> McGill's Psychiatry department was founded in 1943 by Dr. D. Ewen Cameron. Although Cameron continues to be a subject of controversy, there is no doubt that he was a great builder. In 1944, the Allan Memorial Institute opened. The site was Ravenscrag, a stately mansion located on the slopes of Mount Royal, which was renovated to house an institute of psychiatry. Cameron then led both the Allan and the McGill department of psychiatry until 1963. During those years, he attracted faculty with a wide range of interests, so that McGill became a center for research in subjects as diverse as neurochemistry, psychopharmacology, transcultural psychiatry, psychosomatics, and psychoanalysis.... [McGill] became one of the largest psychiatry departments in the world, training a large number of residents coming from all over the world. As a result, many McGill graduates have had leading positions in psychiatry, both in North America and abroad.... Investigations in our department have always been, and continue to be, broad and eclectic. We have strong research programs in almost all areas—alphabetically listed, they are: Addiction Psychiatry, Alzheimer's Disease, Anxiety Disorders, Attention Deficit Hyperactivity Disorder, Autism, Brain Imaging, Child Psychiatry, Community Psychiatry, Consultation-Liaison, Eating Disorders, Expressed Emotion, Geriatrics, Infant Psychiatry, Mood Disorders, Neurochemistry, Obsessive-Compulsive Disorder, Pain, Personality Disorders, Psychopharmacology, Psychotherapy, Schizophrenia, Suicide, and Transcultural Psychiatry.[67]

---

*Both Ban and Healy use the metaphor "brainwashing" without questioning its metaphoric character.

The truth is that Cameron was one of a group of world-famous "patriotic poisoners," psychiatrists and psychologists who, working as covert CIA agents, poisoned and killed unsuspecting persons.[68] The psychiatrists' reaction to the Cameron scandal illustrates the profession's habitual refusal to acknowledge error, admit guilt, apologize for force and fraud, and repudiate manifest evil committed by their own revered members. The episode represents what chemists would call an "aliquot sample": as the analysis of a single drop of sea water reveals the composition of all of the waters in the oceans, so the Cameron affair reveals the nature of all of the history of involuntary-institutional psychiatry.

8

The eighteenth century was a century of revolutions—political and scientific.

The phenomenon physicists call "magnetism" had been observed in antiquity. However, the fabrication of magnets, for sale to scientific investigators and terrestrial navigators, began around 1740. The famous Leyden Jar, a simple electrical capacitator that could be used to give a person a violent, albeit weak, shock, was invented about 1745, by a Dutch physicist at the University of Leyden. This device quickly became a show-business prop and sensation. In 1752, Benjamin Franklin (1706-1790), familiar with the Leyden Jar, invented the lightning rod, a feat that made him world-famous, perhaps the first modern "celebrity." Finally, in 1780, the Italian scientist Luigi Galvani (1737-1798) discovered the electric current and what he mistakenly thought was "animal electricity."[69] It was in this atmosphere of scientific discovery along with medical quackery and popular showmanship that Franz Anton Mesmer (1733-1815), an Austrian physician, "discovered" what he thought was "animal magnetism," a mysterious "force" to which he attributed vast therapeutic powers.[70] Some psychiatric historians—Henri Ellenberger and Gregory Zilboorg among them—trace the origin of modern psychotherapy specifically to Mesmerism.[71] They do so, paradoxically, not because Mesmer made deliberate use of communication as a means of healing, but because, as they saw it, Mesmer's method proves that suggestion ("hypnosis") is a valid method of medical treatment. As I see it, Mesmer's success-and-failure proves the power and extent of human gullibility, based on man's ultimate helplessness as expressed in the adage, "There are no atheists in the foxholes." In the modern secular world, human gullibility is displayed most prominently in the quasi-religious belief in, and submission to, medical authority, the therapeutic state.[72]

The twentieth century, too, has been revolutionary, both in politics and science. In medicine and psychiatry, many of the important discoveries rested on novel uses of electricity and magnetism—for example, computerized axial tomography (CAT scan), positron emission tomography (PET scan), and magnetic resonance imaging (MRI), not to mention radio, television, computers, and the Internet. It is in this atmosphere that modern-day Mesmers discover near-miraculous cures for mental illnesses making use of electrical-magnetic devices, such as vagus nerve stimulation (VNS), deep brain stimulation (DBS), and transcranial magnetic stimulation (TMS).* I shall briefly review Mesmerism and then consider the new electrical treatments, especially those directed toward the control of depression.

Although we live in an age of far greater scientific and technological sophistication than did people in the eighteenth century, this has not in the least diminished human gullibility and the need to believe in, and submit to, authority. Critics of the pharmaceutical-psychiatric complex often complain that advertisements for psychiatric drugs and other novel treatments for mental illnesses mislead the public. All advertisements more or less mislead the public. In our present medical-political system, however, pharmaceutical companies and the makers of medical devices could not mislead the public without their efforts being actively aided and abetted not only by the media but also by the American government, in particular the FDA.

An estimated 1 percent of the general population suffers from epilepsy. In about 30 percent of the patients, seizures cannot be controlled by drugs, or can be controlled only at the expense of unacceptable adverse effects. Ever since the 1930s, physicians have known that vagus nerve stimulation has a direct effect on the brain. In 1988, neurologists performed the first implant of a vagal stimulating device into a human being. The mean percentage of reduction in seizures was 46.6 percent. Adverse effects include hoarseness, due to the proximity of the vagus nerve to the vocal cords, and tingling in the neck when the vagus nerve is stimulated. In 1994, the European Community approved the use of VNS for seizure prevention and control. In 1997, the FDA approved its use for epilepsy, and in 2005 for depression. The mode of action of VNS is not known.[73] Discussion and debate again

---

*VNS, DBS, and TMS are recent "experimental" therapies that, until now, have been used only on voluntary patients with their (presumably informed) consent. I include some brief remarks about them nevertheless, because, should they be regarded at some future time as forming a part of the "standard of care" for mental patients, they will almost certainly be forcibly imposed on involuntary patients.

center on whether VNS works; yet, again, there are no objective criteria or tests to answer that question; and again those who stand to gain by providing the treatment promote it with grand claims for its effectiveness:

> In July 2003, Cyberonics, which manufactures the VNS device, announced that the Vagus Nerve Stimulator is effective in treating severe, treatment-resistant depression.... Researchers say "positive open trial results in a severe, treatment-resistant depression patient group suggest that VNS is a safe and effective treatment for a significant proportion of these patients.... Lauri Sandoval, 42...had suffered from depression for 30 years and was having trouble holding down a job. It took her three months after receiving the implant to feel the change, and 18 months later, she reported feeling dramatically better."[74]

Psychiatric anecdote has replaced pathological evidence as the "scientific" standard of disease. The VNS device costs $12,000 and the cost of surgery to implant it can run as high as $15,000. With millions of depressed patients needing treatment, there is the promise of big money in VNS. The prestigious New York-Presbyterian Hospital/Columbia University Medical Center has lost no time in advertising itself as the first facility in the greater New York City area to offer "Vagus Nerve Stimulation therapy as a long-term treatment specifically approved by the FDA for treatment-resistant depression (TRD)." Its Web site offers the following promotion:

> VNS Therapy is approved as a long-term adjunctive (add-on) treatment for patients 18 years of age and older who are experiencing a major depressive episode and have not had an adequate response to four or more adequate antidepressant treatments.... Major depressive disorder is one of the most prevalent and serious illnesses in the U.S., affecting nearly 19 million Americans every year. Of those, one fifth, or approximately four million people, do not respond to multiple antidepressant treatments. For these people, psychotherapy, antidepressant medications, and even sometimes electroconvulsive therapy do not work, or only work for a short while and stop working over time. VNS Therapy is a newly approved treatment option for these people.[75]

In February 2006, the *New York Times* reported that "a top federal medical official overruled the unanimous opinion of his scientific staff when he decided last year to approve a pacemaker-like device to treat persistent depression.... The device, the surgically implanted vagus nerve stimulator, *had not proved effective* against depression in its only clinical trial for treatment of that illness. As a result, *scientists at the Food and Drug Administration repeatedly and unanimously recommended rejecting the application of its maker, Cyberonics Inc., to sell it as such a treatment.*"[76] Nevertheless, Dr. Daniel G. Schultz, director of the Center for Devices and Radiological Health at the agency, approved it. Why? According to Susan Bro, an FDA spokeswoman, "because many people with persistent depression 'are otherwise on their way to institutionalization, because of the seriousness of their illness'.... Robert P. Cummins, Cyberonics's chairman and chief executive, said...his company's device was 'the only safe and effective treatment option ever specifically developed, studied, F.D.A.-approved and fully informatively labeled for the treatment of chronic or recurrent treatment-resistant depression.'"[77]

Reimbursed for performing procedures, not for healing suffering persons, surgeons are happy to believe that the treatment of depression requires their expertise. Declares Frank J. Veith, M.D., professor of vascular surgery at Montefiore Medical Center, Albert Einstein College of Medicine: "Vascular surgeons possess all the skills and training to perform VNS because of their extensive knowledge and understanding when it comes to operating within the carotid sheath. The vagus nerve lies deep and in between the common carotid artery and the jugular vein."[78] The announcement of a training session for vascular surgeons refers to VNS matter-of-factly as a "treatment [that] requires surgical implantation of a device by a procedure similar to a carotid endarterectomy performed by a vascular surgeon.... The treatment offers hope to the millions who have failed to respond to electroconvulsive therapy (ECT), a combination of antidepressant medications and psychotherapies. ... It is expected that over 80,000 implants will be performed within 4 years." At $15,000 per operation, that adds up to $1.2 billion. "Insurance companies are balking at paying the $20,000 price tag for VNS, claiming it is investigational despite its FDA approval. Patients have, however, been able to appeal some of these denials successfully." The *U.S. News & World Report* story concludes: "And if the medical science turns out to support the continuing technical advances, brain fixes will increasingly rely on plugs instead of just pills."[79]

We must not lose sight of the premise underlying VNS and similar therapies, and of the neurological fantasizing such procedures inspire. It is stated in the title of the article: "Parkinson's, stroke, and depression," boldly bracketing depression with two obvious brain diseases. However, there is no evidence that depression is a disease, much less a disease of the brain.

9

In March 2006, the *New York Times Magazine* published a feature article, titled "A depression switch?", devoted in effect to advertising deep brain stimulation (DBS) as a treatment for "treatment-resistant" depression.[80] David Dobbs, the author, builds the report around a patient, Deanna Cole-Benjamin, whose depression proved "resistant to every class of antidepressant, numerous combinations of antidepressants and anti-anxiety drugs, intensive psychotherapy and about a hundred sessions of electroconvulsive therapy. Patients who have failed that many treatments usually don't emerge from their depressions." Although Deanna had been incarcerated for "ten months straight and for 85 percent of another three years," she was deemed mentally competent to give permission for "a procedure called deep brain stimulation, or DBS, which is used to treat Parkinson's. It involves planting electrodes in a region near the center of the brain called Area 25 and sending in a steady stream of low voltage from a pacemaker in the chest.... Dr. Helen Mayberg, a neurologist, had detected in depressed patients what she suspected was a crucial dysfunction in Area 25's activity. She hypothesized that the electrodes might modulate the area and ease the depression." The results of the operation on Deanna and several other patients—performed by Dr. Andres Lozano, professor of neurosurgery at the University of Toronto—were spectacular. He offered this explanation for how DBS works: "Electroconvulsive therapy is analogous to rebooting your computer. This is very pinpointed, precise.... It was as if the thermostat was set for 120 degrees and you want it to be 70 degrees. This area of the brain [Cg25] is running in overdrive, and it is causing depression..."[81] According to Dobbs, 8 out of the 12 patients Lozano operated on

> felt their depressions lift while suffering minimal side effects—an incredible rate of effectiveness in patients so immovably depressed. Nor did they just vaguely recover. Their scores on the Hamilton depression scale, a standard used to measure the severity of depression, fell from the soul-deadening high 20's to the single digits—essentially normal. They've re-engaged their families, resumed jobs and friendships, started businesses, taken up hobbies old and new, replanted dying gardens. They've regained the resilience that distinguishes the healthy from the depressed. ...many scientists following the trial say they believe it will change how psychiatrists define and treat mood disorders. Mayberg, who speaks of a "paradigm shift," notes that she developed the trial to evaluate not a treatment but a hypothesis. In that sense the trial succeeded. Mayberg's focus on Area 25 tests the emerging "network" model of mood disorders, a new way of looking at psychiatric conditions that isn't restricted by the neurochemical model of mood that has dominated over the past quarter century or so.... Along with redirecting research, the quieting of Area 25 may also change our conception of depression from a condition in which something is lacking—self-esteem, resilience, optimism, energy, serotonin, you name it—to one in which an active agent makes a person sick.... The network model carries profound implications for research and, ultimately, treatment. The Prozac revolution showed everyone that tweaking neurochemistry can dampen and sometimes extinguish depression—but only through a generalized approach, hitting the entire brain. ("Carpet-bombing," one neuroscientist calls it.) And the 50 percent success rate of antidepressant drugs sug-

gests that they aren't hitting depression's central mechanism. The network approach, on the other hand, focuses on specific nodes, pathways and gateways that might be approached with various treatments—electrical, surgical or pharmacological. This small trial appears to confirm this model so emphatically that it's already changing the neuropsychiatric view of the brain and the direction of research.[82]

Dobbs's essay reveals not only the growing media disenchantment with drug treatment for depression, but also the popularity of an astonishing denial that our emotional states have existential meaning and significance. Dobbs reports that Deanna had said: "The worst part for me was not being able to feel anything for my children. To hug them, to have them hug me, and feel nothing." I submit that it is a momentous ethical and philosophical leap to assume that this *feeling* was completely *unrelated to how this woman felt, and what she thought,* about her marriage, her motherhood, her aspirations and hopes for her life, and, most of all, her obligations to her children. Still, let us grant that assumption and take seriously what it implies. *If feeling nothing when we hug our children or they hug us means nothing, then feeling something, such as joy, when we hug them or they hug us also means nothing.* The prospect is enough to prompt even an atheist to recall the Scriptural warning: "What profiteth a man if he gains the whole world, but loses his own soul?"

Moreover, it appears that the DBS treatment hasn't quite cured Deanna: "She now takes standard doses of Effexor, an antidepressant, and Seroquel, an anti-psychotic drug.... All the patients have benefited from coordinated assistance from psychiatrists, social workers and occupational therapists who try to smooth the transition. 'That help is crucial,' says Mayberg, who is now a professor of psychiatry and neurology at Emory University in Atlanta. 'We're just fixing the circuit. The patient's life still needs work.'"

Lastly, it must be emphasized that while doctors and patients prefer to talk about depression, disease, and treatment, the most important issue in many situations such as Deanna's is something more basic and obvious, namely, suicide—not as a symptom of an illness, but as a *solution for a serious existential problem:*

> During the bad periods, which was much of the time, Deanna thought about suicide almost constantly. Through the windows of the locked ward [of the Kingston mental hospital] she could see Lake Ontario, cold and immense.... Deanna thought obsessively of doing the same. "I imagined that all the time," she said. "That I would walk out there and walk into the lake and that would be it." As the months and years passed and all treatments failed, it began to feel as if there were only one way out. "It started to seem like, this is not going to stop," Gary said. "This is our life now. There were times I thought that it was going to end"—he looked across the table at Deanna — "only when you committed suicide."

A year earlier, in March 2005, the *Economist* magazine ran a short piece about DBS performed under the auspices of the same group of physicians. In that report, too, we were told that for the patient, Mr. Matte, whose case was featured, "the next step would have been suicide.... For Mr. Matte and three others, the treatment worked completely. As soon as the electrodes implanted in their brains were switched on, they noticed a difference." Unlike the story in the *New York Times Magazine*, the *Economist* report noted the risks: "There is a price to pay. Not only do patients have electrodes implanted in their brains, they also have a battery implanted into their chests (in the case of men) or their stomachs (in the case of women, to avoid damage to the breast tissue). But that is a small charge for resisting suicide.... If bigger studies prove this new approach to treating refractory depression works on even a fraction of that fraction, neurosurgeons could be in for a busy time."[83] I doubt it.

10

Transcranial magnetic stimulation (TMS), introduced in 1985 as a treatment for depression, involves the passing of a magnetic field through the brain.[84] In contrast to ECT, TMS requires no anesthesia and does not induce a convulsion. The FDA has approved TMS devices for diagnostic, but not for therapeutic, use. In Canada and Israel, however, TMS is approved as a therapy for depression.

In 2003, writing in the *American Journal of Psychiatry,* a group of psychiatrists declared: "TMS shows promise as a novel antidepressant treatment.... In addition to its potential clinical role, TMS promises to provide insights into the pathophysiology of depression through research designs in which the ability of TMS to alter brain activity is coupled with functional neuroimaging."[85] The press needed no prodding to get on the bandwagon. The *Boston Globe* touted TMS under a headline that read, "New depression therapy intriguing." The story began by declaring ECT to be a spectacularly effective treatment for depression: "Roughly 80 to 90 percent of the time, ECT works well, better, in fact, than drugs, which help in 60 to 70 percent of cases. Because of its effectiveness, 50,000 people a year turn to ECT." Then the reader is informed that, "ECT causes confusion after treatments ... mood may improve for only three to six months." But there is hope: "Now, however, brain researchers say they may have found another way to jolt the brain out of depression—TMS, or transcranial magnetic stimulation—that has many potential advantages over ECT."[86] *Science News* was equally uncritical. In a style characteristic of media reporting about psychiatric "breakthroughs," the writer avoids the declarative "is" and instead uses the tentative "may," as in "Magnetic fields that map the brain may also treat its disorders." We read:

Since its invention 15 years ago, TMS has become a relatively simple, noninvasive, and usually painless way to electrically stimulate specific brain regions.... More recently, TMS has also grabbed the attention of physicians and psychologists who predict that it has the potential to treat conditions ranging from epilepsy to stuttering to depression.... By the 1990s, technology had advanced to the point where repetitive TMS, or rTMS, also became available to most researchers. In rTMS, scientists deliver repeated magnetic pulses at frequencies up to 50 times a second (50 hertz).... The finding that rTMS can have lasting effects on the human brain has turned the technology into a potential therapeutic tool for several serious disorders.... rTMS significantly reduced auditory hallucinations experienced by a dozen people with schizophrenia.[87]

TMS researcher Eric Wassermann, M. D., at the National Institute on Neurological Disorders and Stroke (NINDS), expresses hope for the method's curative promise and, in the process, reaffirms the effectiveness of electroconvulsive therapy: "ECT unquestionably works. It's the gold standard for treating depression."[88]

Let's face it. ECT, VNS, DBS, and TMS are signposts that we are in the heart of the darkness of modern quackery. Declares Paul J. Rosch, M.D., co-editor of *Bioelectromagnetic Medicine* and clinical professor of psychiatry at New York Medical College: "[Together with VNS and TMS,] cranioelectrical stimulation, electroporation millimeter wave therapy, pulsed and static magnetic field applications ... [illustrate] theories of mechanisms of action and a new model of communication in the body based on electromagnetic signaling and the concept of an 'electrical circulatory system.'" Bioelectromagnetic medicine is the new panacea:

Some of the disorders covered include far advanced metastatic malignancy, pancreatic cancer, terminal cardiomyopathy, headache and other pain relief, macular degeneration, obesity, insulin resistance, depression, epilepsy, multiple sclerosis, tinnitus, degenerative disk disease, insomnia, anxiety, incontinence, soft tissue and bone healing, paralysis, dystonia and movement disorders, and Parkinson's disease. In many instances, these bioelectromagnetic approaches and devices have proven successful in patients resistant to traditional treatment and much safer and more cost effective than drugs.[89]

11

At the beginning of this book I stated that I shall not be concerned with the alleged efficacy of psychiatric treatments. Nevertheless, I want to note the astonishing variety of interventions psychiatrists peddle, and the press and the public embrace, as treatments. In addition to the procedures mentioned in this chapter, psychiatric researchers also promote, in the pages of the prestigious *British Medical Journal*, "animal facilitated therapy with dolphins": "Animal facilitated therapy with dolphins is an effective treatment for mild to moderate depression, which is based on a holistic approach.... We studied the *effectiveness* of animal facilitated therapy with dolphins in treating mild to moderate depression and in the context of the biophilia hypothesis, controlling for the influence of the natural setting."[90]

It appears that neither psychiatrists, nor the editors of medical and scientific publications, nor the media, nor the public feel the need to reconcile the contradiction of treating the same brain disease with interventions as different as ECT, VNS, DBS, TMS, antidepressant drugs, cognitive therapy, various "talk therapies," and dolphin therapy. At this point, it may be well to recall that the so-called effectiveness of this kind of therapeutic hocus-pocus had been investigated more than two hundred years ago by some of the greatest scientific figures of the time who had no difficulty concluding that the miracle-cure they were examining—Mesmerism—was simply bogus. Just as importantly, they also concluded that because healer and healed are equally deceived and self-deceived, the effectiveness of the hocus-pocus therapy appears real, at least for a while. Then, after they are debunked, they lose their effectiveness and are soon replaced by new miracle cures.

Mesmer first used magnets to cure patients. Then his mere touch turned out to be curative. Finally, he didn't even have to touch patients to cure them—they could cure themselves and each other by means of rituals that utilized the powers of an imaginary magnetic fluid, a property of "animal magnetism." Between 1774 and 1777, in a mere three years, Mesmer rose from obscure physician to world-famous healer, only to be exposed as a quack. Having married a rich widow, he moved his practice to Paris in 1778 and became an instant success there: he had a vast practice, acquired many disciples, became the darling of the nobility, and, in 1782, formed a secret society to safeguard and merchandise his discovery, which he called *Societé de l'Harmonie Universelle* (Society of Universal Harmony).

Scientists and scientifically minded physicians doubted Mesmer's claims and challenged him to submit his method to objective testing. Mesmer was sincere. The first person he deceived was himself. Thus, when in March 1784, Louis XVI appointed a commission to investigate animal magnetism on behalf of the French Academy of Sciences, he was happy to cooperate and expected to be vindicated. Unlike the members of the FDA, the members of the French royal commission included some of the most famous scientists of the time: Antoine Lavoisier, the great chemist; Ignace Guillotin, physician and pioneer euthanasia advocate; Jean Sylvan Bailly, astronomer and statesman; and Benjamin Franklin, grand old man of eighteenth-century rationality and American ambassador to France. Franklin headed the commission.

Exactly what were the commissioners supposed to investigate? Let me emphasize that here we are in the presence of the birth of modern, *empirical-materialistic* science concerned with, as Bailly put it, "physical proofs."[91] This science is interested in the *observable behavior of matter*, not in the *stories of patients obsessed with being ill and doctors obsessed with curing them*. The commissioners' task was to ascertain whether Mesmer's "magnetic fluid" existed. They established that it did not. Just as importantly, they established "that imagination, apart from magnetism, produces convulsions, and that magnetism without imagination produces nothing."[92] In a French at its aphoristic best, they concluded: *"L'imagnation fait tout; le magnétisme nul"* (Imagination does everything; magnetism, nothing).[93]* Margaret Goldsmith, a psychologist and biographer of Mesmer, naively laments: "The Commission's investigation of animal magnetism was entirely materialistic. *These scientists naturally failed, therefore, to become the discoverers of modern psychology."*[94] The terms "animal," "magnet," and "fluid" refer to material things. Goldsmith fails to recognize that the commission did make a discovery, the importance of which is still not fully recognized—namely, that not only is Mesmerism "all in the head," but that, by the same token, psychology and psychiatry are pseudosciences par excellence. Goldsmith's naiveté has a fine pedigree. In 1892, William James (1842-1910) declared, "I wished, by treating Psychology *like* a natural science, to help her to become one."[95]** This is precisely what psychiatrists have done ever since, in the eighteenth century, mad-doctors undertook to "diagnose" and "treat" madness as if it were a disease. When psychiatry became a recognized branch of medicine, in the nineteenth century, psychiatrists consciously set themselves the task of "treating Psychiatry *like* a natural (medical) science, to help her to become one." It's a misconceived task, generating fake diagnoses and fake treatments. Only after we abandon the pretense that mind is brain and that mental disease is brain disease can we begin the honest study of human behavior and the means people use to help themselves and others to cope with the demands of living.

---

*This phenomenon is now often referred to as the placebo effect.
**James was trained as a physician but never practiced medicine. He began his career teaching physiology at Harvard.

In 1784, scientists examined animal magnetism and found it to be a fraud. Today, neuroscientists examine DBS and TMS and find them, like drugs and dolphin therapy, to be effective treatments for depression. There is not a trace of objective evidence that the "condition" psychiatrists, the public, and the media call "depression" and consider a brain disease is a (bodily) disease. Nevertheless, the search for methods of "treating" it by chemical and physical methods continues with ever-increasing fervor. This distortion of medical effort is aided by the distortion of the medical marketplace. Individuals are eager to define their personal suffering as disease for many familiar reasons. Psychiatrists are eager to legitimate this misdefinition for both economic and professional reasons. Pharmaceutical companies and the manufacturers of electrical devices are eager to sell their drugs and devices as therapeutic agents and medical instruments. The government is eager to underwrite this bogus enterprise and thereby enlarge its scope and increase its powers. The result is that the state foots the bill for countless methods that allegedly improve a person's unhappy state of mind, provided the method is officially defined as "health care." A fanatic, said Santayana, is a person who, when he loses sight of his goal, redoubles his effort. The psychiatrist is a medical professional who, when he loses sight of what counts as disease, redoubles his effort to treat nondisease by means of drugs or electrical gizmos reimbursable as health-care services.

6

Lobotomy: Cerebral Spaying

It [killings by gas] was indeed a medical matter, since it was prepared by physicians; it was a matter of killing, and killing, too, is a medical matter.
—*Robert Servatius, defense attorney for Adolf Eichmann (1961).[1]*

1

Murdering mental patients, which doctors in National Socialist Germany called "euthanasia" and "mercy death," is the most extreme form of psychiatric treatment. Mutilating the healthy brains of mental patients—which doctors first called "prefrontal lobotomy" and now call "psychosurgical treatment"—is a close second. With good reason Walter Freeman, the most notorious lobotomist in history, is often compared to Josef Mengele, the emblem of Nazi medical criminality.[2]

Despite the dehumanizing destructiveness of lobotomy, or perhaps because of it, as soon as mental patients were subjected to the procedure the world community of scientists hailed it as a miracle cure.[3] In 1949, Portuguese neurosurgeon Egas Moniz was even awarded the Nobel Prize in Physiology and Medicine for his contribution to humanity's struggle to cure disease.[4]

The neuromythological rationalizations and justifications for lobotomy reflect the blind commitment of Western science and society to the belief that the troublesome behaviors of persons called "mental patients" are due to diseases of the brain, and that the relationship between abnormal brains and abnormal behaviors is of the same kind of cause-and-effect relationship as that between, say, atrophy of the optic nerve and blindness. The term "psychosurgery"—the proper, scientific expression for describing the mutilation of the brains of mental patients—is itself a symptom of this belief. It is a misleading term that must not be allowed to remain unexamined and unchallenged.

When a surgeon operates on the brain of a person *with a brain disease*, he calls it "neurosurgery." When he operates on the brain of a person *without a brain disease*, he calls it "psychosurgery." It is a convenient arrangement, *legitimizing brain surgery regardless of whether the subject has or has not a brain disease.* Inasmuch as most persons destined for psychosurgery are considered legally incompetent because of severe mental illness, the arrangement allows the surgeon to operate regardless of whether his ostensible patient accepts or rejects the operation.

Plastic surgery changes the way a person looks. Psychosurgery changes the way he thinks and behaves. Unwanted physical (facial) appearance (ugliness) and unwanted thoughts and behaviors (mental illness) are not medical diseases; interventions to change them, even if performed by physicians and even if performed with the subject's consent, are not medical treatments.[5]

Seventy years have passed since the introduction of lobotomy, a long period in the brief history of psychiatry. There is a vast literature on the subject, for and against the procedure, which the interested reader should consult. Suffice it to say that the critics' claim that lobotomy causes brain damage is tautological: lobotomy *is* the surgical destruction of healthy brain tissue.

If there is no mental illness, the truth about the therapeutic value of lobotomy cannot be sought in weighing the claims and counterclaims of the contending parties. It must be sought, instead, in understanding the uses and consequences of lobotomy: What problem is the operation expected to remedy? Who decides that a person should have the operation? Who grants permission for it? Who pays for it? Who benefits or suffers from its consequences?

2

The vast majority of mental patients are unwanted persons, rejected by their families or society or both. The most famous lobotomy patient in the world is the late Rosemary Kennedy, the first daughter of Joseph and Rose Kennedy and President John F. Kennedy's sister.[*] What was wrong with Rosemary Kennedy? The official answer is that she was "mildly retarded." When Rosemary died in 2005, at the age of 86, her obituary in the *Washington Post* described her as "the developmentally disabled oldest sister of President John F. Kennedy."[6] This was, at the very least, an exaggeration. It is clear, however, that she displeased and embarrassed her father, and that he rejected her.

---

*Rose Williams, the sister of playwright Tennessee Williams, is another well-publicized victim of lobotomy.

Rosemary Kennedy, born in 1918, was a placid, good-natured child. She grew up to be the most beautiful of the Kennedy women, regularly described as voluptuous. Sheltered by her parents, as were her sisters, Rosemary was said to be "slow," but was normal enough to keep a diary, go to dances, and be presented at the Court of St. James in 1938, when Joseph Kennedy was ambassador to Britain. Kennedy family biographer Laurence Leamer writes: "Rosemary was so voluptuous, sweetly spoken, and demure that during the summers at Hyannis Port, Jack and Joe Jr. had to ward off young men."[7] To young Edward (Teddy) Kennedy, fourteen years Rosemary's junior, she was the "dream of what an older sister should be. 'I just had the feeling of a sweet older sister…who was enormously cheerful, affectionate, loving perhaps even more so than some of the older ones.'"[8]

In 1939, the Kennedy family returned from London. According to Leamer, Rosemary, aged twenty-one, "could have handled a menial job," but that was not an option for her. Instead of going to work, Rosemary was expelled from the family home and placed in a convent school. Chafing at the restrictions of her living arrangement, she became belligerent, "difficult to control," began escaping from her quasi-prison, stayed out at night, and returned "with her clothes bedraggled." The nuns feared that she was picking up men and might become pregnant: "For years, Joe [Kennedy] had left Rosemary's problems largely to Rose, but this was a matter too important to leave to his wife. This was Joe's problem, affecting the family reputation."[9] Rosemary's existence threatened to sully the image of the physical, mental, and moral perfection of the Kennedy children that Joe was crafting to advance his grand political plans for his sons. Joseph Kennedy was not a man to be trifled with.

Joe Kennedy tried to deal with Rosemary as if he were living in France in the days of Louis XVI, when men of aristocratic rank routinely disposed of unwanted wives and daughters by having them incarcerated in convents. That did not work. Rosemary wanted to be free, wanted a life outside the convent. In twentieth-century America, nuns cannot imprison young women. Only psychiatrists can do that. Kennedy turned to psychiatry to dispose of his unwanted daughter.

In 1940, mental illness and new miracle cures for it were already a media staple. According to psychiatrists and the press, the conquest of mental illness was at hand. Rosemary had a "mental problem." Mental problems were diseases cured by doctors. Joe Kennedy was going to cure his daughter and went shopping for lobotomy. First, he sought out a famous neurosurgeon in Boston, whom Kennedy biographers do not identify, who declined to operate and cautioned Kennedy against pursuing that option. Undeterred, Joe took his daughter to the Barnum of lobotomy, Walter Freeman:

> Dr. Freeman, a showboating self-promoter, had repeatedly stated that he performed the operation only when all other approaches had failed.... They had performed only one of their eight operations on a patient younger than Rosemary, and never on an individual with mental retardation.... Having such an operation performed on Rosemary, a mildly retarded young woman with ill-defined emotional problems, was by any definition an extreme measure, but Joe was a pragmatic man who saw life as a series of problems waiting to be solved. He decided to go ahead, convincing the doctors that his daughter was a perfect candidate.[10]

Before the lobotomy, Rosemary had never been called mentally ill and had received no psychiatric diagnosis or treatment. What made her suddenly a "mental patient"? Her father's decision to have her lobotomized and Freeman's eagerness to operate on the daughter of a Very Important Person. Freeman diagnosed Rosemary as suffering from depression and he—and his then partner, neurosurgeon James Watts—proceeded to disconnect Rosemary's frontal lobes from the rest of her brain. The operation was performed under local anesthesia, the surgeon gauging how deeply to cut into the brain by having the patient talk or sing:

> Rosemary viewed the world around her with trust. The more Rosemary cooperated with the doctor, the more she talked, the more she sang, the more Dr. Watts cut. When Rosemary finally grew quiet, the surgeon knew that he had cut enough.... When she woke up, the doctors found that Rosemary had talked too much and sung too long and that Dr. Watts had cut too deep. She was like an infant, capable of speaking only a few words, staring out into a world she did not know or understand. Rosemary loved and trusted her father.[11]

Joseph Kennedy was single-handedly responsible for initiating the events that led inexorably to the horror of the calculated psychiatric butchery of his own daughter. Responsibility for the lobotomy was mainly his. Of course, Freeman and Watts were also responsible, and so, too, was Rose. Rose had rested her married life on her Catholic faith and on closing her eyes to her husband's behavior. She did not want to know about his womanizing. She did not want to know what he did to Rosemary. Only in 1961, twenty years after the operation, did she learn the truth—assuming she learned it rather than merely heard it. "Eunice [Kennedy Shriver] said that she did not even know where her sister was during that decade [following the lobotomy]."[12] The other siblings' role in this lamentable affair, if any, is shrouded in mystery.

There was, however, one person who participated in the lobotomy and quickly recognized its unspeakable horror: "The nurse [who worked for the two doctors] was so horrified by what she saw happening that she left nursing and never returned to the profession ... Over half a century later it was a horror that still kept coming into her consciousness. She might be sitting in a restaurant with her daughter talking about her childhood, and it would come back to her again, and she would talk about the guilt and sadness that never fully left her."[13]

I must interrupt here to observe that Helen Keller had been more severely handicapped and had engaged in more flagrantly aggressive and antisocial behavior than Rosemary Kennedy ever did. But Helen was lucky to have good parents who loved her and did not seek "professional" help—or, *horribile dictu*, psychiatric help—for her. They secured, instead, human and humane help for her, in the person of Anne Sullivan, an exceptionally gifted and tender person to love, care for, and teach their severely handicapped daughter. Unlike the Kennedy clan, the Keller family is unremembered. Helen's parents, Arthur H. and Kate Adams Keller, are not celebrated for advancing the cause of mental health.*

The Kennedys have never acknowledged what they had allowed to be done to Rosemary and have never apologized for it, just as organized psychiatry has never acknowledged its crimes against humanity and has never apologized for them. On the contrary, some of the Kennedys have arrogantly assumed leadership roles in sponsoring new forms of psychiatric barbarisms, promoted and justified by prestigious "institutes of medical ethics."[14]**

3

Apologists for the Kennedys and for psychiatry regularly refer to Rosemary's lobotomy as having been botched. Democratic court historian Doris Kearns Goodwin states that Joseph Kennedy regarded lobotomy "as a miracle treatment...'an obvious solution' to the frustrations she [Rosemary] experienced in trying to find a place for herself in a hard-driving family. *However... 'something went terribly wrong,' and she emerged 'far worse' than ever.'"*[15] Freeman biographer Jack El-Hai writes: "Cer-

---

*Arthur H. Keller, a captain in the Confederate Army, was an attorney, a wealthy farmer, and editor and publisher of a weekly newspaper, *The North Alabamian*. Kate Keller, née Adams, was descended from the Adams family of New England.
**The Kennedy Women includes a photo of President Jack Kennedy and his mother, Rose, in formal attire "at a 1962 dinner of the Kennedy Foundation honoring research in the field of mental retardation" (between pages 650 and 651.) In 1971, the Joseph P. and Rose F. Kennedy Institute of Ethics was established at Georgetown by a grant from the Joseph P. Kennedy, Jr. Foundation.

tainly their [Freeman and Watts's] *most notorious failure* was the case of Rosemary Kennedy, the sister of John F. Kennedy."[16]

Tragically, Rosemary's operation accomplished exactly what Joseph Kennedy, who ordered and paid for it, wanted it to accomplish: it removed Rosemary from the family and from public view. "Rosemary's name was excised from the family and its history and its aspirations.... Joe had turned his eldest daughter into an unmentionable Kennedy, as exorcized from the family dialogues as if she had been condemned to a biblical shunning."[17] Following the operation, Rosemary was housed in private psychiatric clinics. Then, in 1949, Joe created a special place for Rosemary at the St. Coletta School for Exceptional Children in Jefferson, Wisconsin. The institution was recommended to him by Archbishop Richard Cushing. It was a Catholic "home"—established in 1904 and called St. Coletta Institute for Backward Youth—run by the Sisters of St. Francis of Assisi.[18] Joe Kennedy richly endowed St. Coletta, where Rosemary had a cottage all to herself—a handsome, cream-colored brick house, which the nuns called "the Kennedy Cottage." There, Rosemary was well cared for by the nuns. In 1958, nine years after placing his daughter in the home in Wisconsin, Joe wrote to Sister Anastasia Mueller, the superintendent at St. Coletta's: "I am still very grateful for your help. After all, the solution of Rosemary's problem has been a major factor in the ability of all the Kennedys to go about their life's work and to try to do it as well as they can."[19] What *work*?

After John F. Kennedy was elected president in November 1960, the Kennedys proceeded to take personal and political advantage of Rosemary's tragedy. The family donned the mantle of protectors of the mentally ill and mentally retarded, as if these two terms referred to similar conditions or diseases. They do not. In 1962, Eunice Kennedy—with the consent of her parents and the president—published an essay in the mass circulation *Saturday Evening Post* titled "Hope for Retarded Children." Leamer reports:

> It was not simply the coming out of the Kennedys, but an attempt to use Rosemary's condition to further the evolution of concern about the developmentally disabled and their treatment. By any measure, the article represented the Kennedys at their most exemplary, taking this deep family tragedy and turning it into activities of the highest social usefulness.... Eunice avoided any suggestion of Rosemary's lobotomy by saying simply that the doctors had said "that she would be far happier in an institution...." Many health professionals, especially psychiatrists, linked mental health and mental retardation together, considering retardation a disease, not a condition.[20]

Then, for the first time in history, the leader of a great nation—the President of the United States—took up the cudgels for the mentally ill,

creating a Camelot of Quackery. In January 1963, Kennedy devoted a part
of his State of the Union Message to lecturing the American people on
mental health. With insolent hypocrisy, John F. Kennedy—whose sister
had been involuntarily lobotomized and incarcerated since 1941—hec-
tored the nation about its callous "abandonment of the mentally ill and
the mentally retarded to the grim mercies of custodial institutions."[21] A
month later, Kennedy delivered a special message to Congress, entitled
"Mental Illness and Mental Retardation"—once again bracketing mental
illness and mental retardation—proposing the establishment of Community Mental Health Centers (CMHCs) and calling for "a bold new
approach" in the war against mental illness. "It has been demonstrated,"
declared the president, "that two out of three schizophrenics—our largest
category of mentally ill—can be treated and released within six months."[22]
Where did Kennedy think the released schizophrenics would go? Home?
But they had no homes. Did anyone want them in his home? No. Did the
Kennedys want Rosemary in their home? No.

The gravesite inscription on John F. Kennedy's tombstone reads in
part: "With a good conscience our only sure reward / With history the
final judge of our deeds..."[23] Just so. No one knows what is in another
person's conscience. Many people don't even know and want to know
what is in their own consciences. Did the Kennedys know? "In this family
where all the important events of the day were discussed over the dinner table," writes Leamer, "surely it was time to confront Joe with what
he had done, to have it out, to discuss, to cry, to ask God's mercy and
forgiveness, and then go on? But it did not happen."[24]

It did not happen and it could not have happened. Leamer's scenario
rests on the premise that Joe acted wrongfully in having Rosemary lobotomized. However, it appears that neither he nor his family ever acknowledged or recognized this. Joe had donned the apparel of innocence. He
was a solicitous father who had tried to secure the best possible medical
treatment for his sick daughter. There was nothing to repent, nothing for
which to ask God's forgiveness.

This is not Leamer's view. He assumes that Joe and the Kennedy family
recognized the horror of what they had done and allowed to be done to
Rosemary: "[I]t is here that the Kennedy pattern of denial is implanted
in the psyches of the children. The truth becomes a form of betrayal. The
mumbling inarticulateness with which many of them discuss personal
history has its beginnings here."[25] Perhaps so. However, this interpretation
is inconsistent with the Kennedys' references to Rosemary in connection
with their championing of the cause of mental illness and mental retar-

dation: "For Eunice the [*Saturday Post*] article was just one weapon in her single-minded attack on mental retardation."[26] When Rosemary died, her surviving siblings—Eunice, 83, Patricia, 80, Jean, 76, and Senator Edward Kennedy, 73—provided the following statement to the *Washington Post:* "Miss Kennedy was 'a lifelong jewel to every member of our family,...her mental retardation was a continuing inspiration to each of us, and a powerful source of our family's commitment to do all we can to help all persons with disabilities live full and productive lives.' Her sister Eunice Shriver is known as the founder of the Special Olympics, and some accounts describe Rosemary as an inspiration for the athletic competition aimed at those with intellectual disabilities."[27]

Did the Kennedys recognize that they had sinned against Rosemary and then *denied* it, as Leamer suggests? That interpretation is contradicted by what Joseph and Rose Kennedy and their adult children knew, and could have known, about lobotomy *before Rosemary's operation.* Had they used their considerable intelligence, common sense, and access to a variety of first-class medical opinions, they would have realized that an operation that involves destroying a part of the frontal lobes of the brain is to be avoided at all cost. With a little effort they could have discovered that many prominent psychiatrists and neurologists bitterly opposed the operation. Indeed, one of the Kennedy children, Kathleen, born in 1920, did investigate the procedure.

After returning from England in 1939, Kathleen met John White, a star reporter for the *Times-Herald* newspaper. Without telling him why she was curious, Kathleen asked White what he knew about lobotomy. It so happened that White was writing a six-part series on St. Elizabeths Hospital and the new experimental brain surgery being carried out there. White told Kathleen that the results were "not good...that afterwards the patients 'don't worry so much, but *they are gone as a person, just gone.*'" Leamer also tells us that lobotomy "violated the church's belief in the sacredness of each human life."[28]

Nor is this all. The Kennedys had ready access to anti-lobotomy information but were not interested in it. From 1903 to 1937, the superintendent of St. Elizabeths Hospital in Washington, D.C., was William Alanson White (1870-1937), one of the most distinguished and most honored psychiatrists of his day, who happened to be also one of the bitterest critics of lobotomy. White had been president of the American Psychiatric Association (1924-25), president of the American Psychoanalytic Association (1928), and professor of psychiatry at the medical schools of George Washington and Georgetown universities. He was the author of the most widely used psychiatric text for medical students, which progressed through fourteen editions from 1906 to 1936.[29] Needing patients on whom to perfect his technique, Freeman asked White for permission to lobotomize patients incarcerated at St. Elizabeths. Replied White, "It will be a hell of a long while before I'll let you operate on any of my patients."[30] In 1937, White died. Winfred W. Overholser (1892-1964), the new superintendent, threw the doors of St. Elizabeths wide open to Freeman's depredations.

Interestingly, Sherwin Nuland goes out of his way to falsify this period of psychiatric history. He writes: "Superintendents and medical staff initially saw lobotomy as a potential route toward cure or at least discharge to a community environment.... And there is also no question that many people not only benefited from the procedure but were actually cured, at least in the sense of being able to resume normal life."[31] The truth lies elsewhere. The tragedy of Rosemary Kennedy shows us, in microcosm, the kinds of family problems that lead persons other than the denominated patient to seek psychiatric help, and the kinds of psychiatric interventions that ensue. The practice is not always as barbaric as lobotomy, but the intent is always the same—making life easier for the family.

4

Prima facie, lobotomy is the destruction of a human being qua person. This evil is rendered absolute by the fact that, virtually without exception, the procedure has been imposed on persons without their knowledge or consent. Indeed, the typical patient deemed a proper subject for lobotomy was considered so seriously mentally ill that he was, *eo ipso*, incapable of consenting to the operation. Again, this is not the way scientists, physicians, psychiatrists, scientific and medical organizations, and science writers saw lobotomy in the 1940s or see it today. El-Hai writes: "The popular press...uncritically accepted the theories of Freeman and Watts. An Associated Press report...in 1941 called lobotomy a 'personality rejuvenator'.... The surgery held little danger, the article maintained.... [Lobotomy is] only a little more dangerous than an operation to remove an infected tooth."[32]

This comment is typical of science reporting about psychiatry: it is not merely ill-informed and irresponsible, it is biased in the way that religious reporting about religion is biased. The reporter's "findings" invariably confirm his and society's basic premises: mental illness exists. Media support for psychiatry is now more solid than it has ever been. For example, *Publishers Weekly* describes *The Lobotomist* as a chronicle of "Freeman's crusade to help millions of asylum patients who might otherwise remain incarcerated indefinitely." The reviewer for *Booklist* concludes: "Generally, lobotomy was considered to have improved the lives of many but damaged those of many others."[33]

Freeman became a lobotomy enthusiast not because there was evidence that the procedure helped patients, but because of his favorite metaphor, which he took as literal truth: "If a person had a strangulated hernia the only cure was surgical. What these psychotic patients were suffering from was a strangulated Oedipus complex."[34] The idea that mental illnesses are brain diseases was nothing new; it has always been the basic belief of organized psychiatry. What was relatively new was the use of this belief to justify surgical brain mutilation as a treatment. The "goal *to benefit society by returning to usefulness some of its most seriously lost causes*," Freeman declared, justified lobotomizing patients incarcerated in state mental hospitals.[35] Nazi psychiatrists sought to benefit German society by euthanizing mental patients they viewed as "useless eaters."

Freeman was a neuropsychiatrist, not a neurosurgeon. Yet he operated on thousands of patients, anesthetizing them not with drugs but by electroshocking them into obliviousness. In his review of *The Lobotomist*, sociologist Andrew Scull writes:

> [Freeman] insisted that in pediatric cases, "maximal operation"—a particularly extensive standard lobotomy—"is the only effective procedure and necessarily leads to a rather vegetative condition." For adults he preferred the transorbital operation, because it was so much simpler and quicker. Whereas a standard lobotomy might take several hours, the operation via the eye sockets took less than six minutes, including time out to photograph the ice picks in place. El-Hai notes that Freeman delighted in demonstrating his prowess before an audience. Wearing no gown, mask or gloves, he treated the occasion almost as a circus act, spearing the brain and twisting his hands back and forth to make identical cuts behind each eye. He once managed to perform 228 of these procedures in the space of only 12 days, courtesy of the superintendents of the West Virginia state hospitals, who gave him unlimited access to their charges.[36]

In the sixty years that have elapsed since then, the psychiatric coercion of the patient and the psychiatrist's extravagant therapeutic claims have remained constant. Only the psychiatric technology has changed. Declared Freeman, "...we have found a safe and permanent cure for this dreadful malady [involutional depression]."[37] A similar claim is made today for ECT and antidepressant drugs.

Freeman was a driven man. His motto might well have been: "Only the unexamined life is worth living." He suffered from what he called "nervous breakdowns" and wrote a paper subtitled, "On the Advantages of a Nervous Breakdown in Certain Men Under 40." He treated himself with manic professional and recreational activities and with barbiturates he procured for himself: "What Walter Freeman prescribed for himself was...recreation and distraction.... He began swallowing Nembutal... which he continued using for most of the rest of his life. 'I am dependent on it but do not consider myself addicted since I have rarely needed more than three capsules a night,' he wrote."[38]*

Freeman enjoyed the support of some of the most influential men in the field. Adolf Meyer, professor of psychiatry at Johns Hopkins University Medical School, publicly declared: "The available facts are sufficient to justify the procedure in the hands of responsible persons. ... At the hands of Dr. Freeman and Dr. Watts I know these conditions will be lived up to."[39] Other psychiatric leaders also lavished praise on Freeman, perversely lauding his "therapeutic courage."[40] El-Hai concludes that Freeman was a "medical genius," qualified as "maverick."[41] Assuredly, Freeman was not a medical genius. He was a genius con-man, a master of self-promotion. Although El-Hai's well-researched book may not have been intended as a hagiography, the result, once again, is psychiatric apologetics: fraud and force—permanent features of lobotomy and most somatic treatments—disappear in a text couched relentlessly in the language of illness, diagnosis, treatment, cure, complications, and so forth.

A report of lobotomy practices in Sweden, featured in the *Sunday Telegraph* (London), illustrates the pervasiveness of this misleading medicalized language. "Sweden is rocked by scandal of forced lobotomies," read the headline, implying that there had been unforced lobotomies as well. A television program broadcast in 1997 revealed that Swedish authorities were facing "huge claims for compensation after revelations that up to 4,500 mental patients were made to undergo lobotomies [between 1944 and 1964] in an officially approved programme that lasted almost 20 years."[42] In 1940, the population of Sweden was 6.5 million. The total number of lobotomies performed in the country may have been even higher. But even 4,500 lobotomies in a population of 6.5 million is an extraordinarily large number. The population of the United States in 1940 was approximately twenty times that of Sweden. Had lobotomies been performed here at the same rate as in Sweden, there would have been 90,000 such operations, three times as many as had actually occurred.

---

*The normal dose of Nembutal, a relatively long-acting barbiturate, was one capsule for a maximum of 7-10 days.

A man named Sixten Karlsson, sixty-four when the article was published, had been lobotomized when he was thirteen. He was confined "for more than 30 years. 'Where they put me wasn't a hospital but a prison... I was a child locked up all day. Do you call that a hospital?'" That is precisely what not only psychiatrists but the World Health Organization, the United Nations, and all people in societies that harbor psychiatrists call the institutions in which persons are forcibly detained, brains are mutilated, and souls are tormented—in the name of mental healing. Calling such places "hospitals" is essential for maintaining the integrity of psychiatry as a medical specialty.[43]

In England, the most enthusiastic supporter of lobotomy—and other somatic treatments—was William Walters Sargant (1907-1988), founder and director of the Department of Psychological Medicine at St Thomas's Hospital in London, and a consultant to the British Secret Intelligence Services (MI5/MI6). Rarely has an author paraded his own sadism as unabashedly as did Sargant in his autobiography, *The Unquiet Mind*. About his early experience as a psychiatrist, he wrote: "Threats of suicide were always a main preoccupation of ours.... Among a group of patients handed over to me on my first day at the Maudsley, was a man who took a single look at me, walked out and immediately killed himself."[44]

Sargant loved lobotomy (leucotomy in the United Kingdom) for its help to psychiatry, not the patient: "Leucotomy started to be used... psychiatry had at last taken on a medical and surgical character."[45] After interviewing a lobotomized patient, he commented: "I came away in a state of great excitement; the [lobotomized] alcoholic commended the operation highly; he said he could now drink half his ordinary amount of whisky and get twice as high!... We had, in fact, witnessed a preliminary skirmish in a surgical attack on the supposed 'soul' of man."[46] Jesus Christ, Sargant suggested, "might simply have returned to his carpentry following the use of modern [psychiatric] treatments."[47] He was not jesting.

Sargant also loved shock treatment: "L. J. Meduna, who first suggested convulsion treatment...should certainly have been awarded the Nobel Prize for his discovery.... [P]sychiatry should be as direct in its approach as general medicine, and that the mind (conceived merely as the brain) would, in the end, be treated as practically as the liver, the lungs, and similar organs."[48]

In 1947, Sargant visited the Tuskegee State Hospital in Alabama and proposed to "rescue Negro patients" from it by mass lobotomy: "Patients were specially chosen...permission was obtained from all the relatives concerned...Professor Freeman even volunteered to come down and perform all the operations himself without fee. The sequel was calamitous. The Veterans' Hospital Administration in Washington put a sudden ban on the use of this treatment. The whole Negro-rescue plan had to be canceled."[49] Perhaps not entirely coincidentally, Tuskegee was the site of the United States Health Service's infamous experiment of withholding treatment from African American patients suffering from syphilis. An unknown number of the persons Sargant proposed to cure by lobotomy might have been rendered disabled by their untreated syphilis.[50]

5

In 1895, Alfred Nobel wrote in his testament: "The capital of my estate shall constitute a fund, the interest on which shall be annually distributed in the form of prizes to those who, during the preceding year, shall have conferred the greatest benefit on mankind."[51] In 1949, the Nobel Foundation honored Egas Moniz as a physician who has "conferred the greatest benefit on mankind." Moniz, however, had violated the First Commandment of Medical Ethics: *Primum non nocere*! (First do no harm!).

Sensing that its award to Moniz was not wearing well, in 1998 the Nobel Foundation compounded its mistake. Ignoring the wisdom of the French adage, *Qui s'excuse, s'accuse* (He who excuses himself, accuses himself), the Foundation did something unprecedented: it published a public defense of the decision to bestow the award on Moniz. The defense—written by Bengt Jansson, a professor of psychiatry affiliated with the Nobel Institute—is a long article accompanied by many illustrations and references, entitled "Controversial Psychosurgery Resulted in a Nobel Prize."[52] Jansson began by emphasizing the lack of effective treatment for schizophrenia in the 1930s and contrasted that sorry state with the present happy state due to discovery of chlorpromazine:

At that time [1935] there did not exist any effective treatment whatsoever for schizophrenia, and the leukotomy managed at least to make life more endurable for the patients and their surroundings. The treatment became rather popular in many countries all over the world and Moniz received the Nobel Prize in 1949. However, by this time the treatment had had its most successful period and in 1952 the first drug with a definite effect on schizophrenia was introduced, chlorpromazine, our first neuroleptic drug.... Since about 1960 lobotomy, with a strongly modified technique (more discrete incisions), has been used only when there are very special indications such as in severe anxiety, and compulsive syndromes which have proved to be resistant to other forms of therapy. Perhaps about five operations a year are now being performed in Sweden. However, I see no reason for indignation at what was done in the 1940s as at that time there were no other alternatives!

Moreover, Moniz deserved the Award because of his work on angiography: "One reason why Moniz's operations gained better acceptance than the earlier trials mentioned above was evidently the fact that he was internationally respected for having developed cerebral angiography." This is gauche, implying that the work on lobotomy per se did not justify the award. Nevertheless, Jansson defended it:

> Moniz's first twenty cases all survived and did not develop any serious morbidity. The leukotomy soon achieved a good reputation.... Moniz strongly believed that the potential benefits of surgical lesions in the frontal lobes, even allowing for some behavioral and personality deterioration, outweighed the debilitating effects of severe psychiatric illness.... Moniz's conclusion was this: "Prefrontal leukotomy is a simple operation, always safe, which may prove to be an effective surgical treatment in certain cases of mental disorder."

The history of medicine is full of quacks who believed in the effectiveness of their harmful therapeutic methods.[53] The point at issue here is that the Nobel Committee believed it when it should have doubted it, and still believes it.

True to psychiatric form, Jansson called the most obvious effects of lobotomy "side effects." Under the subtitle, "Side Effects on Personality," he stated: "Negative effects on personality were observed as early as the end of the 1930s. In 1948, Swedish professor of forensic psychiatry Gösta Rylander, reported a mother as saying: 'She is my daughter but yet a different person. She is with me in body but her soul is in some way lost.'"[54*] Some side effect.

Jansson continued: "Initially operations were performed on a majority of patients with affective disorders, i.e. various types of depression, such as involutional depression, agitated depression and so on.... As a rule, severity was a more important factor than diagnosis, i.e. consideration was taken to suicidality and dangerousness, among other things." Again we meet the most conventional "reason" for calling persons "mentally

---

* The notion of "soul murder" has a long history in psychiatry, psychoanalysis, and religion. According to Zvi Lothane, author of *In Defense of Schreber: Soul Murder and Psychiatry*, the origin of the term dates back to a thirteenth-century papal bull where heretics are called "soul murderers." Lothane states: "I first encountered the word in Grimm's 1854 Deutsches Wörterbuch where it was defined as omicidio spirituale dell'anima, a spiritual, i.e., moral killing, i.e., destruction of the soul. It is used in this same meaning in Shakespeare.... Luther used it too when fulminating against the Catholics. Finally, Schreber used it in the same sense: as an impropriety committed against him by Flechsig." (Personal communication, November 28, 2005. I thank Dr. Lothane for this information.) Judge Daniel Paul Schreber (1842-1911) was a famous mental patient whose "case" was "analyzed" by Freud. Dr. Paul Flechsig (1847-1929) was a prominent German neuropsychiatrist who had incarcerated Schreber.

ill" and punishing them with medical tortures called "treatments"—dangerousness to self and others.

Jansson asked, "Why Was Psychosurgery so Popular in the 1940s?" and answered: "First, there were no alternative therapies available for chronically institutionalized patients. Second, during and following World War II there was an alarming increase in the number of admissions to psychiatric institutions in the United States...." He then cited statistics about the therapeutic effects of lobotomy. A study of 9,284 lobotomized patients in England and Wales from 1942 to 1954 "showed that 41% had recovered or were greatly improved while 28% were minimally improved, 25% showed no change, 2% had become worse and 4% had died. Not surprisingly, patients with an affective disorder showed the best prognosis with 63% recovered compared to 30% among schizophrenic patients."

Finally, Jansson touched on the problematic ethics of involuntary lobotomy and was forced to look into the moral abyss in which psychiatrists labor: "Lobotomy is an ethically dubious treatment if carried out against the patient's wishes, but this is always a difficult question in severely psychotic patients who totally lack insight about their illness—what is it exactly that such a patient wants?" What, indeed? He wants *not* to be incarcerated, *not* to be treated as a mental patient, *not* to be lobotomized. In conclusion, Jansson asked, "Did Moniz Deserve the Nobel Prize?" and offered this pathetic answer:

> Moniz, who was born in 1874, was shot in the leg by a patient and had to spend the rest of his life in a wheel chair (he died in 1955). Moniz had problems with his hand and did not very often hold the knife himself. However, there is no doubt that it really was Moniz who initiated and managed to inspire enthusiasm for the importance of prefrontal leukotomy in the treatment of certain psychoses. The more sophisticated surgical methods, however, were developed by other people, primarily by Freeman and Watts but also by Lyerly-Poppen, Strecker and others. Moniz's main interests were evidently encephalography and cerebral arteriography. Already in the 1920s Moniz succeeded in making cerebral arteriographies possible by injections of a contrast agent containing iodine, an invention which made it possible to diagnose tumors and vascular deformities. Actually, I think there is no doubt that Moniz deserved the Nobel Prize.

Swedish neuroscientist and Nobel laureate Torsten Wiesel disagreed. In an editorial in *Science* in 2001, celebrating the one hundredth anniversary of the Nobel Prizes, Wiesel stated: "Historical records fail to explain some astounding errors of judgment. Witness the 1949 prize in physiology or medicine, shared by neuroscientist Antonio Egas Moniz for his development in 1935 of the prefrontal lobotomy.... It was a terrible mistake that caused permanent damage to thousands of patients."[55]

Christine Johnson, an American and founder of the web site <psycho-surgery.org> also disagrees. Offended by Jansson's statement, in April 2004 Johnson protested to the Nobel Foundation:

> It is difficult to describe how painful your posted article on Egas Moniz is to us. In our years of talking to victims we have found no one who was helped by these operations.... These doctors hurt us, they did not help us in any way.... The worst part of the article is the claim that it was only used when there were, "very special indications such as in severe anxiety, and compulsive syndromes which have proved to be resistant to other forms of therapy." This is not true. One boy was lobotomized when he was 12 years old for delinquent behavior.... My own grandmother was lobotomized in 1954 and was still held in a psychiatric hospital for twenty years. Obviously there was no great cure there.[56]

In July, Johnson received a reply from Agneta Wallin Levinovitz, executive editor, Nobel e-Museum, the Nobel Foundation, defending both Moniz's Nobel Prize and Jansson's representation of it:

> The purpose of the essays on the Nobel e-Museum is, amongst other things, to inform the general public about previous Nobel Prizes, to give some background information and to describe the history that led to the awarding of the prizes. The essay "Controversial Psychosurgery resulted in a Nobel Prize" by Bengt Jansson, a former Professor of Psychiatry, who lived and worked during the time when this controversial therapy was introduced and practiced, is such an example. The Nobel archives are kept closed for 50 years after the awards have been made. It has therefore not been possible until recently (1999) to comment publicly on the prize to Egas Moniz (1949) based on information in the archives. When the archives were made accessible, the editorial board of Nobel e-Museum found it important to invite a knowledgeable expert to write an essay on this controversial and heavily criticized prize.... The opinions expressed in the essays are those of the author and not the editorial board. However, the editorial board thinks that the essay in a fair, critical and balanced way recapitulates the history and the period following the gradual abandoning of lobotomy. We therefore are unwilling to remove it from our repertoire of essays. We have also consulted Professor Jansson who has read your e-mail and decided not to change the text. We sympathize with your views expressed in your letter regarding the long-term, negative consequences of lobotomy. Fortunately, *thanks to continuous research efforts which have led to the development of new neuroleptic drugs, the medical profession can today offer much more humane and effective therapies for the severely mentally ill patients.*[57]

In short, the Nobel Foundation continues to embrace psychiatric slavery and now hails chemical lobotomy with the same uncritical enthusiasm with which it had hailed surgical lobotomy fifty years ago. Note also that, unlike Jansson, the Nobel Foundation regards the use of psychiatric fraud and force as so morally unproblematic that its spokesperson does not even acknowledge its existence.

In August 2004, John Sutherland, a columnist writing in the British newspaper *The Guardian*, suggested that Moniz be posthumously stripped of the Nobel Prize. The title and subtitle of his essay are framed as questions: "Should They De-Nobel Moniz?: What Happens When a Nobel Prize Winner is Subsequently Exposed as a Fraud?" Sutherland answers: "Nothing, apparently":

> In the British army, when an officer was drummed out, his epaulettes would be ceremonially ripped from his uniform. Priests are defrocked and enter the secular world in their underpants. Lawyers are disbarred and doctors struck off. But no one, as far as I know, has ever been de-Nobelled—stripped, that is, of the Nobel prize. Like the Soviet government (as Solzhenitsyn wryly put it), Stockholm's motto is: "We never make mistakes." In one egregious case, the committee did err. And, if the campaign to de-Nobel Egas Moniz succeeds, Portugal...will lose one of its two laureates (the other, novelist Jose Saramago, seems safe enough). Moniz invented human lobotomy in 1935. American surgeons had earlier observed that if you hacked the frontal lobes off chimpanzees' brains, the primates stopped jumping round the monkey house.... [Moniz] went to work on the (unconsenting and mainly female) inmates of Lisbon's asylums. As with the chimps, the results were dramatic. Moniz trumpeted to the world the beneficial effects of lobotomy. He duly got his Nobel prize in 1949. He was, the committee said, "a wonderful man."

Sutherland continues with the lurid story of Freeman's lobotomy orgy and concludes by referring to the campaign to strip Moniz of his Nobel Prize "led by Christine Johnson, who had a close relative destroyed by lobotomy and has mobilized on her web site (psychosurgery.org) a powerful lobby of victims and their families.... Should they de-Nobel Moniz? A no-brainer, I'd say."[58]

6

On November 16, 2005, National Public Radio's "All Things Considered" program featured the story of a twelve-year-old boy lobotomized by the "father of lobotomy," Walter Freeman. "The operation," explained the *New York Times*, "was originally intended as a last resort for intractable patients, especially those in mental institutions before the advent of drugs like Thorazine made such patients easier to manage. But Dr. Freeman eventually expanded his practice to include patients who suffered from nothing more than migraine or postpartum depression. All told he performed some 3,000 lobotomies, including some on children as young as 4, whom he believed to be suffering from the early onset of schizophrenia."[59]

After noting that Freeman's most famous patient was Rosemary Kennedy who was twenty-three at the time of the operation in 1941 and required full-time care until her death in 2005, the program switched to the case of "a crew-cut 12-year-old Californian named Howard Dully." Today Dully is "a huge, barrel-shaped 56-year-old" man, thrice married, "twice happily," with a grown-up son and a job driving a tour bus. Except for his family and a few close friends, no one knew he had been lobotomized. Dully, for his part, tried to ignore his lobotomy and his memory of it. About two years ago he began to look into it and what he discovered eventually led to the NPR program.

In researching his story, Dully visited Freeman's son, relatives of patients who underwent the procedure, the archive where Freeman's papers are stored, and his own father, to whom he had never spoken about the lobotomy. "If you saw me you'd never know I'd had a lobotomy," Dully says. "The only thing you'd notice is that I'm very tall and weigh about 350 pounds. But I've always *felt* different—wondered if something's missing from my soul. I have no memory of the operation, and never had the courage to ask my family about it. So two years ago I set out on a journey to learn everything I could about my lobotomy."[60]

Dully's mother died of cancer when he was five. His father remarried. Dully says, "My stepmother hated me. I never understood why, but it was clear she'd do anything to get rid of me." In Freeman's files archived at George Washington University, Dully found the answer:

> According to Freeman's notes, Lou Dully said she feared her stepson, whom she described as defiant and savage looking. "He doesn't react either to love or to punishment," the notes say of Howard Dully. "He objects to going to bed but then sleeps well. He does a good deal of daydreaming and when asked about it he says 'I don't know.' He turns the room's lights on when there is broad sunlight outside." On Nov. 30, 1960, Freeman wrote: "Mrs. Dully came in for a talk about Howard. Things have gotten much worse and she can barely endure it. I explained to Mrs. Dully that the family should consider the possibility of changing Howard's personality by means of transorbital lobotomy. Mrs. Dully said it was up to her husband, that I would have to talk with him and make it stick." Then on Dec. 3, 1960: "Mr. and Mrs. Dully have apparently decided to have Howard operated on. I suggested [they] not tell Howard anything about it...." Dully says that when Lou Dully realized the operation didn't turn him "into a vegetable, she got me out of the house. I was made a ward of the state. "It took me years to get my life together. Through it all I've been haunted by questions: 'Did I do something to deserve this?, Can I ever be normal?', and most of all, 'Why did my dad let this happen?'"

A horrifying personal and family tragedy is laid bare before us. "For more than 40 years, Howard Dully had never discussed the lobotomy with his father. In late 2004, Rodney Dully agreed to talk with his son about the operation."

> "So how did you find Dr. Freeman?" Howard Dully asks. "I didn't," Rodney Dully replies, adding that Lou Dully was the one. "She took you...I think she tried some other doctors who said, '...there's nothing wrong here. He's a normal boy.' It was the stepmother problem." Why would a father let this happen to his son? "I got manipulated, pure and simple," Rodney Dully says. "I was sold a bill of goods. She sold me

and Freeman sold me. And I didn't like it...." Howard Dully's two-year journey in search of the story behind his lobotomy is over. "I'll never know what I lost in those 10 minutes with Dr. Freeman and his ice pick," Dully says. "By some miracle it didn't turn me into a zombie, crush my spirit or kill me. But it did affect me. Deeply. Walter Freeman's operation was supposed to relieve suffering. In my case it did just the opposite. Ever since my lobotomy I've felt like a freak, ashamed."

This a heart-rending story. It shows us the horrifying psychiatric abuse of this particular child, in this particular family. At the same time, it displays the anatomy of the psychiatric child abuse we call "child psychiatry"—that is, the ease with which a parent can collude with a psychiatrist in the destruction of a helpless youngster. What happened to Howard Dully happens to every child whose parents take him to be "fixed" by a psychiatrist. Sometimes the consequences are less serious, sometime more serious.

This was not the conclusion that the producers of the program drew from the story, nor was it the lesson they wanted the audience to draw from it. One of the voices included in the broadcast was that of Angelene Forester whose mother had been one of Freeman's patients. Forester was satisfied with the results of the operation: "She [her mother] was absolutely violently suicidal beforehand. After the transorbital lobotomy there was nothing. It stopped immediately. It was just peace. I don't know how to explain it to you, it was like turning a coin over. That quick. So whatever he did, he did something right."

7

Psychiatrists, psychiatric historians, and even some so-called psychiatric critics continue to treat lobotomy as a legitimate treatment for "severe mental illnesses." Thus, they validate, however unwittingly, the core concepts of psychiatric mythology and deny the lobotomy holocaust. Thousands of persons the world over were the victims of coerced lobotomy. The fact is that lobotomy was not, and could never be, a legitimate treatment, even with the operation performed by competent and respected surgeons, just as euthanasia and physician-assisted suicide are not, and can never, be legitimate treatments, even if carried out under medical auspices.[61]

Elliot S. Valenstein, professor of psychology and neuroscience emeritus at the University of Michigan, titles his book on psychiatric tortures, *Great and Desperate Cures: The Rise and Decline of Psychosurgery and Other Radical Treatments for Mental Illness*.[62] In the title and subtitle and throughout the text, Valenstein refers to "mental illnesses," "cures," and "treatments"; he accepts that everyone whom a lobotomist called "patient" had a bona fide disease and that the psychiatrists and psycho-surgeons were interested in helping him. This is typical of the writings of psychiatric apologists.

Valenstein's book is a simplistic rehash of the history of modern psy-chiatry and a defense of its latest practices. For example, in a chapter entitled, "The Treatment of Mental Illness," he writes: "Not only had chlorpromazine and other psychoactive drugs provided a simple and inexpensive alternative [treatment], but it had also been discovered [sic] that these operations [lobotomies] were leaving in their wake many seriously brain-damaged people."[63] It is absurd to call the brain damage deliberately caused by lobotomy a "discovery." Lobotomy is synonymous with brain damage: it is intentional brain damage, just as cutting-off the hands of pickpockets is intentional hand damage. Valenstein's account obscures that Freeman himself maintained that it was precisely the dam-age that was therapeutic: "[T]he greater the damage, the more likely the remission of the psychotic symptoms. Surpassing the shock methods in terms of demonstrable injury is the lobotomy. It has been said that if we don't think correctly it is because 'we haven't brains enough.' Maybe it will be shown that a mentally ill patient can think more clearly and more constructively with less brain in actual operation."[64] Paul Hoch (1902-1964)—long-time New York State Commissioner of Mental Health, professor of psychiatry at Columbia University, and one of the most powerful psychiatrists of his day—agreed: "This brings us for a moment to a discussion of the brain damage produced by electroshock.... Is a certain amount of brain damage not necessary in this type of treatment? Frontal lobotomy indicates that improvement takes place by a definite damage of certain parts of the brain."[65]

Valenstein buys into the classic psychiatric canard about new treat-ments saving taxpayer funds. He endorses chemical straitjackets as an "inexpensive alternative" to lobotomy, forgetting that, as he himself notes later in his book, the same argument was used to promote lobotomy: "In 1948, John Fulton remarked that if only 10 percent of the patients occupying neuropsychiatric beds could be sent home, 'it would mean a savings to the American taxpayer of nearly a million dollars a day.'"[66*]

---

* John Farquhar Fulton (1899-1960), professor of physiology at Yale, was a famous scientist. He--and Carlyle Ferdinand Jacobsen (1902-1974), a physiological psycholo-gist, later president of the State University of New York's Upstate Medical Center (now Upstate Medical University)--had done some of the original experimental work on lo-botomy in monkeys that inspired Moniz. Jacobsen did not support lobotomy.

Whether naively or in consciously bad faith, psychiatric experts continue to recommend new psychiatric services on economic grounds, that is as policies to save the taxpayer's money. The argument is economically nonsensical. Diabetics would cost the taxpayer less if there were no insulin. The longer people live, especially people with chronic illnesses, and the more medical services they consume in the present, the more medical services they will consume in the future. The most cost-effective way for the state to save money on taxpayer-funded medical care is to pay for less or no care.

Wrapped as a critique of lobotomy, Valenstein's book is an elaborate panegyric to psychiatry: "The great breakthrough in *the treatment of mental illness* seemed to have arrived in the 1930s with the introduction of four radical somatic therapies: three modes of shock treatment and one surgical procedure."[67] In psychiatry, every therapeutic claim supported by the powers of pharmacracy is a "breakthrough."

As long as medical scientists and medical ethicists insist that mental illness is a bona fide disease located in the brain, the rationale for psychosurgery, and other somatic treatments, is secure. Fred Ovsiew, professor of psychiatry at the University of Chicago, and British psychiatrist Jonathan Bird assert that "psychosurgery is an invaluable intervention for certain kinds of seriously disordered patients who have not responded to other forms of treatment, and they insist that failure to provide this intervention to those who need it would be ethically questionable."[68] Not even Moniz and Freeman went so far as to call the "failure to provide" psychosurgery for mental patients "ethically questionable." Once enough psychiatrists decide that the failure to provide a service—say, coerced drugging—is ethically questionable, providing it becomes the "standard of care," and failure to provide it qualifies as medical negligence (malpractice). *Thus does psychiatric non-coercion become a civil offense.*

In a similar vein, Joseph J. Fins, medical ethicist at Cornell University, declares: "Our society uses words like 'malignant' to describe cancer, but severe mental illness is the most malignant disease you can have. These are horrifying illnesses and, as doctors, we have an obligation not only to protect patients but to investigate procedures that might benefit them.... *Modern psychosurgery is a legitimate science* that shouldn't be tainted by the 'moral blindness' of its early practitioners."[69]* Fins is a careless

---

* Joseph J. Fins, M.D., F.A.C.P., is chief of the Division of Medical Ethics at Weill Medical College of Cornell University and also professor of medicine, professor of public health, and professor of medicine in psychiatry.

writer. Psychosurgery is the destruction of healthy brain tissue. It is not, and cannot be, a science. Fins states that modern psychosurgery is carried out only with the consent of the patient. Some time ago I showed that, as long as we live in a society with coercive mental health laws, there can be no such thing as a voluntary psychiatric intervention.[70] Moreover, even if a patient requests a lobotomy, his consent to the procedure is not the sole ethical consideration. The desire to alter one's physical appearance by amputating healthy body parts is familiar to psychiatrists, plastic surgeons, and people knowledgeable about the varieties of human experience.[71] Suppose a person asks an ophthalmologist to remove his healthy eyes? Or an orthopedic surgeon to remove his healthy hands?

I believe that competent adults ought to have the right to engage in all kinds of mutually consensual relations—sexual, pharmacological, or medical-psychiatric. That means that the government ought not to prohibit such relationships. It does not mean that all such relationships are morally praiseworthy or professionally appropriate. Personally, I oppose voluntary psychosurgery for the same reasons that I oppose voluntary physician-assisted suicide or voluntary sex between physicians and patients—because I regard such interactions as ethical violations of the boundaries between a medical-professional relationship and everyday human relations.[72]

Not surprisingly, psychosurgery continues to be practiced, albeit without the sensationalism of the Freeman era. In 1997, a notice posted on an Internet web site advertised: "We at Massachusetts General Hospital perform a type of limbic system surgery called bilateral stereotactic cingulotomy. The primary indication for which this procedure is considered is medically intractable obsessive compulsive disorder.... Some people who suffer from chronic pain syndromes, refractory depression, and addictive disorders may also be candidates for the procedure."[73] The old terms "lobotomy" and "psychosurgery" are replaced with fresh, technical-euphemistic terms such as "cingulotomy," "limbic leucotomy," and "stereotactic surgery."[74] *Plus ça change...*

7

Psychopharmacology I: Psychiatric Drugs

I believe that most mental diseases are molecular diseases, the results of a biochemical abnormality in the human body. I think that the mind is a manifestation of the structure of the brain, that it is an electrical oscillation in the brain supported by the material structure of the brain.

—*Linus Pauling (1901-1994)[1]**

1

Webster's defines pharmacology as "the science of drugs" and "the study of the properties and reactions of drugs especially with relation to their therapeutic value."

Psychopharmacology—a branch of pharmacology—is then the science of drugs that act on the psyche or mind. Whether the use of particular drugs is permitted or prohibited by religion or law, or is considered socially proper or improper, are matters that fall outside the scope of psychopharmacology as a science. Such matters belong in the domains of religion, ethics, law, criminology, and politics.

Yet, psychopharmacology is political through and through. The term "psychotropic drug" was coined by Ralph Waldo Gerard (1900-1974), an American physiologist, socialist, and scientific front-man for organized psychiatry. In 1955, Gerard and James Grier Miller (1916-2002), founded the Mental Health Research Institute at the University of Michigan.** The Institute's goal was to "integrate"—that is, conflate and confuse—biology, medicine, sociology, and politics, in an effort to make the burgeoning psychiatric-therapeutic state appear in the guise of hard science. According to Thomas A. Ban, Gerard used the term "psychotropic drug" to refer to "all drugs with an effect on mental activity and human behavior." This is not true. Gerard used it to refer to "psychiatric drugs," a fact we learn from Ban himself: "The first set of six psychotropic drugs consisted of...

---

* Pauling is the only person to individually receive two Nobel Prizes, the first in chemistry, the second a Peace Prize.
** It is now called the Molecular and Behavioral Neuroscience Institute.

neuroleptics, i.e., chlorpromazine and reserpine...; antidepressants, i.e., iproniazid...and imipramine...; an anxiolytic, i.e., meprobamate...; and a mood stabilizer, i.e., lithium carbonate."[2]* All of these drugs were introduced in a six-year period, 1949-1957. Note that chlorpromazine heads the list and that not one of these drugs is a substance a healthy person uses, or would want to use, as a recreational drug. Moreover, a list of "all drugs with an effect on mental activity and human behavior" would have to include alcohol, nicotine, opium, cocaine, and cannabis—as well as barbiturates, sex hormones, steroids, and many other drugs, none of which are mentioned by Ban. The truth is that psychopharmacology is an arm of the modern therapeutic state: the discipline is supported and regulated by the government; its practitioners serve primarily, or solely, the interests of the psychiatric profession and / or the pharmaceutical companies, both, in effect, agencies of the state.

2

For millennia, people have used religion to change personal conduct, their own or that of others. Since the decline of faith, modern Western governments have prohibited religious coercion and replaced it with medical (psychiatric) coercion.[3] Today, drug prohibition and forced drugging are two of the commonest forms of (medical-political) coercion.

A person can have drugs enter his body in two ways, voluntarily by choice, or involuntarily by coercion. (I am disregarding accidental ingestion.) Along with fearing, worshiping, and generally ceremonializing drugs, most Americans have come to view some drugs as satanic destroyers, others as God-like saviors. Accordingly, they have deputized their lawmakers to prohibit and criminalize the voluntary use of the former drugs, and to authorize the forcible medical use of the latter. This has made mental-health professionals especially dangerous: in addition to possessing the power to forcibly confine innocent persons, they now also possess the power to forcibly drug healthy persons in the name of psychiatric treatment.

The use of drugs to change a person's behavior, one's own or another's, is fashionable today. Most people believe that the drug treatment of mental illnesses is a modern scientific breakthrough. Nothing could be further from the truth. For thousands of years, people have coped with

---

*A neuroleptic drug is a "tranquilizer used to treat psychotic conditions when a calming effect is desired." An antidepressant drug is "any of a class of drugs used to treat depression."http://thefreedictionary.com/neuroleptic+drug; http://thefreedictionary.com/antidepressant+drug.

the vicissitudes of life by the use of drugs: opium, coca, hemp, fermented grapes and grains (alcohol), tobacco, coffee, tea, and others. During the nineteenth century, bromides, chloral hydrate, morphine, heroin, and barbiturates were developed. All of these substances were sold in the open market like other commercial products. There were no prescription laws, self-medication was the rule, and the drug user decided whether or not a drug worked. Stefan Zweig painted this moving scene of the "homeless" Nietzsche in his barren rented room: "... on a tray innumerable bottles and jars and potions against the migraines, which often render him all but senseless for hours...against his stomach cramps, against spasmodic vomiting, against the slothful intestines, and above all the dreadful sedatives against his insomnia, chloral hydrate and Veronal. A frightful arsenal of poisons and drugs, yet *the only helpers* in the empty silence of this strange room in which he never rests except in brief and artificially conquered sleep."[4]

It is important to keep in mind that what is new about the psychopharmacological era is *not the use of drugs as remedies for madness*. What is new about it is the elimination of the drug user as a judge of what works, and the assumption of that role by psychiatrists and bureaucratic agents of the government. The results include the prohibition of many drugs people want (because they may be "abused"); the pathologization of self-medication as "drug abuse"; the forcible drugging of vast numbers of persons with drugs they do not want; a politically powerful and profitable pharmaceutical industry closely allied with the government, medicine, and "private" lobbies supporting the increased use of forced drugging;[5] a new academic and medical discipline, "psychopharmacology"; and the Food and Drug Adminstration, Drug Enforcement Agency, and the Supreme Court as the arbiters of what count as therapeutic, recreational, and forbidden drugs. To understand the history and present state of psychopharmacology we must view the subject not as a new medical approach to the treatment of mental illnesses, but as a new political approach to the chemical control of unwanted behaviors and persons.

The pharmacological-physiological effects of drugs are independent of how they enter the body. An antibiotic combats infection, and a beta blocker slows the heart rate and lowers blood pressure, regardless of whether a person takes the drug voluntarily or is forcibly injected with it. This is true for psychoactive drugs as well. However, the ingestion of a drug of one's choice is an *act by the drug-taker*, whereas the injection of someone with a drug against his will is an *act by the drug-giver*. The person who uses a drug voluntarily is an agent; the person who takes drugs under duress or is forcibly drugged is an object or victim. Today these phenomena are not supposed to be described this way. Neither medical professionals nor journalists describe them in this way. Voluntary ingestion of a psychiatrist-prescribed psychoactive drug is called "treatment compliance"; refusal to ingest such a drug is "treatment noncompliance" or "treatment resistance"; use of the drug differently than directed is "prescription drug abuse"; and use of a controlled substance acquired without a prescription is classified and managed as both a crime and a disease—a violation of the drug laws, and a symptom of the disease called "substance abuse." At the same time, the forcible injection of another person with a controlled substance he does not want—that is, poisoning him—is classified and accepted as "psychiatric treatment." In short, some of the same chemicals are used voluntarily by "addicts" in the pursuit of pleasure, and coercively by "therapists" in the pursuit of profit. Logic requires that we conclude that what makes certain psychoactive drugs "therapeutic" is medical coercion, not pharmacological action.[6]

As I have noted in *Ceremonial Chemistry* and *Our Right to Drugs*, the distinction between drugs and foods is legal and political, rather than medical or scientific. Nevertheless, physicians, especially psychiatrists, play a large role in the crafting and enforcing of drug laws. They define what legally counts as a drug; they decide whether a drug is "addictive" or "dangerous"; and they recommend legislation about which drugs should be sold over the counter, which by prescription, and which not at all. They are also intimately involved in the enforcement of drug laws. With an enormous existential and economic stake in statist drug regulation, physicians, especially psychiatrists, are zealous supporters of pharmacratic social controls and the therapeutic state.[7]

Medical licensure provides doctors with a state-protected monopoly over the practice of medicine. Prescription laws and drug regulations extend and strengthen this monopoly. Yet, physicians tend to be astonishingly unaware of the powers they possess, and psychiatrists, who possess the most power, are the most unaware. Jonas Robitscher—a professor of psychiatry at Emory University in Atlanta and one of the few psychiatrists who has paid attention to the power of psychiatry—observed: "They [psychiatrists] do not define or fully conceptualize the power they exert,...psychiatrists generally have been oblivious to the extent of the power they exercise in society."[8] Although forensic psychiatrists might be expected to know better, they do not: they are taught, and learn, how better to rationalize the power to coerce as the "duty to care."

Prior to the nineteenth century, doctors were dangerous because, as Voltaire (1694-1778) famously observed, they "pour drugs of which they know little for diseases of which they know less into patients about whom they know nothing." Today, doctors are potentially dangerous for additional reasons as well: because they prey on the weak and defenseless, forcibly administer drugs to persons who do not want them, deprive persons of the drugs they want, and deny the vital distinction between the voluntary ingestion of a drug and the coerced drugging of another person.

The legally authorized and psychiatrically implemented drugging of mental patients thus brings us full circle, back to coercion as the practical basis, social function, and fundamental characteristic of psychiatric practice. Consistent with my plan to consider coerced psychiatric interventions only, I focus on so-called drug treatments of mental illnesses that are imposed on persons against their will or are administered to them without their consent. I say "so-called" because just as coerced hospitalization is imprisonment, not hospitalization, and coerced sex is rape not love, so coerced psychiatric drugging is poisoning, not treatment.

3

In medicine, there are interventions to treat diseases. In psychiatry, there are interventions called "treatments," but there are no diseases. There are only persons to please and displease by psychiatric interventions, and persons who are pleased or displeased by them. The disanalogy between bodily disease and mental disease generates countless confusions, illustrated by the popular analogy between antibiotics and antipsychotics.

It is reasonable to ask whether an antibiotic drug, say penicillin, cures *gonorrhea*, because there are objective criteria to determine whether a person has or does not have gonorrhea. But it is not reasonable to ask whether an antipsychotic drug, say Zyprexa, cures schizophrenia, because there are no objective criteria to determine whether a person has or does not have this alleged disorder. Hence, it is futile to debate whether psychotropic drugs "work." All we can know and say is whether particular mental patients or most mental patients like or do not like to take a particular psychotropic drug; whether particular family members or family members in general like or do not like their "loved ones" to receive a particular psychotropic drug; whether particular psychiatrists or most psychiatrists like or do not like to prescribe, or compel patients to ingest, a particular psychotropic drug; and so forth.

Today in the West, clerical-religious coercion—exemplified by coerced worship—is regarded as evil independently of its theological consequences. *Mutatis mutandis*, we have a choice between regarding clinical-psychiatric coercion—exemplified by coerced drugging—as good because it is "therapeutic," or as evil regardless of its "therapeutic" consequences. In my view, the ultimate arbiter of whether or not a psychotropic drug helps or harms the patient must be the patient himself. And the best way to determine whether a person thinks a psychoactive drug *helps or harms him* is by attending to his behavior: if he seeks the drug and pays for it, then it helps him; if he avoids the drug and is unwilling to pay for it, then it harms him. To call entire classes of drugs "therapeutic" or "toxic" is foolish and misleading, as drug effects depend on dose, user, and social context. This is why psychiatrists regard the same drug—for example, Ritalin—as therapeutic if they prescribe it for a child said to be suffering from "attention deficit hyperactivity disorder," and as toxic if a child said to be suffering from drug abuse buys it from other children and self-medicates with it. From an economic and psychological point of view, psychiatric drugs may be divided into two groups, those that people want to take (and pay for), and those that people do not want to take (and do not pay for). Barbiturates and benzodiazepines, such as Seconal and Valium, and amphetamines, such as Ritalin, fall into the first group.[*] The major antipsychotic drugs, such as Thorazine, Haldol, and Zyprexa, fall into the second group. It is clear that these drugs cause serious metabolic and neurological damage.[9][**]

My criteria for assessing whether a drug helps a mental patient are not the psychopharmacologists' criteria. Thomas Ban explains: "The need for a methodology for the demonstration of the therapeutic effectiveness of new [psychotropic] drugs was met by the development of sensitive rating scales; the replacement of an idiosyncratic classification of mental illness by consensus based classification with glossary of definitions and operationalized diagnostic criteria; and replacement of single center,

---

[*]Of course, these drugs, too, may be, and often are, administered to people against their will or without their informed consent.

[**]Most psychotropic drugs used to treat so-called psychotic illnesses damage the extrapyramidal motor system and cause complex metabolic derangements. Herewith a brief definition of two key terms. The pyramidal motor system controls voluntary movements. Injury to this system, for example by poliomyelitis or spinal cord trauma, results in paralysis. The extrapyramidal system--phylogenetically older that the pyramidal system--maintains muscle tone and truncal stability and controls voluntary but not consciously modulated behavior, such as walking. Injury to this system, for example, by Parkinsonism or neuroleptic drugs, results in so-called movement disorders.

isolated clinical trials by centrally coordinated clinical, investigations with sample sizes determined by power statistics."[10] This is psychiatric gobbledygook at its finest. The "method" Ban endorses consists of the familiar consensus of psychiatrists who share the same prejudices. Not surprisingly, Ban ignores coerced psychiatric drugging. For him the important thing is that "by the end of the 1970s, pharmacotherapy became the primary treatment modality in psychiatry."[11]

Because drugs affect the brain and the brain affects our behavior, the use of neuroleptic and other psychiatric drugs has proved to be a bonanza not only for pharmaceutical companies, psychopharmacologists, and personal-injury lawyers, but also for psychiatrists eager to testify in tort litigation concerning mental illness, drug treatment, and their esoteric insight into people's "dangerousness to self and others"(self-mutilation, suicide, assault, and murder).

- The pro-drug psychiatrist claims that psychotropic drugs treat mental diseases, often manifested by suicide and homicide. When a patient does not take his "prescribed medication" and then kills himself or others, he blames the patient's behavior on "untreated mental illness." The pro-drug psychiatrist attributes agency to mental illness, and non-agency to the persons he calls "mental patients"—and testifies in court that the patient was not legally responsible for his lawless acts.
- The anti-drug psychiatrist claims that psychotropic drugs predispose to (cause) suicide and murder. When a patient takes his "prescribed psychiatric" medication and then kills himself or others, he blames the patient's behavior on the psychotropic drug. The anti-drug psychiatrist attributes agency to certain psychotropic drugs (but not to others, such as alcohol and nicotine), and non-agency to persons whom he considers victims of psychiatric malpractice—and testifies in court that the patient was not legally resposible for his lawless acts.

Members of the two groups resemble one another in that neither treats the patient-subject as a motivated actor, a moral agent. There is, finally, the most hypocritical psychiatrist of all, the expert who maintains that he is neither pro-drug nor anti-drug: sometimes, he testifies that a psychiatric drug has caused suicide, another time that it has not. David Healy is such a psychiatrist. He writes:

> Before proceeding, it is worth putting the issue of expert witnessing in context. In over 90% of the SSRI [selective serotonin reuptake inhibitors] cases on which I have been approached, I have given the view that the injuries in question have not been caused by the SSRI. I have charged nothing for the great majority of these reports, or nothing for any reports I have offered to coroners' courts for the purposes of inquests. Moreover, regarding actions by plaintiffs in general, far from being plaintiff friendly,

I have been used as an expert by the National Health Service in the United Kingdom, and in that capacity have offered reports favoring the defense rather than plaintiffs in, again, over 90% of cases. It should also be noted that I have no interests in any competing treatments. *I use antidepressants, including SSRIs, to treat both adults and children, and, as a former secretary of the British Association for Psychopharmacology, convened a consensus conference and authored the ensuing guidelines on the issue of treating children with psychotropic drugs. These guidelines endorsed the cautious use of such drugs, a position I maintain to this day.*[12]

Healy does not tell us how, faced with the story of a suicide, he knows that Jones killed himself of his free will, while Smith did so because he took a particular psychotropic drug. He has no way of knowing. And, regardless of Healy's unpersuasive posturing about his economic purity, the doctors in malpractice litigation earn big fees, some becoming famous hired guns.[13] To demonstrate his "scientific" impartiality, or moral naiveté, Healy tells us that he "has been a consultant for, clinical trialist for, speaker for, chairman of symposia for, or engaged in other capacities for Astra-Zeneca, Eli Lilly, Pfizer, SmithKline Beecham, Sanofi-Synthelabo, Janssen-Cilag, Lundbeck, Organon, Pharmacia & Upjohn, Pierre-Fabre, and Roche, and has also been an expert witness for plaintiffs in a series of SSRI-related suicide, homicide, and physical dependence cases, and for defense in a series of LSD-therapy cases." He laments his rejection by Pfizer: "Clearly, at one point Pfizer thought me a creditable scientist in the area of psychopharmacology."[14] Or perhaps a "useful idiot," in Lenin's memorable phrase.

Only satire can satisfactorily expose the absurd deceits and hypocrisies of psychiatric courtroom testimony, as the following example illustrates. In the New Mexico Legislature's 1995 session, Senator Duncan Scott, a Republican from Albuquerque, proposed this amendment to a psychologist-regulatory bill:

When a psychologist or psychiatrist testifies during a defendant's competency hearing, the psychologist or psychiatrist shall wear a cone-shaped hat that is not less than two feet tall. The surface of the hat shall be imprinted with stars and lightning bolts. Additionally, a psychologist or psychiatrist shall be required to don a white beard that is not less than 18 inches in length, and shall punctuate crucial elements of his testimony by stabbing the air with a wand. Whenever a psychologist or psychiatrist provides expert testimony regarding a defendant's competency, the bailiff shall contemporaneously dim the courtroom lights and administer two strikes to a Chinese gong.

The bill passed the Senate by voice vote and cleared the House 46-14. Governor Gary Johnson vetoed the legislation.[15]

I maintain that neither mental illness nor psychiatric drugs cause suicide or murder. Self-killing and the killing of others are voluntary acts for which the actor is responsible. We must distinguish between a drug's, say a barbiturate, causing sleep, and a drug's, say Thorazine, "causing" suicide. Sleep is a biological condition. Suicide is an action. To be sure, an antipsychotic drug may cause involuntary movements and tormenting inner tensions, which may "drive" some people to kill themselves, as also may the loss of loved ones, bad marriages, and stock market crashes. Coerced drugging, as I have stated, is an evil, even if it has no biologically harmful effects. If it does, the evil is compounded.*

4

The modern age of psychopharmacology begins in 1952, with the serendipitous discovery of the first antipsychotic drug, chlorpromazine (Largactil in France, Thorazine in the United States). Jean Thuillier, an on-the-scene observer as an intern in Sainte-Anne, the largest mental hospital in Paris, identifies Henri Laborit (1914-1995), a surgeon, and Pierre Huguenard, an anesthesiologist, as the discoverers.[16] Laborit had been doing research in what he called "artificial hibernation for surgical anesthesia." In 1951, he contacted the pharmaceutical company, Rhône Poulenc, for a better compound than promethazine to include in his "lytic cocktail." The result was chlorpromazine. In 1952, Laborit suggested that chlorpromazine be used in psychiatry for sedation and to "potentiate barbiturate sleep therapy." Several French psychiatrists tried the drug on persons they called "psychotic patients" and declared its therapeutic effects to be spectacular.[17] Laborit characterized the effect of the drug as "a veritable medicinal lobotomy."[18] Was that praise or criticism? I don't know. Many people regarded and still regard lobotomy as an effective treatment.

The phrase "medicinal lobotomy" turned out to be no mere figure of speech. Once again, a somatic treatment for an imaginary brain disease proved to be the cause of a real brain disease: chlorpromazine causes a kind of Parkinsonism, called "tardive dyskinesia." The scope of the epidemic of this iatrogenic neurological disease has dwarfed the incidence of the brain-damaging consequences of insulin shock, electric shock, and lobotomy combined.

Brought to the United States in 1953, chlorpromazine was tried on about 100 psychiatric patients and declared to be an effective antipsychotic. It was approved for the American market in 1954.[19] The drug has turned out to be one of the biggest bonanzas in pharmaceutical history.

---

*If a person ingests a drug voluntarily, he is and ought to be held responsible for his drug-influenced behavior. If a person is drugged against his will, the poisoner ought to be held responsible for the poisoned person's drug-influenced behavior.

It has also inspired the foundational drama of psychiatry's most recent legend. In 1998, a PBS television docudrama recreated the Thorazine story. Flois, a female reporter, interviews Laborit in 1952.

F: I understand that you discovered a pill that cures mental illness.

L: *Oh mon dieu!*—I could never honestly make that claim. What I did was find a drug that would calm my patients before surgery. ...two years ago, in 1950, I began a search for a drug that would reduce my patients' need for an anesthetic—you know, before I operated on them.... Yes, something to render them unconscious. Anyway, I thought that an antihistamine—something used to treat allergies and asthma—might, as you say, "do the trick."

F: And did it?

L: With remarkable success. My patients, they did not need as much anesthesia. But something else there was, too. They no longer were anxious. They no longer were afraid. You could even say they no longer had a care in the world....

F: And this is where mental illness comes into the picture.

L: *Précisement!* Since the drug calmed my surgical patients, I reasoned that it could calm psychiatric patients, especially those who needed to be restrained.... I believed that one antihistamine in particular would prove useful to psychiatry—the name of this drug is chlorpromazine. But trying to convince psychiatrists of the chlorpromazine's potential was not easy. Finally, there were two who tried an experiment—Dr. Jean Delay [1907-1997] and Dr. Pierre Deniker [1917-1998].

The action then moves to Sainte-Anne's Mental Hospital. Flois talks with Dr. Deniker. "F: Dr. Deniker, tell me about the first time you used the drug recommended by Dr Laborit. / D: We first tried chlorpromazine on ten uncontrollable patients. Almost immediately the patients seemed less agitated. They no longer needed straitjackets or to be kept in isolation rooms. / F: It must have seemed like a miracle."

Later, Flois is typing her story: "...and so psychiatrists have a new treatment at their disposal. A treatment that takes care of a mental disease in the same way that an aspirin takes care of a headache."[20] And so another psychiatric myth is created, set appropriately in Paris, re-enacting Pinel's "liberation" of the madman. Veritably, Psychiatry has replaced Christianity, but is worshiped more catholically. The Christian Passion Plays celebrate man's liberation from sin by the sacrifice of a man-God. That myth has been replaced by the Psychiatric Passion Plays that celebrate man's liberation from mental illness by the prescription of a psychiatric miracle drug.

5

For me, the story of psychopharmacology is not historical in the same sense that nineteenth-century psychiatry is: it relates to events I have witnessed or played a part in. In 1957, I had called antipsychotic drugs "chemical straitjackets." In 1968, French critics of antipsychotic drugs began to use the same term, *"camisole chimique."*[21] In the course of his interviews of prominent psychopharmacologists, David Healy asks a group of French pioneers: "...how could a treatment which was so liberating in 1952 become by 1968, only 16 years later, such a symbol of state oppression that when the students revolted, one of the key things they did was to sack the office of Jean Delay, who was forced to retire? In Tokyo, they occupied the department of psychiatry for 10 years. Herman van Praag, in Holland, had to have a police escort because biological psychiatry was seen, for some reason, by the public as being very dangerous and an instrument of oppression."

Paul Brouillot, a Rhône-Poulenc chemist, replies: "In the USA and England, it was a movement for liberation...it had become forbidden to forbid.... That was the contention, that these drugs were another kind of straitjacket into which we were putting the patients. But this was entirely wrong."[22] No, it is Brouillot who is entirely wrong. He ignores or is ignorant of the fact that "drugs" became the flag under which marched the legions of American prohibitionists, the "forbidders" whose absence he laments, that in America a war against drugs was raging with great ferocity and the passion to forbid was reaching new heights in "politically correct" speech. Healy's question falsifies the facts. The "persecuted" psychiatrists were autocrats and coercers of the first rank. They treated patients against their will, and that is probably why they were attacked. The issue was pharmacracy, not pharmacology—forced drugging, not fake liberation.

Later, Healy himself raises the issue of Delay's personality and maligns him with psychiatric diagnoses: "I've heard that, toward the end, Delay was very phobic, very obsessional. Is this true?" French psychopharmacologist Pierre Lambert replies: "He was most concerned with his own honor and standing. It was for this reason that the students ransacked his office. ... He had no feeling for the needs of others.... After that [the events of May 1968] he never worked again."[23]

Healy returns to the Paris student revolts of 1968 in his interview with Jean Thuillier. "Lots of things happened in 1968,"says Healy, "... chlorpromazine, which had so recently *liberated people from their chains,* was seen by many radicals as a means of state control, or something like that..." Thuillier replies: "People did not know, or did not remember, what the real state of mad people had been before 1953, and because of this they were able to claim that people had been turned into vegetables by neuroleptics."[24]

How many times did Parisian mental patients need to be liberated from their chains? If they were still in chains in 1952, as Healy states, then Pinel ought to be removed from the pantheon of psychiatric liberators. Healy blames it all on the pharmaceutical manufacturers: "Companies now are not simply confined to finding drugs for diseases. They have the power to all but find diseases to suit the drugs they have. The effective incidence of depression, of obsessive-compulsive-disorder, of panic disorder and social phobia have all grown a thousandfold since 1980."[25] The manufacture of madness is primarily a psychiatric business. Healy engages in the fashionable scapegoating of Big Pharma. True, the drug companies mislead the public, but they could not do this if psychiatrists did not engage in the manufacture of madness by manufacturing psychiatric diagnoses, equating them with brain diseases, and writing prescriptions for psychiatric drugs. Long before drug companies profited from the creation of new mental illnesses, psychiatrists were busy creating mental illnesses, such as drapetomania, nymphomania, masturbatory insanity, and homosexuality.[26]

Healy consistently distorts the discourse about antipsychotic drugs by failing to distinguish between drugs people want and drugs people don't want, between voluntary medical treatment and involuntary psychiatric treatment. "The discovery of chlorpromazine by Delay and Deniker," he declares, "was the discovery of a drug that acted on a disease in order to *restore* a person to their place in the social order. In contrast, Henri Laborit's discovery of chlorpromazine the previous year, which led to artificial hibernation, was the discovery of a drug which *produced* an indifference, so that taking this kind of drug taxi drivers drove through red lights."[27] This is rubbish. Healy detaches moral agency from persons and attaches it to drugs. Delay and Laborit did not make two different discoveries; they used the same drug to bring about two different results. This can be done with most drugs. Barbiturates may be used to help individuals sleep better or enable them to commit suicide painlessly and non-violently—and also to help the criminal justice system to carry out the death penalty.

"I happen to believe," Healy continues, "that Prozac and other SSRIs can lead to suicide. These *drugs may have been responsible* for one death for every day that Prozac has been on the market in North America."[28] Healy ignores the ethical and political dimensions of giving and taking drugs. His game is to blame Big Pharma, with Big Tobacco as the cardboard villain: "There has been a change from companies run by physicians and chemists to companies run by business managers who rotate in from Big Oil or Big Tobacco. The companies are advised by the same lawyers who advise Big Oil and Big Tobacco and other corporations."

Where does Healy stand on the value of psychiatric drugs and the nature of "mental illness"? His critical asides notwithstanding, Healy is a psychopharmacological enthusiast. On the dust jacket of *The Creation of Psychopharmacology* we read: "Healy argues that the discovery of chlorpromazine (more generally known as Thorazine) is as significant in the history of medicine as the discovery of penicillin, given the worldwide prevalence of insanity within living memory."[29] Exuberantly, he declares: "The year, 1952, in which chlorpromazine was discovered is a key year in the modern calendar."[30] Joseph Schildkraut's paper, "The Catecholamine Hypothesis of Affective Disorders," published in 1965, Healy explains, "defined the psychopharmacological era. ...the paper was foundational, the 1960's equivalent to Freud's *The Interpretation of Dreams*."[31] A Massachusetts Mental Health Center Web site lauds the paper for advancing "ideas [that] eventually reached the popular culture and helped lessen the stigma of psychiatric illness, emerging as the view that depressions are medical illnesses and that many mental disorders are related to 'chemical imbalances.'"[32] The *Wikipedia Encyclopedia* soberly explains: "Chemical imbalance theory is not a scientific theory, but refers to the lay conception of an idea generated by the use of the term 'chemical imbalance.'"[33]

Laborit, let us remember, called the action of chlorpromazine "medicinal lobotomy." It is that and more: the drug and other antipsychotics subsequently developed and declared to be superior are also diabetogenic, in part by stimulating both appetite and lassitude. One in every five patients on an antipsychotic drug develops diabetes. "This is a little-recognized surge," states a 2006 feature report in the *New York Times*. "Psychiatrists are literally watching patients balloon up before their eyes," said Dr. Gail Daumit, an assistant professor of medicine at Johns Hopkins Medical School. "This has been especially true since the advent of so-called atypical antipsychotic drugs in the early 1990's.... For decades, psychiatrists have worried primarily about patients' mental states, making sure they did no harm to themselves or others ... Far more of the mentally ill, however, die today from diabetes and complications like heart disease than from suicide."[34]

Thanks to the regime of drugs-and-deinstitutionalization, masses of impoverished mental patients have not only been burdened with iatrogenic diabetes, they have also been "confined" in "adult homes" with disastrous consequences: "With numerous mental institutions emptied, patients often live in lightly supervised settings. Many occupy adult homes that...are poorly equipped to treat diabetes." One such "profit-making adult home" in New York City where thousands of the mentally ill live is Surf Manor. Drugged into sleepiness, lacking work, interests, and motivation, "the men and women eat, sleep, smoke, watch TV, sleep, then do it all over again." Diabetic residents cannot give themselves insulin because "needles are considered perilous.... 'I'll be honest with you, I don't understand diabetes,'" says one of the residents. Another resident, a woman who receives Haldol by injection and Zyprexa orally "has seen her weight soar to 241 pounds from 150. When she gets her Haldol infusion every three weeks, all she wants to do is sleep. 'It's my favorite activity,' she said."

"'I'm not a doctor, but we're very helpful,' said Mordechai Deutscher, the case manager at Surf Manor, who said he did not think the home had many diabetics. The people here are doing very well.'" Dr. P. Murali Doraiswamy, head of biological psychiatry at Duke University, explains: "'These drugs are enormously beneficial.' Without the drugs, psychiatrists believe, many high-functioning patients would find themselves in institutions or jail."

Schizophrenia is modern psychiatry's foundational fiction, its "sacred symbol."[35] Its "treatment" with toxic drugs constitutes one of psychiatry's cruelest hoaxes. An Editorial in the March 2006 issue of the *American Journal of Psychiatry* comes close to acknowledging the looming bankruptcy of the psychopharmacological-therapeutic enterprise: "The hope that other new antipsychotics with fewer metabolic side effects might offer a similar effect was not fulfilled. ...the side effect outcomes are staggering in their magnitude and extent and demonstrate the significant medication burden for persons with schizophrenia.... Sky-high drug discontinuation rates were seen, suggesting rampant drug dissatisfaction and inefficacy.... Much remains to be learned."[36] Even more remains to be unlearned.

6

"If you miss the first buttonhole," remarked Goethe, "you will not succeed in buttoning up your coat."[37] There are times, however, when missing the first buttonhole is the socially correct thing to do, when persons who make a profession out of fastening garments incorrectly but with the pretense of "scientific" sophistication are rewarded, while those who look for the first buttonhole before beginning the process are dismissed as unscientific. The modern psychopharmacologist is like the man who inserts the first button on his coat into the second buttonhole and then tries to make the garment fit. What is the first buttonhole? The nature of the problem for which people take, or are forced to take, psychotropic drugs. *That* is the buttonhole the modern psychiatrist avoids. Instead, the "new" biopsychosocial psychiatrist begins with the second buttonhole, marked "mental illness," proceeds methodically down the rest of the coat, and, when the mental patient takes the psychotropic drug prescribed for him, declares the garment fitting perfectly.

Modern psychopharmacological research and the subsequent practice of psychopharmacological treatment must be situated in their proper legal-social context—a context in which the moral legitimacy of psychiatric coercion and statist drug regulation—drug prohibition, prescription laws, and the criminalization of self-medication—are taken for granted. The parameters they set cannot be questioned, indeed cannot even be noted. Psychopharmacologists accept the conceptual premises and coercive practices of psychiatry: mental illness is a medical illness like any other, the imprisonment of the mental patient is a medical treatment like any other. Not surprisingly, everything psychopharmacologists have said and done has validated psychiatry as a medical specialty and psychiatric drug treatment as a type of medical chemotherapy. This allows them to pretend that a patient with mental disease stands in the same relation to an antipsychotic drug as a patient with an infectious disease stands to an antibiotic drug. This is absurd. A person forcibly subjected to psychiatric drugging stands in the same relation to the psychopharmacologist's drug as a woman forcibly subjected to coitus stands to the rapist's sexual fluids.

Reminiscing about the introduction of chlorpromazine into American psychiatry, Jonathan Cole, a leading psychopharmacologist, relates this revealing anecdote: "Al Kurland ... was research director at Springfield State Hospital in Maryland and he tried it [chlorpromazine] on six or eight patients and said, 'gee, this stuff does something I've never seen done before.' He put a second mortgage on his home and bought stock in Smith Kline and French and made a fair amount of money out of it, as a matter of fact."[38]

Donald Klein, professor of psychiatry at Columbia University College of Physicians and Surgeons, has a similar recollection: "So they [psychiatrists at the Lexington, Kentucky U. S. Public Health narcotics 'hospital'] had this ward with prisoners and volunteers and they gave this guy a shot of chlorpromazine and asked him an hour later 'how is it' and he said 'doc, I don't know what that shit is, but it will never sell.'"[39] He was only half right. Chlorpromazine was not intended to be the kind of drug that persons who wanted drugs to fill their empty lives would be interested in using. He failed to recognize that chlorpromazine was a first-rate chemical straitjacket and would sell splendidly to the people who want to use drugs to subdue mental patients. Chlorpromazine/Thorazine and the other leading antipsychotic drugs, such as Haldol and Zyprexa—the drugs that are the pride and joy of psychiatrists—were never intended to be sold to mental patients or the public. They were intended to be sold, have been sold, and are being sold to the patients' keepers, just as mechanical straitjackets once were.

From July 1954 to July 1956, I was serving my required military tour of duty at the National Naval Medical Center in Bethesda, Maryland. I well remember seeing, in late 1954 or early 1955, what must have been one of the first films promoting chlorpromazine. Produced by Smith, Kline and French, the pharmaceutical company that patented the compound in the United States as Thorazine, the film showed monkeys, rendered irritable and aggressive by starvation and crowding, being injected with the drug and becoming "tranquilized." The term was new then. This, we were told, was the new cure for schizophrenia. I did not like what I saw and wrote the following:

> The widespread acceptance and use of the so-called tranquilizing drugs constitutes one of the most noteworthy events in the recent history of psychiatry.... These drugs, in essence, function as chemical straitjackets.... When patients had to be restrained by the use of force—for example, by a straitjacket—it was difficult for those in charge of their care to convince themselves that they were acting altogether on behalf of the patient.... Restraint by chemical means does not make [the psychiatrist] feel guilty; herein lies the danger to the patient.[40]

This was the glorious—but unacknowledged and unacknowledgeable—psychopharmacological breakthrough: the insane person could now be controlled with a chemical straitjacket, rendering the mechanical straitjacket obsolete. Restraint could be put *in* the patient instead of *on* him and be defined as "drug treatment."

If official bodies that, *de jure* or *de facto*, represent the state—such as the Supreme Court, Food and Drug Administration, American Medical Association, American Psychiatric Association—declare that a condition is a disease, then it's a disease, and if they declare that an intervention is a treatment, then it's a treatment. These judgments cannot be appealed. Only the official bodies themselves can change them, as they did when they reclassified homosexuality from severe mental illness to fundamental human right.

It was obvious from the start that neuroleptic drugs benefit psychiatrists, not patients. Even when the officials acknowledge this, it does not impair their determination to define drugging patients against their will as a bona fide medical treatment. In 1990, investigators solicited the opinions of both patients and psychiatrists about neuroleptic drug treatment of schizophrenia; they concluded: "From the present study, then, it appears that neuroleptic treatment of schizophrenia is most defensible from an institutional perspective. Unlike Szasz, we do not believe that an institutional justification for neuroleptics is wrong, *ipso facto*. There are many legitimate reasons for families and society to prefer that schizophrenic patients receive such therapy. Nevertheless, a conflict between individual and institutional utilities complicates treatment decisions, and *our results suggest that schizophrenic patients and society differ in their treatment priorities.*"[41]* That's putting it mildly.

There are drugs people seek, and drugs people avoid. And there are drugs whose use the government permits, and drugs whose use it prohibits. These elementary distinctions have complex economic, political, and medical consequences. Prohibition of a desired drug, such as marijuana, inspires many people to defy the ban, and it creates a black market in the prohibited product. Medicalization of a desired drug, making it available only with a physician's prescription—as for example opiate analgesics—corrupts law, medicine, and mores. During Prohibition, 1920-1933, "Whiskey was available by prescription from medical doctors. The labels clearly warned that it was strictly for medicinal purposes and any other uses were illegal, but even so doctors freely wrote prescriptions and druggists filled them without question, and the number of 'patients' soared. Authorities never tried to restrict this practice, which was the way many people got their booze."[42] Ironically, now we call this sort of drug use "prescription drug abuse" and treat it as a form of mental illness. Physicians call persons who obtain prohibited drugs in this way "sick," diagnose their alleged illness as "addiction," and eagerly participate in incarcerating and treating them against their will. Lastly, if lawmakers, urged by psychiatrists, declare certain chemicals to be effective treat-

---

* The same argument had been made for lobotomy. See chapter 6.

ments for mental diseases, it then becomes lawful for physicians to compel persons deemed to be mentally ill and dangerous to themselves or others to take such drugs and, if they refuse, to forcibly introduce the unwanted drugs into their bodies. In this process, the psychiatrist too loses his freedom: he cannot reject the role of coercive state agent and remain a psychiatrist. If he fails to forcibly medicate the mental patient, he risks being considered "medically negligent," that is, of engaging in medical malpractice.[43] Psychopharmacologists and psychiatrists have enthusiastically embraced this web of drug prohibitions, drug persecutions, and forced druggings.

"The desire to take medicines is perhaps the greatest feature which distinguishes man from animals," observed William Osler (1849-1919).[*] In this book, I am not concerned with that vast subject. I am concerned only with the use of prescription drugs foisted on persons as a form of psychiatric control and punishment, defined as treatment. Were Osler alive today, perhaps he would supplement his remark about the distinctive human desire to take medicines by observing that human beings have an equally powerful desire to reject medicines foisted on them by psychiatrists, a desire psychiatrists define as a symptom of mental illness: "Nonadherence to antipsychotic medication regimens is a grave and pervasive problem in the clinical management of schizophrenia.... A lack of awareness of mental illness is common among patients with schizophrenia who are nonadherent to antipsychotics. Such nonadherence tends to be especially disruptive and unresponsive to simple commonly used psychological interventions."[44] As noted earlier, psychiatrists now attribute refusal to submit to psychiatric despotism to "anosognosia," a symptom of brain damage.

Determined to resist their tormentors, heretics were called "obdurate," a term *Webster's* defines as "stubbornly persistent in wrongdoing." Persecuted by psychiatrists who want them to embrace the faith of neuroleptic-drug worship, some mental patients assume a similar posture, obdurately refusing psychiatric medication. The priest hunting heretics was satisfied with destroying his adversaries' bodies by burning them at the stake. The psychiatrist has higher aspirations: true soul-murderer, he denies his adversaries' capacity to possess moral agency. The "patient" who refuses psychiatric drugs does so because he suffers from anosognosia.

---

* Osler was one of the founders of the Johns Hopkins Medical School and later Regius Professor of Medicine at the University of Oxford.

7

What manner of men were this new breed of American psychopharmacologists? Researching the story of psychopharmacology, I am struck to find that many of the leaders in the field display a special affection for psychiatric coercion, utterly oblivious of their intoxication with psychiatric power. Donald Klein, for example, began his psychiatric residency at the notorious Creedmoor State Hospital in Queens, New York, in 1953. As late as 1959, Creedmoor housed 7,000 mental patients. After arriving at the hospital and reporting to his supervisor, Klein proudly relates that he received the following training: "'Yes, Klein, here's this little book which is going to teach you how to do a mental status. You'll be admitting 20 patients a week and there are 300 patients to take care of.' That was the extent of my psychiatric education. That was all I got and it was okay...I was being thrown into a snake pit. It was just terrific."[45]

Jonathan Cole, too, loved the snake pits. "I enjoyed going to State Hospitals," he tells Healy. "In fact, I enjoyed it so much that when I got frustrated with some things happening in the NIMH (National Institute of Mental Health], and I got offered the job of superintendent at the State Hospital in Boston I took it because I thought it might be fun. It was fun for about five years..."[46] Cole was in good company. He notes that while the early psychopharmacologists "were mainly State Hospital types," the psychoanalysts in the 1950s and 1960s didn't "care much what happened at the State Hospitals."[47] Indeed so. There is worse. Cole seems to think it funny that young psychiatrists in training were charged with the task of forcibly subduing crazy people. He tells Healy: "The psychiatric resident and the nurse would go out to the house, if they heard there was somebody crazy out there. They would drive out to the house, park the car in front of the driveway so the patient couldn't escape on wheels, go in, often backed up by the police, and offer to give the guy a shot of depot prolixin, if he didn't want to go the hospital with that nice man in blue standing right behind.... *So it [the State Hospital] was a nice comfortable place. All the patients were locked up* so they couldn't fail to come back for their interviews. There was almost no outpatient experience. It was probably good training for my future."[48]

The history of psychiatry is a chronicle of how "nice and comfortable" state mental hospitals were for sadistic psychiatrists: They could commit horrendous crimes there and not only get away with them but be hailed as humanitarian healers.

Herman van Praag, a Dutch psychiatrist and psychopharmacologist who has worked in the United States, laments the relaxation of commitment laws: "Recently, in Holland a new law was passed that makes it extremely hard, much harder even than before, to admit psychiatric patients. Again—whose interests are we serving this way—certainly not those of the patients. ... I think this is terrible, absolutely terrible that you cannot admit patients who are floridly psychotic but not genuinely dangerous. Is this ethics? This is anti-ethics, ethics upside down."* And he adds: "I know it sounds a bit pathetic, but our profession is truly dear to my heart."[49] My country, right or wrong. Van Praag, a Jew, survived three years in Nazi concentration camps. Yet, neither that experience nor the roles of psychiatrists in the Holocaust has created doubts in his mind about the dangers of psychiatric power, or aroused his compassion for the self-defined interests of the inmates of psychiatric hospitals. Perhaps that is because Van Praag confuses and equates diagnoses with diseases. "Psychiatric diseases are what we study," he asserts, and then complains: "There has been an exponential increase in the number of diseases from DSM-II, to DSM-III, to DSM-IIIR, to DSM-IV; the number tripled. What a nonsensical state of affairs."[50] The adjective "nonsensical" applies to Van Paag's views as well. He believes it is useful to regard schizophrenia as similar to a tumor: "Actually, the tumor metaphor makes a certain, though limited, sense. ...a concept like tumor and a concept like schizophrenia share the qualities of being a 'diagnostic basin.' One can carry the analogy even one step further. Apart from surgical interventions, tumors are nowadays treated with a variety of compounds slowing down cell division; those are in a way comparable to the present neuroleptic treatment of schizophrenia."[51] Van Praag's "schizophrenia is like a tumor" analogy is singularly inept and offensive. Nazi physicians used the same analogy: "In a 1936 lecture...the SS radiologist Professor Hans Holfelder in Frankfurt showed students...a slide on which cancer cells were portrayed as Jews (the same slide depicted x-rays launched against these tumor-Jews as Nazi storm-troopers.) Jews were often characterized as tumors within the German body."[52]

Van Praag believes that it is ethically imperative that psychiatrists forcibly treat patients who decline antipsychotic drugs, and he exults at the passing of individual psychotherapy: "I witnessed a second revolution in psychiatry:...the de-individualization of psychotherapy...

---

* According to Dutch psychiatrist Jan Pols, this is false. Pols writes: "In the past ten years [1995-2005], the number of involuntary commitments has tripled, from about 2000 to 6000 per year."Http://janpols.net/Epilogue/9.html.

I thought, people are living together, why isolate them in treatment? Family and group therapy were for me a refreshing revelation."[53] Van Praag also dwells on his Jewishness, telling Healy, "As I said, I've been a Zionist all my life." Healy then says: "I was teetering on the brink of asking you a question I've asked one or two people, which is why has psychopharmacology been Jewish? Not completely but if you look at the names—Kety, Axelrod, Snyder, Kline..."[54] Van Praag's reply is long and convoluted, and its racially self-congratulatory reference is unseemly: "First of all, psychiatry has been a Jewish profession for many years... Jewish Rabbis encouraged critical analysis of data." Surely, the notion of rabbis as Popperian critics, engaged in the falsification of fictions, is a bit of a stretch.

Joel Elkes's views provide another shocking example of psychiatric insensitivity, perhaps even brutality, by a Jewish psychiatrist. Born in Germany, Elkes lost his father and much of his family in the Holocaust. He grew up in Lithuania, received his medical education in England, and had a brilliant career in the United States. He was professor of psychiatry and chairman of the department at Johns Hopkins University medical school, and is often described as "the acknowledged founder of the science of psychopharmacology."[55] Elkes's wife, Charmian, was also a psychiatrist. Elkes spoke with Healy about his early experiences with drug trials in state mental hospitals: "This included the selection of patients—we decided to err on the heavy side and chose some overactive and disturbed patients...Charmian, and to a much lesser extent, I, were faced with the realities of working in a chronic mental hospital ward.... *A chronic 'back' ward thus became a rather interesting place to work in.*"[56] Did Elkes have any more right to *select, for medical experiments, persons imprisoned in mental hospitals* than had Mengele to *select, for medical experiments, persons imprisoned in concentration camps?* Louis Lasagna, for many years a distinguished professor of pharmacology at the University of Rochester medical school, puts it mildly: "We were so ethically insensitive that it never occurred to us that we should get consent...we trampled on the rights of people who didn't know they were in a study."[57]

The theme of the Jewishness of psychopharmacology arises again in Healy's interview with Merton Sandler, an English professor of chemical pathology and the author of books on the biology of alcoholism and aggression. Sandler reminisces: "I am a little provincial Jewish boy from Manchester...I think I met Seymour Kety first in 1961 when I first went to the United States of America. Seymour, at that time chief of the lab of clinical science at NIH, gave me lunch and had all his disciples around him—what a galaxy they were. Julie Axelrod, Irv Kopin, Joe Schildkraut, Sol Snyder, Dick Wurtman, Joe Fisher.... It was funny because sitting around the table, there were 11 or 12 of us and we were all Jewish."[58]

Finally, there was the inimitable Nathan Kline (1916-1982), in the 1970s and 1980s one of America's most famous and flamboyant psychopharmacologists. Kline seriously suggested putting lithium in the drinking water: "Since we are already putting chlorine and fluorine in the water supply, maybe we should also put in a little lithium. It might make the world a little better place to live in for all of us."[59] The Nathan S. Kline Institute for Psychiatric Research, an agency of the New York State Office of Mental Health, on the campus of the Rockland Psychiatric Center, honors Kline, as "a pioneer in the pharmacological treatment of mental illness."[60]

I find these scenes sad rather than funny. Here were all these men who identified themselves as Jews scheming about novel methods for torturing mental patients with drugs, even treating the whole population as mad and drugging it with lithium. Apparently it never occurred to them that they were acting in the same capacity towards their "patients" as did Nazi psychiatrists towards their "patients," namely as brutal coercers acting with complete disregard for the humanity and self-defined interests of the denominated patients. "To see what is in front of one's nose needs a constant struggle," observed Orwell.[61] Psychiatrists are not interested, cannot afford to be interested, in that kind of struggle: seeing what is in front of their noses would destroy their raison d'être.

Still one more black mark must be added to the brief against the psychopharmacologists: many of their leaders have eagerly participated in CIA-funded and sponsored "experiments," poisoning unsuspecting victims with psychotropic drugs. One of the most famous among these medical criminals was Paul H. Hoch, M.D. (1902-1964). A Hungarian emigré, Hoch was professor of psychiatry at Columbia University College of Physicians, director of the New York State Psychiatric Institute, New York State Commissioner of Mental Hygiene, and confidant of four-term New York State Governor Nelson Rockefeller. Hoch had played a leading role in introducing the European somatic therapies of the 1930s to American psychiatry and was, between the early 1940s and the time of his death, one of the best known and most powerful psychiatrists in the country.[62] After my publication of *The Myth of Mental Illness* in 1961, Hoch led the campaign to have me declared unfit to be a psychiatrist and fired from my tenured professorship at the State University of New York College of Medicine at Syracuse.[63]

In 1953, in the course of a CIA-sponsored experiment, Hoch and James P. Cattell, then a young psychiatrist, surreptitiously injected Harold Blauer—a New York tennis professional who had sought Hoch's help as a patient—with a psychoactive agent. Blauer jumped to his death while being "cared for" by Hoch's team in a New York hotel. After the CIA-sponsored psychiatric scandal was exposed, Cattell casually remarked to John Marks, author of *The Search for the "Manchurian Candidate": The CIA and Mind Control:* "We didn't know whether it was dog piss or what it was we were giving him."[64]

In Germany, psychopharmacologists (physicians were not yet called that) used their professional expertise to kill people with psychoactive drugs (chemicals were not yet called that). In the United States, psychopharmacologists used their professional expertise to poison people with psychoactive drugs. Quantitatively, the comparison is not valid. Qualitatively, it is.

American psychiatrists and psychopharmacologists have never apologized for the de facto crimes of their colleagues who participated in the state-sanctioned "abuse" of psychopharmacology. On the contrary, the poisoners have become revered figures, prominent in the pantheon of American psychiatry. As noted earlier, a large psychiatric research institute is named in honor of Nathan Kline. Paul Hoch is posthumously lauded as "an outstanding figure in the field of psychopharmacology. The psychomimetic drugs, such as the old mescaline and the new LSD-25, were applied to various types of psychiatric disorders. There was a fortuitous combination of these studies with simultaneous work in psychosurgery. In these clinical areas he and his coworkers were the first to shift emphasis and indications for psychosurgery from the deteriorated schizophrenic to the most promising groups of nondeteriorated psychiatric illnesses (sic)."[65] *Res ipsa loquitur.*

8

Contract is the great equalizer: everyone is free to engage in, or eschew, any particular exchange relationship. In contrast, coercion is the great unequalizer: force impacts and injures the weak more than the strong. Not surprisingly, most of the individuals subjected to coerced psychopharmacological treatments are captives: mental patients, prisoners, old people, children, and the disabled. Writers on psychopharmacology never acknowledge this important fact. They are shockingly oblivious of the social context in which they operate and of the powers they wield over coerced populations whose members they conveniently label as "patients."[66]

During the past half-century, psychiatrists have inserted themselves into every nook and cranny of modern society, claiming to be indispensable for the management of human life from the cradle to the grave, from the kindergarten to the hospice. The key to the psychiatric occupation of life is the psychiatrist's ostensibly empirical claim of having discovered a high incidence of "psychiatric morbidity"—that is, mental illness—in the target population.

In chapter 1, I showed how, in the course of the drugging and deinstitutionalizing of mental patients, psychiatric and correctional institutions became commixed—psychiatric hospitals serving as prisons, and prisons serving as mental hospitals. A few additional remarks on this subject should suffice here. The United States has the highest per capita prison population in the world. The American rate is five to eight times the rate of Western European nations and Canada. In the United States in 2000 more than 2 million persons were housed in prisons. About 60 percent of the inmates of federal prisons were serving time for violating drug laws. About 12 percent of all black males in the United States between the ages of 20 and 39 were in prison, compared to 4 percent of Hispanic males and 1.6 percent of white males.[67] Inasmuch as it is psychiatric dogma that criminal behavior is a form of mental illness, psychiatric experts diagnose many prison inmates as suffering from mental illnesses, requiring psychotropic medication.

In September 2000, Reginald A. Wilkinson, director of the Ohio Department of Rehabilitation and Correction and vice president of the Association of State Correctional Administrators, testified before Congress: "Mental health care is a constitutional right.... Like anyone with a mental illness, offenders benefit from regular participation in a psychopharmacology regimen. Mood altering and stabilizing drugs often make the difference between an offender co-existing normally in confinement or in the community and committing serious harm to others or to him or herself."[68] Prison personnel, Wilkinson explains, must be skilled psychiatric diagnosticians: "For years, corrections personnel have attempted to discern the difference between prisoners who are 'mad' versus those who are 'bad.' For both security and health care reasons, we need to know whether offenders are demonstrating purposeful, negative behavior as opposed to those who are 'acting out' because of a mental illness."

Persons confined in prisons, like anyone else except perhaps more so, may wish to kill themselves. The managers of modern madhouse-prisons fear this ever-present possibility more than they fear prison rebellion. Why? Because psychiatric science teaches them that suicide is always the result of depression or some other serious mental illness, and that it is the duty of the imprisoners to treat such diseases and thus prevent suicide: "Suicide, and suicide attempts, are stark examples of the consequences of unknown or unattended deterioration. Accordingly, prevention and amelioration of mental health related problems, from an administrative and clinical perspective, must be a conscious, ongoing mission."

Today, prisons are de facto mental hospitals: "Operating a comprehensive mental health service delivery system for offenders is one of the biggest challenges faced by correctional administrators. There is a long history in our nation's quest to address mental illness in prisons and jails. Duties include assessment, treatment, staffing, training, resources, and continuity of care. The goal of providing a holistic mental health system is becoming increasingly compromised by evolving budget limitations." The recommendation is predictable: More drugs for the imprisoned and more money for the imprisoners.

Professional publications, newspaper articles, and television shows reprise the triumphalist, carceral-chemical rhetoric of contemporary psychiatry. The ideal doctor-patient relationship to which this dehumanized psychiatry appears to be aspiring is represented by so-called telepsychiatry with prisoners. Telepsychiatry makes personal contact between patient and doctor unnecessary: they meet only on the TV screen. "Growing prison populations have a lot to do with the trend," explains Don McBeath, director of telemedicine and rural health at the Texas Tech University Health Sciences. "Since reimbursement for prison care is easy and safety issues for doctors are significant, many telemedicine programs, notably an ambitious one in Texas, started there.... Basically, doctors can do, surprisingly, almost everything. The difference is they can't touch you..."And that, according to telepsychiatrist Sara Gibson, has, at least when it comes to psychiatry, proved to be a good thing. "Being physically in the presence of another human being, she said, can be overwhelming.... Initially we all said, 'Well, of course it would be better to be there in person. But some people with trauma, or who have been abused, are actually more comfortable. I'm less intimidating at a distance....' 'It's hard for me to trust any other doctor,' said Mr. Kueneman, who attended a telesession in the St. Johns clinic in leg shackles and handcuffs, accompanied by an Apache County sheriff's deputy."[69]

The prison cell has replaced the mental hospital bed. "Prisons: The nation's new mental institutions," reads the headline of a report in the *New York Times*. Fox Butterfield, the reporter, states: "The Los Angeles County Jail...is the nation's largest mental institution. On an average day, it holds more than 1,500 inmates who are severely mentally ill, most detained on minor charges, essentially for being public nuisances....' The inmates we see in jail today are the same people I used to see in psychiatric hospitals,' said Dr. Eugene Kunzman, the former medical director of the mental health program at the Los Angeles jail."[70] The problem, Butterfield explains, began in the 1960s, when "new antipsychotic drugs made medicating patients in the community seem a humane alternative to long-term hospitalization." It is a lie that antipsychotic medications worked *humanely*. Henri Laborit, the physician who discovered Thorazine, himself said so when he called the effect of the drug a "medicinal lobotomy." The claim that neuroleptic drugs benefit schizophrenic patients is the foundational lie of psychopharmacology: it is the falsehood that psychiatrists refuse to admit and journalists refuse to recognize. "I was not wrong that antipsychotic medications were good," says Dr. Richard Lamb, a professor of psychiatry at the University of Southern California School of Medicine. Lamb worked in a state hospital in the 1960s and was among those pushing for the treatment of people outside hospitals. "But I was wrong about discharging so many people with severe problems."

Butterfield concludes: "But the drugs work only when they are taken, and when they work, patients are tempted to stop, because of the unpleasant side effects." The fact that most patients forced to take antipsychotic drugs stop taking them as soon as they can speaks for itself: they and their behavior are the ultimate definers of what works. Predictably, the reader is reminded that "Suicide is a risk: 95 percent of those who commit suicide in jail or prison have a diagnosed mental disorder, according to a study in the *American Journal of Psychiatry*." The remaining 5 percent no doubt have an undiagnosed mental illness.

9

"An aged man is but a paltry thing, / A tattered coat upon a stick...,"wrote William Butler Yeats (1865-1939). Not so, says the American Psychiatric Association. Its *Diagnostic and Statistical Manual* in effect asserts, An aged man is a happy man, but for the effect of clinical depression, a treatable disease. According to a Department of Health and Human Services (DHHS) report on *Psychotropic Drug Use in Nursing*

Homes, "The prevalence of psychiatric disorders in long-term care facilities is formidable, and nursing homes have become de facto mental health facilities."[78] Here we are face to face with one of the ugliest acts in the vast repertoire of obscene psychiatric scenarios: the defining of old people as wards of the psychiatric system.

Geriatric psychiatry is a modern invention. In the 1940s, when I was a young physician, doctors did not talk about depression in old folks. If the person was sad, the physician suggested that he drink some wine or whisky. Why the emphasis on the "diagnosis" now? Because the psychiatric diagnosis of depression now leads quasi-automatically to (coerced) treatment with antidepressant drugs. In a well-documented study, "The origin of old age psychiatry in Britain in the 1940s," Claire Hilton states: "It [old age psychiatry] has been a specialty recognized by the [U. K.] Department of Health only since 1989. A conference in March 2003 of the Faculty for the Psychiatry Old Age of the Royal College of Psychiatrists claimed to celebrate 30 years of old age psychiatry..."[72] That makes 1973 the date of origin of geriatric psychiatry in the United Kingdom. Strikingly, Hilton notes that an examination of the records of fifty patients confined at the Tooting Bec Hospital in London in 1943—which then housed "over 2000 elderly mentally ill patients"—showed that "All admissions had an organic diagnosis, and none were diagnosed with depression..."[73] The frequent diagnosis of depression in old people today, like the frequent diagnosis of attention deficit hyperactivity disorder in young people—and no longer in young people alone—is driven by psychopharmacology, not neuropathology.

In the modern West, old people are often unhappy, an emotional state that psychiatrists diagnose as depression. Negative emotions, according to psychopharmacological dogma, are neurochemical brain states, not existentially meaningful experiences. "[I]f affective states represent a balance between central cholinergic and adrenergic activity," writes Ban, "with depression being a disease of cholinergic dominance, and central anticholinergic receptor blockade is an essential feature in the action mechanism of antidepressant drugs, the lower therapeutic response rates encountered in meta-analyses with some of the newer antidepressants might be explained by the lesser affinity of some of the newer drugs to muscarinic cholinergic receptors."[74] This dehumanized conception of "melancholia"—validated by law and medicine as a disease—governs how old people as a group are now treated in the United States.[75] Consider this "Position Statement on Psychotherapeutic Medications in the Nursing Home," issued jointly by the American Geriatrics Society, the American

Association for Geriatric Psychiatry, and the American Psychiatric Association: "Research demonstrates that there is a high prevalence of psychiatric illnesses that can respond to psychotherapeutic medication and that these disorders have been underdiagnosed and undertreated. ...nursing home residents with psychiatric disorders are *entitled to the full benefits of treatment* with the broad spectrum of therapeutic options available to *clinicians responsible for their care.*"[76] This sermon is preached from every psychiatric and political pulpit in the land. *Cui bono?*

One authority on the "diagnosis and management of late-life depression," explains: "Depression is not a normal consequence of aging*.... Late-life depression remains underdiagnosed and inadequately treated."[77] Another declares: "Notwithstanding a lack of knowledge about the origins of depression in the oldest old,...it is clear that more active case-finding is warranted, as treatment of depression in the oldest old is as potentially rewarding as in younger people."[78] In 1999, the Senate Special Committee on Aging "studied the extent to which psychotropic drugs are being used in nursing homes as inappropriate chemical restraints," and concluded that "in general, these drugs are being used appropriately." Having thus reassured themselves that all is well in nursing-home care, the writers acknowledged some problems: "Mental disorders are present in a large percentage of the nursing home population. ... Historically, antipsychotics and benzodiazepines have been used excessively...in nursing home residents, *often solely for the convenience of staff.*... Meanwhile, antidepressants have been underutilized because depression is often overlooked as a cause of behavioral disturbances in this population."[79] Note that the psychopharmacologists lamenting the "underutilization" of antidepressants in old people recommend more liberal use of these drugs as if the drugs were harmless. That, of course, is not the case. According to the drug experts themselves, psychotropic drugs accelerate the onset of dementia and increase the risk of death in this population.[80]

In advanced societies, the incidence of suicide has always been highest among old people. The psychopharmacologists use this as further ammunition in their campaign to immobilize old people with psychotropic drugs. "Depression is a major risk factor for suicide in the elderly, who account for about 13 percent of the United States population, but for nearly 24 percent of all completed suicides.... Elderly men have the highest suicide rate: 25 per 100,000 compared with 4 per 100,000 for older women.

---

* Depression is assuredly a normal consequence of being in a standard nursing home, even if the person is only a visitor.

White men age 85 or older have the highest rate of completed suicide, 55 per 100,000." The notion of suicide as a human right is absent from the vocabulary of psychiatry, especially geriatric psychiatry. And so, too, is an existential perspective on a person's wanting to end his life voluntarily, especially when its naturally ordained and probably painful end is near. "Late-life depression" is a disease with a specific etiology, "Damage to frontal subcortical circuitry ...."[81] The correct treatment for old-age depression is "monotherapy.... Long-term treatment may be necessary to prevent recurrence. ... ECT is used more frequently in the elderly than in younger patients, and may be effective for the older patient who is intolerant of medications or not responding to adequate medication trials."[82] Is it any wonder that many candidates for nursing home care prefer suicide?

Geriatric psychiatry and forensic psychiatry are growth industries. Psychiatric authorities, warning against underdiagnosis and undertreatment, fan the flames of diagnosis and treatment. No one resists the *furor therapeuticus*—not the denominated patients, not their relatives, not ex-patient groups, and, sadly, not physicians. Again, the problem is "Who shall guard the guardians?" It is a rhetorical question. Says the Inspector General of the U. S. Department of Health and Human Services: "In this context, groups representing providers with expertise in this area must take responsibility for developing and disseminating a statement of the clinical principles that define appropriate treatment with psychotherapeutic medications."[83] *Nursing home inmates are wards of their keepers who have a vested interest in drugging them.* Some experts acknowledge that "there is considerable evidence that these medications have frequently been overused and misused in the nursing home," only to lend weight to their overarching claim, that mental diseases in the elderly are either underdiagnosed and undertreated or, as here, that they are overused and misused. The Department of Health and Human Services report quoted earlier provides further evidence: "Four of the 10 nursing homes we visited specifically target psychiatric patients. All four have psychotropic drug usage rates that are above the national average. These nursing homes actively seek out such patients..."[84]

Finally, psychiatrists have managed to invade the last sanctuary of the dying, the hospice. In a Position Statement titled "Psychiatric aspects of excellent end-of-life care," the Academy of Psychosomatic Medicine declares:

> Studies show that psychiatric morbidity in the setting of terminal illness is exceptionally high.... Psychiatric problems and issues commonly seen at the end of life include anxiety symptoms and anxiety disorders, depressive symptoms and depressive disor-

ders, delirium and other cognitive disorders, *suicidal ideation*, consequences of low perceived family and other social support, personality disorders or personality traits that cause problems in the setting of extreme stress, questions of capacity to make informed decisions, *grief and bereavement, and general and health-related quality of life*.... Good end-of-life care requires explicit attention to these matters.[85]

A psychiatrist describes the hospice as "*a laboratory for the understanding of death, loss, and mourning,*" and adds: "*... these issues can be studied fruitfully at the hospice because of the accessibility to dying patients and the bereaved, both before and after the death of their loved one.*"[86] As is usually the case, attention to the psychiatrist's rhetoric reveals his motives and values. The hospice is a "laboratory." Dying patients and their relatives are "accessible." There is no evidence that patients who seek hospice care or their relatives want psychiatric help. However, they are a vulnerable and exploitable population and the hospice psychiatrist preys on them: "Many of the problems special to the hospice relate to loss, mourning, and death. Psychiatric diagnostic input has been helpful in the treatment of organic and functional psychiatric disorders including the treatment of the emotional components of pain and disordered grief which is manifest as depression.... The psychiatric consultant to a hospice is helpful in establishing and maintaining a sensitive therapeutic system of care for the patient and family.[87] In psychiatry, self-praise is often accepted as evidence of "sensitivity" or "therapy."

Dying before the Age of Psychopharmacology, Yeats saw "the aged man" as a person, not patient. The full stanza of the poem with which I began reads: "An aged man is but a paltry thing, / A tattered coat upon a stick, unless / Soul clap its hands and sing, and louder sing / For every tatter in its mortal dress." The remedy for the "aged man" is meaning, not medication.

10

The mass drugging of American children with stimulants and antidepressants has been a media staple for decades. The ready availability of information about child drugging makes it unnecessary to rehash the conflicting claims and contrived "studies" of the supporters and opponents of the practice. A few recently reported facts and figures should suffice to indicate the present state of affairs.

The administration of psychotropic drugs to children, like all psychiatric-therapeutic interventions, rests on belief in mental illness and the legitimacy of therapeutic coercion: children, and often their parents, too, are unable to reject the authorities wielding psychiatric diagnoses and treatments. Children are captives *par excellence*: they are the prisoners of their parents, parent surrogates, schools, the medical and social service professions, and, overseeing them all, the therapeutic state.[88] Some children are more imprisoned than others and it is instructive to see if the degree of their captivity correlates with the frequency with which they are drugged.

It is reasonable to assume that children cared for by strangers are, on the whole, considered more unwanted—and hence more troublesome and more mentally ill—than are children cared for by parents or relatives. Andrés Martin, a leading child psychopharmacologist—yes, there is such a psychiatric subspecialty!—set out "to determine the prevalence, patterns, and demographic correlates of multiple psychotropic pharmacotherapy in a statewide sample of low-income children and adolescents in community-based clinical care." Predictably, Martin found that the degree of child captivity directly correlated with the frequency of child drugging, the most unwanted children being the most frequently drugged. Minors in state custody represent 4.7 percent of the Medicaid population, yet account for 17.8 percent of the psychotropic drug consumption. "This 4.5-fold higher rate emerged as the single strongest predictor of psychotropic drug use in our study," Martin reported. "Given that children in state custody are a vulnerable group at high risk of *serious psychopathology*, this is not an entirely surprising finding."[89]

The children most abused by fate are also the most abused by psychiatrists. In Massachusetts in 2003, "almost two-thirds of children in DSS (Department of Social Services) care—that is, children in foster care and guardianship programs—were receiving psychotropic drugs."[90] In 2004, Texas State Comptroller Carole Keeton Strayhorn launched an investigation into charges that children in foster care "are being given psychiatric drugs so they're more docile, or so doctors and drug companies can make a buck.... 'Children as young as 3 are receiving powerful, mind-altering drugs,' she said.... 'It is not uncommon for some [foster] children to have up to 14 different prescriptions'.... Commission spokeswoman Jennifer Harris said it has launched a two-track review of whether poor children on Medicaid—including foster children—*receive proper medicine for mental illness.*"[91]

On January 4, 2006, the *Washington Times* reported: "Drug prescriptions meant to counter depression, anxiety and mood or attention disorders in teens increased by 250 percent between 1994 and 2001, according to a Brandeis University study.... Teenage boys are particularly targeted: one out of every 10 who visits the doctor leaves with a prescription to treat a mental condition." Cindy Parks Thomas, who led the Brandeis study, stated: "There is an alarming increase in prescribing these drugs to teens...*despite the fact that few psychotropic drugs, typically prescribed for attention deficit hyperactivity disorder (ADHD), depression and other mood disorders, are approved for use in children under 18.*"[92]

Although the drugging rage unleashed by ADHD and Ritalin affects Americans the most, people in England and Europe are not immune. Frustrated in their attempts to cope with growing lawlessness, law enforcement agencies in the UK are redefining youth violence as ADHD and trying to control it by means of coerced drugging. "The aggressive behavior associated with attention deficit disorders can sometimes land children in trouble with the law," reports the BBC. "Police in east Lancashire have launched an initiative to help such vulnerable children avoid the risk of getting involved in crime. ...there are currently 350 children in this area receiving treatment for Attention Deficit Hyperactivity Disorder (ADHD), although police believe there could be *many others whose condition is undiagnosed.*" In short, the justificatory rhetoric in the UK is virtually identical to that in the US: "The National Attention Deficit Disorder Information and Support Service (ADDISS) welcomes the scheme. ADDISS director Andrea Bilbow declared: 'I think it's a very important project. It's recognizing that ADHD is *a legitimate condition...* and a very serious public problem.... *The earlier we treat children with this condition, the better their development is going to be.*'"[93] There is no evidence to support that claim.

Periodically, newspapers run stories that they and the public foolishly regard as "exposés." These pseudo-exposés reinforce the standard psychiatric premises that are at the root of the problem. A feature article in the *Columbus Dispatch*, sensationally titled, "Drugged into Submission: Forced Medication Straitjackets Kids," is typical. A 15-year-old girl is reported to have complained that she "slept for four days and was in a drug-induced fog for a week after being subdued with three shots of a powerful drug at a Dayton treatment center. Now she is at a Columbus center, but her mother worries about the number of medications she takes daily—14, compared with two when she went into treatment two years ago." A 16-year-old boy "endured drugs that made him sleep 18 hours a day, gain 50 pounds and become hyper before doctors found the one to treat his bipolar disorder." The official conclusion: mental diseases are real diseases and psychotropic drugs are effective treatments—but it requires superior psychiatric competence to make the correct diagnoses and use the right drugs.

Legal groups advocate the imposition of "stricter rules to limit the use of medications.... *Both sides agree that psychiatric drugs can help kids suffering with anxiety, depression or a host of other mental illnesses. The question in these cases is whether medications are being used to treat children or as a chemical straitjacket.*" Who is to decide and on what grounds? Lawyers appoint themselves to the job:

> Legal Rights, an independent state agency, has examined nearly 500 cases involving chemical restraints during the past five years, including:
> * A 5-year-old boy who was so doped up that he couldn't stop batting the air...
> * A 10-year-old boy who was chemically restrained 69 times over 80 days...
> * A 12-year-old girl who was injected six times over nine months with high doses of Thorazine.... She also was physically restrained 31 times by as many as three men, despite a history of being physically and sexually abused.
>
> It is scandalous that medications are used to subdue kids...as punishment for bad behavior.... State officials say Ohio law prohibits chemical restraints except in emergencies.... "It's been outlawed," said Thomas Wood, chief of licensure and certification for the Department of Mental Health.[94]

It does not matter whether using drugs as restraints is in-lawed or outlawed. In psychiatry, the only law is the law of the psychiatric jungle: "Critics say the state's [Ohio's] 52 private residential centers often skirt the law by calling the restraints emergency medications.... 'No one wants to call it a chemical restraint because it is too emotionally charged a term,' said Curtis Decker, executive director of the National Association of Protection & Advocacy Systems in Washington.... 'It happens underground all the time,' said Steve Eidelman, executive director of the ARC of the United States, a national advocacy group for the developmentally and mentally disabled."[95]

As I write this, a minor backlash against psychiatric drugging, especially of children, appears to be developing. It is not based on clear thinking about the connections between the introduction of psychotropic drugs and the invention of an epidemic of childhood mental illnesses. Instead, it is based on the well-founded fear that psychotropic drugs are harming children. Given the nature of these drugs—designed to alter brain function—this contingency ought to have been suspected, a priori. "More Kids Are Getting Anti-Psychotic Drugs," states an Associated Press report dated March 16, 2006:

The annual number of children prescribed anti-psychotic drugs jumped fivefold between 1995 and 2002, to an estimated 2.5 million, the study said. That is an increase
from 8.6 out of every 1,000 children in the mid-1990s to nearly 40 out of 1,000. But
more than half of the prescriptions were for attention deficit and other non-psychotic
conditions ... The increasing use of anti-psychotics since the mid-1990s corresponds
with the introduction of costly and heavily marketed medications such as Zyprexa
and Risperdal. The packaging information for both says their safety and effectiveness
in children have not been established. The drugs, which typically cost several dollars per pill, are considered safer than older anti-psychotics—at least in adults—but
they still can have serious side effects, including weight gain, elevated cholesterol
and diabetes.[96]

An Associated Press release, dated May 3, 2006, warns, "Antipsychotic drug use among kids soars: Report raises concerns that mind-altering pills are being overprescribed": "The number of children taking
antipsychotic medicines soared 73 percent in the four years ending in
2005, far outpacing the increase in adults, according to a Medco Health
Solutions Inc. report.... Use of the new class of drugs known as atypical
antipsychotics by people 19 and younger skyrocketed 80 percent in the
same time period...the atypical antipsychotics aren't approved for use in
children.[97]

I have long maintained that *child psychiatry is child abuse*. This is
glaringly obvious in the case of child psychopharmacology. Every child
given a psychoactive drug by a doctor and is ordered to take it by a parent,
parent surrogate, or school authority is, by definition, forcibly drugged.*
How do forcibly drugged children view their psychopharmacological
rape? Here is the account of one such victim, Amber Smidebush, an 18-
year-old college student and writer for *Sprawl Magazine.*

I've been on psychiatric medications since I was 10 years old. Today, I take six prescribed medications a day, plus three over-the-counter pills. Doctors seem to think
that medications are the cure for everything, and because of that, I am stuck in a trap.
A lot of people use drugs recreationally to feel better. I do that every day with my
meds and hate it. How would you like to remember that you have to take three orange
ones, a blue one, a white one, a red one and one that changes color every time they
up the dose? If I forget one dose, I feel like crap.... Withdrawals from these can be
worse than withdrawals from street drugs. When and where will this stop?... I have
been on so many different psychiatric medications over the years it makes my head
spin.... When my doctors told my Mom I was bipolar, they automatically gave me a
bunch of pills to take. Wellbutrin, Neurontin, Seroquel, Depakote, Effexor, Inderal,
Trileptal, Paxil, Zyprexa, Lamictal, Abilify—I've taken them all. I call them happy
pills; they call them "chemical balancers." At one point I was on a type of speed,
much like Ritalin, that messed me up really bad.... The doctors prescribe the pills to
"make me happy." The pills just don't allow me to think. I don't have a chance to be

---

* Mutatis mutandis, every child who engages in an act of self-medication is, ipso facto,
guilty of drug abuse and exhibits a symptom of mental illness.

happy or upset—I'm just...there.... I see commercials each day about this "change your life forever, and you'll never feel better," but I look at them and laugh. Especially because, nine times out of 10, I've taken the medication they're advertising. They never show the people who can't get out of bed, or the children taking their handful of pills each night before Mom tucks them in. They don't show the people who cry each day because they don't know what's going on and their meds make them worse than they were.[98]

None of this stops psychiatrists from relentlessly escalating their claims about the frequency of mental illness in children and other captive populations and the efficacy of psychopharmacological treatments for them. Aided and abetted by the media and by national and international health organizations and governments—from the American Medical Association to the World Health Organization—the psychiatrization of life is now a veritable crowd madness.

A small flood of articles and books critical of the psychiatrization of childhood has done nothing to stem the tide.[99] Most parents remain unaware of the dangers that child psychiatrists, child psychologists, and school counselors pose to their children. The only people who can save children from the professional "child savers" are their parents. All too often, parents do not protect their children, for the many reasons with which we are all too familiar.

8

Psychopharmacology II: Psychedelic Drugs

We regard state monopoly of the press as a characteristic of a totalitarian society, and state monopoly of the pharmacopoeia as a characteristic of a free society.

—*Thomas Szasz*[1]

1

People have been familiar with substances we now call "mind-altering," "hallucinogenic," or "psychedelic" "drugs" since ancient times. These drugs are the natural products of a variety of plants and belong, from a chemical viewpoint, in the class of organic compounds called "alkaloids." From a medical viewpoint, the most familiar and most important alkaloids are apomorphine, atropine, cocaine, codeine, heroin, hyoscine, morphine, quinine, scopolamine, and strychnine. The use of these drugs predates the distinction between religion and medicine, between what is sacramental and what is therapeutic. In the American social-political context, the most important such substance is peyote, with mescaline as its active ingredient. For native-Americans, peyote is both sacramental and medical. For the FDA, it is neither. No historical review of psychopharmacology would be complete without at least a brief consideration of psychedelic-psychotomimetic substances, qua recreational, psychiatric, and prohibited drugs.[2]*

The story begins in Switzerland in 1938, when Albert Hofmann (1906-), a chemist working at Sandoz Pharmaceuticals in Basel, first synthesized lysergic acid diethylamide, or LSD. Five years later he accidentally ingested some of it and discovered its hallucinogenic properties. From 1943, when Hofmann first experienced the effect of LSD, until 1967, when its sale, possession, and use were prohibited in the United States, LSD was a legal drug. Sandoz Laboratories, the drug's sole pro-

---

* The term "psychotomimetic" emphasizes and falsely implies that there are fundamental similarities between LSD-induced delirium and a so-called psychosis, especially schizophrenia. The term "hallucinogenic" refers to the property of the drug to induce hallucinations, delusions, or other symptoms of a psychosis.

ducer, began marketing LSD in 1947 under the trade name "Delysid." Introduced into the United States a year later, it was distributed liberally to physicians interested in investigating its potential therapeutic uses. "During a 15 year period beginning in 1950, research on LSD and other hallucinogens generated over 1,000 scientific papers, several dozen books, and 6 international conferences, and LSD was prescribed as treatment to over 40,000 patients."[3] When LSD was legal, psychiatric research into its alleged therapeutic value was fashionable and useful for advancing a psychiatric career. After it was banned, investigation of "LSD abuse" became the royal road to psychiatric fame and fortune.

The first American psychiatrists to try LSD on patients were Robert Hyde and Max Rinkel. "We noticed," they wrote in 1951, "predominantly changes similar to those seen in schizophrenic patients. The subjects exhibited preeminently difficulties in thinking, which became retarded, blocked, autistic, and disconnected."[4] For establishment psychiatrists LSD produced retarded and blocked thinking; for anti-establishment psychiatrists, it expanded consciousness and artistic inspiration. LSD proved to be a perfect screen onto which psychiatrists, politicians, social observers, and critics could project their prejudices.

As soon as LSD became available, it attracted the attention of two groups—the military, as a potential chemical weapon for disorienting people and making them susceptible to suggestion (the "Manchurian Candidate" fantasy); and the rock and youth culture, as a magical substance for producing chemical enlightenment (the secular-pharmacological "peace on earth" fantasy). For some twenty years, during the 1950s and 1960s, the CIA in the United States and MI6 in Britain subsidized clandestine LSD experiments. At the same time, LSD became a popular recreational drug, and it has remained so. Eventually, disenchantment set in, and in 1967 the FDA classified LSD as a Schedule I drug, "having high abuse potential and no accepted medical use." The possession and sale of Schedule I drugs are felonies, and their use constitutes "drug abuse" par excellence.

The comic saga of psychedelic-hallucinogenic drugs complements the tragic saga of psychotropic-neuroleptic drugs. The web site featuring Hofmann's book, *LSD: My Problem Child,* is headed by a photograph showing the elderly Hofmann in a posture of clowning. Exhibitionism, frivolity, grandiosity, sensationalism, mysticism, ersatz religion, and pseudoscience have characterized the psychopharmacology of LSD use from its beginning to the present. Hofmann's naive philosophizing illustrates the prevailing style: "Instead of all the energy and effort directed at the war to end drugs, how about a little attention to drugs which would end war?"[5] Hofmann explained:

> Of greatest significance to me has been the insight that I attained as a fundamental understanding from all of my LSD experiments: what one commonly takes as "the reality," including the reality of one's own individual person, by no means signifies something fixed, but rather something that is ambiguous—that there is not only one, but that there are many realities, each comprising also a different consciousness of the ego.... The true importance of LSD and related hallucinogens lies in their capacity to shift the wavelength setting of the receiving "self," and thereby to evoke alterations in reality consciousness. This ability to allow different, new pictures of reality to arise, this truly cosmogonic power, makes the cultish worship of hallucinogenic plants as sacred drugs understandable.... I see the true importance of LSD in the possibility of providing material aid to meditation aimed at the mystical experience of a deeper, comprehensive reality. Such a use accords entirely with the essence and working character of LSD as a sacred drug.... The existence of LSD was even regarded by the drug enthusiasts as a predestined coincidence, it had to be discovered precisely at this time in order to bring help to people suffering under the modern conditions.[6]

Hofmann wrote this in 1980, many years after LSD got off to a poor start: fanatics, mystics, and celebrities of all kinds—cold-war zealots, psychiatric poisoners working for the CIA, research psychiatrists attributing schizophrenogenic properties to LSD, beatnicks and peacenicks and pranksters—rushed to embrace it as their signature drug. The following is a partial Who's Who of LSD advocates, "researchers," and users.[7]

- Lt. General William Creasy, chief officer of the U.S. Army Chemical Corps during the 1950s. Preached the gospel of an LSD-based "war without death"; called for testing hallucinogenic gases on subways in major American cities.
- Sidney Gottlieb (1918-1999), a.k.a, Joseph Schneider. American chemist, CIA operative, oversaw the secret CIA-sponsored MK-ULTRA program, which sought to develop LSD into a mind control weapon.
- Paul H. Hoch, M.D. (1902-1964). Psychiatrist. His activities noted in chapter 7.
- Harris Isbell (1910-1994), psychiatrist, director of the notorious U. S. Public Health Service "Narcotics Farm" (Addiction Research Center). Ran extensive drug experiments for the CIA at the "hospital," where addicts were supplied with heroin in exchange for their participation in secret LSD tests.
- Ronald D. Laing (1927-1989), Scottish psychiatrist, psychoanalyst, anti-psychiatrist. Used LSD, gave friends and patients LSD, was authorized by U.K. government to conduct "clinical experiments" with LSD. Forcibly restrained and injected patient/friend Clancy Sigal with Thorazine.[8] More about Laing to follow.
- Timothy Leary (1920-1991). Jesuit-educated, lapsed Catholic, defrocked psychologist, counterculture icon. Coined the phrase "Turn on, tune in, drop out." Preached a narcissistic, nihilistic, and pathetic

message, addressed to the young faced with the task of growing up and joining the world of responsible adulthood. Mystic and pseudomartyr, replaced the Eucharist with LSD, and the solemnity of the Lord's prayer with the frivolity of drug-fueled exhibitionism. Cooperated with the FBI's investigation of the Weathermen, becoming an informant who implicated friends and helpers in exchange for a reduced sentence.

- Humphry Fortescue Osmond (1917-2004), British-born psychiatrist. Coined the term "psychedelic" in 1957; promoted LSD as a cure for alcoholism. More about Osmond to follow.
- Louis Jolyon ("Jolly") West (1925-1999), showman show-off professor of psychiatry, UCLA. Killed a zoo elephant in experiment with LSD; conducted hallucinogenic drug tests for the CIA; anti-cultist devotee of the brainwashing myth; gave expert psychiatric testimony that Jack Ruby and Patty Hearst were mentally ill and not responsible for their crimes.

***

- William Burroughs (1914-1997), American author of *Naked Lunch* and numerous other works. Scion of a distinguished and wealthy family. Used morphine, heroin, marijuana, LSD, and other mind-altering drugs.
- Bob Dylan (1941-), born Robert Allen Zimmerman. American songwriter, singer, poet, musician, rock star, recreational drug user.
- Allen Ginsberg (1926-1997), American "beat" poet. Buddhist, mystic, socialist, anti-establishment guru. "Our goal was to save the planet and alter human consciousness.... The only thing that can save the world is the reclaiming of the awareness of the world.... Pot is fun."
- Aldous Huxley (1894-1963), British author of *Brave New World* and other works. In later years strongly influenced by Eastern mysticism and advocate of psychedelic drugs. Requested, as he lay dying, that he be given LSD and his wife gave him an intramuscular injection of 100 micrograms of the drug. He died peacefully.
- Ken Kesey (1935-2001), American author of *One Flew Over the Cuckoo's Nest* and other works. In 1959, volunteered to take part in experiments with LSD, mescaline, and psirlocybin at the Menlo Park (California) Veterans Administration Hospital and became advocate of psychedelic drugs and marijuana. Cultural icon, link between the "beat generation" and "hippies."

***

- Charles Manson (1934-), one of America's most famous mass murderers by proxy. Child of a 16-year-old woman who abandoned him. Spent most of his youth in prison. Hippie, Beatles fan, drug user. In 1969, the "Manson Family" committed a series of grisly murders in the Los Angeles area, allegedly under the influence of ("due to") LSD. The crimes are often described as "LSD murders."

2

Ronald David Laing is usually thought of as a psychoanalyst and anti-psychiatrist, someone who does not believe in mental illness and rejects psychiatric coercion. This is not true. In his autobiography, he states:

> Mental hospitals and psychiatric units admit, routinely, every day of the week, people who are sent "in" for non-criminal conduct, but for conduct which their nearest and dearest relatives, friends, colleagues and neighbors find insufferable. This is our society's only resolution to this unlivable impasse. If they refuse to go away, or can't or won't fend for themselves, it is our only way to keep people out of the company that can't stand them.... To say that a locked ward functions as a prison for non-criminal transgressors is not to say it should not be so. Our society may continue to "need" some such prisons for unacceptable persons. As our society functions at present such places are indispensable. This is not the fault of psychiatrists, not necessarily the fault of anyone.[9]

This is not the writing of a psychiatrist who rejects involuntary mental hospitalization. It is the writing of a psychiatrist who rejects responsibility, and hence freedom. Moreover, Laing believed in the notion of chemically induced "model psychosis," used LSD himself, gave it to his patients as part of their "therapy," and, on at least one occasion, forcibly drugged a "patient" with chlorpromazine. Laing's use of LSD illustrates the enormous appeal—even for existential psychologists and philosophers—of drugs and "chemistry" as scientific explanations for problems of human existence and as a convenient means of "fixing" them.

Laing began his personal use of LSD in the early 1960s, when it was still legal in the UK. He loved it. Laing hagiographer John Clay writes: "LSD opened up new vistas, new fields of experience for him, and he was to use it more and more.... With LSD he found he could 'travel through time in a way that the past wasn't simply at a distance but co-present.'"[10] The LSD mystique was right up Laing's alley, and so also was its appeal to his craving to violate boundaries as a therapist: "He took it experimentally *with* patients at Wimpole Street [his office]." Clay quotes Laing: "I now usually take a small amount of it myself if I give it to anyone, so that I can travel with them."[11]

In 1964, while lecturing in the United States, Laing sought to meet Leary. They met at Bill Hitchcock's legendary estate in Milbrook, New York, where Leary was then staying. Leary recounted what happened: "I groaned. Another dreary, platitudinous psychiatrist.... I told him that medical-therapeutic talk about LSD was a fake. I was interested only in the mystic aspects of the drug. His move. He said that the only *doctor who could heal was the one who understood the shamanic, witchcraft mystery of medicine.*"[12] This, indeed, was the real Laing—the shamanic-mystical, all-powerful "doctor." Laing proposed that he and Leary wrestle. They did and Laing quickly conceded. Later, in London, Laing took LSD with Richard Alpert, a psychologist and former colleague at Harvard. "Alpert recalls Laing's fragility under LSD. He seemed 'very vulnerable and very much in need of protection'.... Laing was not surprised to hear this later and often experienced going back to his earliest childhood during LSD sessions—even once or twice re-experiencing his birth trauma and getting stuck half-way."[13] Laing's penchant for self-dramatization was boundless. He was an inveterate, natural deceiver, because he was a self-deceiver and show-off even to himself.

Adrian Laing's sympathetic biography of his father furnishes more information about Laing's dalliance with drugs. "It was not until 1960 that Ronnie took his first acid trip, smoked his first joint and experienced the particular heights of the hallucinative drugs psilocybin and mescaline. He tried heroin, opium, and amphetamines, but they were not to his liking. Cocaine was fine if you could afford it. LSD was a drug which intrigued Ronnie and for which he was given permission by the British Government, through the Home Office, to use in therapeutic context.... Ronnie used the drug in therapy sessions both at 21 Wimpole Street and, at a later stage, in Kingsley Hall."[14] Obeying the law was for other people, not Laing. Laing deceived the Home Office when he applied, as he must have, for special permission to use LSD "in a therapeutic context," and then used it himself. He also deceived all those who believed him when he declared that mental disorders were disturbances in human relationships, not disorders of brain chemistry, and then proceeded to use a chemical with powerful effect on the brain to "treat" his "patients." I regard Laing's deception, as well as the deception of the psychiatrists who testify that psychotropic drugs *cause* suicide and murder, as fundamentally similar to the deceptions of the biological psychiatrists whose practices Laing criticized.

Laing accepted that LSD produced a "model psychosis," hence that psychosis was a chemical disorder, a bona fide brain disease. Chemicals were both the origin and the cure of the disease: "Under the Misuse of Drugs Act 1964, a qualified doctor was entitled to prescribe LSD to patients.... The actual effects of LSD mimicked a psychotic breakdown.... [In a BBC interview] Ronnie extolled the virtues of lysergic acid, mescaline, psilocybin, and hashish..." and referred to the notion of chemically induced model psychosis as if it were a fact.[15] Laing's interest in and consumption of mind-altering drugs, in addition to alcohol, cannot be overemphasized. Adrian writes: "...as far as Ronnie was concerned, the principal area into which he felt the need to expand during 1966 was drugs and, in particular, LSD, hashish, and mescaline.... From 1960 until 1967, Ronnie's intake of substances, legal and otherwise, increased considerably, and there was clearly a steady increase in his personal consumption during 1965 and 1966, which coincided with his living at Kingsley Hall."

Although Laing denied, and his followers still deny, that Laing was a drug guru and the high priest of "super-sanity," Adrian quotes one of his lectures: "An LSD or mescaline session [sic] in one person, with one set in one setting, may occasion a psychotic experience. Another person, with a different set and different setting, may experience a period of super-sanity.... The aim of therapy will be to enhance consciousness rather than to diminish it. Drugs of choice, if any are to be used, will be predominantly consciousness expanding drugs, rather than consciousness constrictors—the psychic energizers, not the tranquilizers." In short, Laing saw himself as a psychopharmacologist using "uppers" instead of "downers," cocaine- and amphetamine-type drugs instead of neuroleptic drugs. Adrian refers to the Laing of 1967 as "a practicing psychoanalyst and LSD therapist."[16] How does an LSD therapist differ from a Prozac or Thorazine therapist? Each has his favorite drug and uses his medical credentials, medical powers, and medical privileges to *prescribe* it to his patients.* Laing's psychopharmacological claims about LSD prefigure Peter Kramer's similar claims about Prozac, the Eli Lilly Company brand name for fluoxetine: the revised edition of *Listening to Prozac* carries the modest subtitle, *The Landmark Book About Antidepressants and the Remaking of the Self*.[17] These claims remind one of Freud's claims about cocaine, made a century earlier.

In 1976, Laing's luck ran out. His house in London was burglarized, an event he reported to the police. Adrian writes: "To Ronnie's utter amazement the police reappeared shortly after, not to inform him of the results of their investigations but to arrest and charge him with possession of LSD. During their 'routine' check of missing items, they had inexplicably forced open a locked cabinet and found ninety-four ampules of LSD-25. Unknown to Ronnie, the Misuse of Drug Acts 1973 restricted

---

* This may be a good place to point out that when Laing refers to the effects of LSD as a psychosis, he uses the term incorrectly. The correct term is "drug-induced delirium." The Merck Manual: "Delirium is a sudden, fluctuating, and usually reversible cognitive disorder characterized by disorientation, the inability to pay attention, the inability to think clearly, and a change in the level of consciousness."

the possession of the drug to specific prescribers and he, at that stage, was not one."[18] This time, Laing suffered no legal consequences from his lawbreaking. Much could be made of Adrian's choice of words here and his assumption that, in fact, his father—an expert on LSD—did not know that he had lost his dispensing privileges, but I shall refrain from doing so here. Instead, it seems appropriate to let Sigal—who wrote a book about Laing's LSD-fueled "therapy," which Laing prevented from being published in England—have the last word:

> We began exchanging roles, he the patient and I the therapist, and took LSD together in his office and in my Bayswater apartment.... Laing and I had sealed a devil's bargain. Although we set out to "cure" schizophrenia, we became schizophrenic in our attitudes to ourselves and to the outside world. Our personal relationships in the Philadelphia Association became increasingly fraught.... That night, after I left Kingsley Hall, several of the doctors, who persuaded themselves that I was suicidal, piled into two cars, sped to my apartment, broke in, and jammed me with needles full of Largactil [Thorazine], a fast-acting sedative used by conventional doctors in mental wards. Led by Laing, they dragged me back to Kingsley Hall where I really did become suicidal. I was enraged: the beating and drugging was such a violation of our code. Now I knew exactly how mental patients felt when the nurses set about them before the doctor stuck in the needle.... Before I could fight back—at least four big guys including Laing were pinning me down—the drug took effect. The last thing I remember saying was, "You bastards don't know what you're doing..." They left me alone in an upstairs cubicle overlooking a balcony with a 30-foot drop. I had to figure a way to escape from this bunch of do-gooders who had lost their nerve as well as their minds.... In 1975, 10 years after I broke with Laing, I completed a comic novel, Zone Of The Interior, based on my experiences with schizophrenia. Published to widespread notice in the US, it was stopped cold in Britain by Laing's vague threat of a libel action.[19]

Lotus-sitting, long-haired, bare-footed Laing made a sport of betraying every promise and trust, explicit and implicit—to wives, children, friends, and patients. What Laing did to Sigal was more reprehensible than what psychiatrists do when they forcibly drug patients. Psychiatrists distinguish between friends and patients, do not promise to eschew coercion, and their interventions are, at least *pro forma*, legitimated by law. Laing addressed serious moral issues, but lacked—indeed, mocked—moral seriousness. The following sentence from *The Politics of Experience* is illustrative: "If I could turn you on, if I could drive you out of your wretched mind, if I could tell you, I would let you know."[20]

With his LSD-laced "therapy," Indian junket, faux meditation, and alcohol-fueled lecture-theatrics, Laing managed, for a while, to con people into believing that his boorish behavior was a badge of his superior wisdom. Then, as quickly as he built it, his house of cards collapsed of its own featherweight.

3

Jolly West, another publicity-seeking, exhibitionist psychiatrist, was both like and unlike Laing. Both were grandiose self-promoters. Laing cultivated the image of anti-establishment guru, yet sought establishment approval as a medical doctor. West was an establishment psychiatrist who cultivated the image of a fearless "cult-fighter" protecting society from dangerous deviants.

West, a large bear of a man—friendly and outgoing—had a meteoric career. In 1953, at the age of 29, he was appointed professor and chairman of the department of psychiatry, neurology, and behavioral science at the University of Oklahoma. In 1969, he became professor and chairman of the department of psychiatry at the University of California School of Medicine in Los Angeles. In her review of West's career, Rebecca Lemov writes: "The larger-than-life 'Jolly' West ... was chief psychiatrist of the university's 250-bed hospital...headquartered for many years in a suite of offices, with a trio of secretaries and a university car at the ready."[21] In the mid-1950s, when stories of Korean brainwashing were the rage, West—like many other prominent psychiatric coercers, such as D. Ewen Cameron and Paul Hoch—began to do "research" for the CIA. Like most psychiatrists in most countries, West felt imbued with an excess of patriotic loyalty for the best interests of his society, as those interests were defined by the government in power. "He [West] envisioned a future science of human biosocial engineering that would work prophylactically and preemptively. Potential criminals, juvenile delinquents, schizophrenics, and drug addicts would be monitored through remotely sensed electrodes implanted in their brains. 'The prediction of dangerousness'—the likelihood that a person would commit a violent crime in the future—'will be increasingly refined and quantified,'... West wrote."[22]

West's first publicity stunt—many others followed, such as his sensational attacks of cults and his failed, mendacious psychiatric defense of Patty Hearst—concerned the publicity drug LSD. Seeking to study the effect of LSD on an elephant, he accidentally killed the animal, and managed to have an account of his bungling published in the prestigious magazine *Science*. Instead of hanging his head in shame for this foolishness, he shamelessly presented it as a scientific experiment. After insipidly concluding, "It appears that the elephant is highly sensitive to the effects of LSD," he intoned: "LSD has been increasingly and sometimes irresponsibly administered to humans as a putative adjunct to psychotherapy. The possibility of suicide or even homicide by LSD cannot be ignored."[23] Translation: access to LSD must be restricted to physicians.

In the early decades of the twentieth century, psychiatrists saw epilepsy and schizophrenia first as similar, then as antagonistic; the latter perception provided rationale for iatrogenic seizures as therapy. There is no schizophrenia. Psychiatrists, eager to rationalize their aggression as therapy, "see" many kinds and patterns of human behaviors as mental diseases. In his studies of brainwashing, West and his colleagues coined the phrase "DDD syndrome," the acronym standing for debility, dependency, and dread. The mistreating of captives—of children by their parents, of patients by their psychiatrists—while at the same time also providing for their needs tends to create a state of DDD. The CIA researchers regarded this well-known phenomenon as a new discovery: "...as West's group pointed out, DDD was analogous to other extreme states of consciousness and bore an 'interesting resemblance' to post-lobotomy syndrome...it was also akin to certain drug-induced states of mind, such as those resulting from LSD and sodium amytal. Of further interest was brainwashing's resemblance to schizophrenia and hypnosis. All these conditions—whether induced by chemicals, surgery, madness, trance, or coercion—appeared similar."[24] To schizophrenia researchers, the world consists of two parts—things that resemble schizophrenia, and things that do not. One is reminded of the joke about psychoanalysts for whom, too, the world consists of two parts—things that look like penises, and things that look like vaginas.

The results of studying persons as if they were not persons are predictable—they become "conditions," "mental diseases," or animals. In the course of his CIA-sponsored experiments, West studied hippies: "To study them in their *natural habitat*, we established an apartment or 'pad' as a laboratory in the Haight-Asbury district of San Francisco."[25] While Laing took advantage of his gullible patients, West took advantage of his gullible colleagues and the CIA. Both ended up entertaining megalomaniacal dreams/nightmares of human "betterment." Laing's utopia was fueled by LSD and alcohol. West "linked his vision of a truly unified behavioral science that combined insights from neuroscience, pharmacology, electronics, sociology, psychology, and cultural anthropology to a dream of access to total knowledge: he spoke of building a massive databank of consciousness itself, which would consist of bioelectric recording—gathered through electromyography, electro-oculography, rheoencephalography, and CAT scans—subsequently analyzed and coded, then stored in a centralized location such as the National Institute of Mental Health or the National Medical Library."[26]

Schizophrenics have "grandiose delusions." Famous psychiatrists "engage in research."

4

As we have seen in connection with the development of shock thera- pies, psychiatrists are eager to "see" a connection between epilepsy and schizophrenia—either similarity or antagonism. The introduction of LSD and other hallucinogens into psychiatry reignited the psychiatric imagi- nation: psychiatrists began to "see" a similarity between the effects of LSD and schizophrenia. Two of the earliest observers of this mirage were Humphry Osmond and John Smythies. They proposed this view in 1951, in Britain. Disappointed by its cool reception there, in 1952 Osmond and Smythies immigrated to Canada to join the staff of the provincial mental hospital in Weyburn, Saskatchewan. Osborn assumed the post of clinical director at this traditional snake pit. Since this is where Osmond did the work on LSD for which he is remembered, it behooves us to be aware of the kind of psychiatric Auschwitz that was the Weyburn hospital. In 2005 a Canadian Broadcasting Corporation report described the place as follows: "The Weyburn Mental Hospital opened in 1921 and quickly became one of Canada's most notorious psychiatric institutions. It was the site of lobotomies, electric shock therapy, and some of Canada's controversial LSD experiments. It was here that Dr. Humphrey Osmond coined the word 'psychedelic.'"[27]

Osmond and Smythies were not interested in the inmates.* They were interested in proving that schizophrenia was a brain disease due to toxic chemicals produced by the patients' own bodies, as demonstrated by the "model psychoses" produced by LSD. Anticipating Laing's LSD sessions with patients, Osmond and Smythies asserted that "No one is really competent to treat schizophrenia unless he has experienced the schizophrenic world himself. This is possible to do quite simply by taking mescaline."[28] If you believe that schizophrenia is a brain disease, this is a non sequitur. Countless diseases—diabetes, hyper- and hypothyroid- ism, pheochromocytoma, pituitary tumors—give rise to altered mental states, but it would make no sense to suggest that effective treatment of these diseases requires that the physician, too, experience the patient's symptoms. Osmond and his ilk wanted it both ways: they were scien- tific physicians demonstrating that schizophrenia is a brain disease, and existential philosophers possessing special insight into the inner life of

---

* See chapter 1 for Osmond's remarks about the Weyburn hospital.

the schizophrenic. It is noteworthy that they could never detect a longing for liberty there.

Osmond introduced Aldous Huxley to LSD and was proud of his friendship with the great writer. They exchanged witticisms about hallucinogens. Entranced by the beneficial potentialities of hallucinogens, Huxley sent Osmond this rhyme: "To make this trivial world sublime, take half a gram of phanerothyme." Osmond responded with: "To fathom Hell or soar angelic, just take a pinch of psychedelic."[29]

Osmond also began to claim that LSD was an effective treatment for alcoholism and that he had successfully treated "Bill W.", the co-founder of Alcoholics Anonymous. Canadian psychiatrist Abram Hoffer (1917-) has a different version of these events. Hoffer had worked with Osmond not only on LSD but also on niacin, also called vitamin B3. Bill W. was given huge doses of niacin and attributed his recovery to it. Hoffer's entrance onto the scene brings us to the story of so-called orthomolecular psychiatry, which he defined by contrasting it with standard psychopharmacological psychiatry:[*]

> Orthomolecular psychiatry is one of two branches of psychiatry currently advocating chemotherapy for schizophrenia. The other branch is toximolecular psychiatry. There are vast conceptual differences between the two and great differences in efficacy for the patient. Toximolecular psychiatry advocates the use of sublethal doses of agents not normally found in the body. Their use has not significantly improved patient recovery rate over that occurring naturally, and demands a terrible price from the patient in the form of incapacity to work and irreversible toxicity.... In this approach, a drug is promoted and required for patient maintenance. Modern psychiatry generally depends on this system of drug use. Orthomolecular psychiatry, on the other hand, emphasizes a system of treatment, not any one drug or chemical. The schizophrenic is given optimal amounts of materials that are necessary for good nutrition and optimal functioning—vitamins, minerals, fats, carbohydrates, and amino acids. *The orthomolecular program requires full patient participation in changing lifestyle and discontinuing faulty eating habits....* In many cases, megadoses of the essential factors are required, and patients are eventually maintained in a normal state by nutritional therapy alone. Such patients relapse much less frequently than those maintained on drugs alone.[30]

This passage ought to be of special interest to students of the history of psychiatry: it squarely pits the heterodox, anti-establishment psychopharmacology quacks against the orthodox, establishment psychopharmacology quacks. Both assume that schizophrenia is a biochemically caused "mental illness." The orthomolecularists call the APA-approved drugs "toximolecular," the dispensers of which in turn dismiss the orthomolecularists as charlatans. Easily missed in the scuffle may be Hoffer's

---

* The term "orthomolecular psychiatry" was coined by Linus Pauling in 1968.

specification that orthomolecular treatment must be fully consensual, a condition that removes it from the remit of my history of psychiatry. It must be noted, however, that when establishment psychiatrists encounter schizophrenics, they find most of them to be suffering from anosognosia, a brain lesion that makes them refuse psychiatric treatment. In contrast, when orthomolecular psychiatrists meet schizophrenics, they find them willing to "fully participate" in treatment. Neither Osmond nor Hoffer tells us where or how they found these patients. They could not have found them at the "hospital" where Osmond was clinical director.

Orthomolecular therapy has all the classic earmarks of quackery: Its one method—megadoses of vitamins, especially niacin and ascorbic acid (vitamin C)—cures everything from alcoholism to the common cold to cancer and schizophrenia, in short everything but a wooden leg. Identified as having "collaborated with Linus Pauling on several aspects of orthomolecular medicine but especially the anticancer actions of vitamin C," and as being "known for his use of nutritional and vitamin therapies in the treatment of schizophrenia, cancer, and other diseases," Hoffer has served as the director of Psychiatric Research for the Saskatchewan Department of Public Health in Regina, is affiliated with the Huxley Institute for Biosocial Research, and is editor-in-chief of the *Journal of Orthomolecular Psychiatry*.[31]

The contrast between the stories of psychedelic drugs and psychiatric drugs highlights the fact that modern psychopharmacology is primarily a political-social phenomenon, albeit invariably portrayed as a medical-therapeutic discovery. Allied with pharmaceutical companies and the state, psychiatry promotes neuroleptic drugs that people do not want to use, makes them readily available to the public, and authorizes psychiatrists to use force to introduce them into the bodies of unwilling "patients." At the same time, psychiatry, allied with the criminal justice system, demonizes psychedelic and recreational drugs that many people want to use, makes them unavailable to the public (forcing them into a black market), and punishes their users as "addicts" and "drug abusers." In sum, the contrasting legal and societal attitudes toward different types of mind-altering drugs reveal, once again, that psychiatry is concerned with the social control of behavior, not the medical treatment of disease.

Conclusion: Psychiatry—A House United

Falsehood flies and the truth comes limping after; so that when men come to be undeceived it is too late: the jest is over and the tale has had its effect.
—Jonathan Swift (1667-1745)[1]

1

From the founding of the American Colonies in the seventeenth century, until the early decades of the nineteenth century, chattel slavery was the norm: the practice of holding people in bondage and forcing them to submit to their owners was supported by the laws of all of the Colonies and all of the states.[2] Gradually, the tension between liberty and slavery increased. After the Civil War, slavery was abolished.

From the emergence of mad-doctoring/psychiatry as a medical specialty in the eighteenth century, until the late 1950s, psychiatric slavery was the norm: the practice of holding people in bondage and forcing them to submit to their psychiatrists was supported by the laws of every civilized nation. After World War II, tension developed, especially in America and Britain, between consensual psychiatry and coercive psychiatry. Reminiscent of that brief period of confrontation is the remark by Manuel Trujillo, professor of psychiatry at New York University School of Medicine: "One of the problems is the ideological division within the psychiatric profession. When Larry Hogue came to Bellevue, I had problems with the first doctor assigned to the case because he was a follower of Thomas Szasz. He didn't even believe in the existence of mental illness."[3] (Hogue was a "homeless crack addict" who lived on the streets of New York and annoyed the city's mental health authorities.[4]) Those days are long gone. The conflict between free psychiatry and slave psychiatry has been resolved by the *de facto* abolition of contractual relations between "mental patients" and "therapists." Since the 1980s, the DSM, psychopharmacology, outpatient commitment, and the "duty to protect" have defined the "standard of care" in psychiatry. Deviation from it is punishable by tort litigation and delicensing.

In a famous speech in Springfield, Illinois, on June 16, 1858, Abraham Lincoln said, in part: "A house divided against itself cannot stand.

I believe this government cannot endure permanently half slave and half free. I do not expect the Union to be dissolved—I do not expect the house to fall—but I do expect it will cease to be divided. It will become all one thing, or all the other."[5] This was Lincoln's most extreme statement against slavery. He received the Republican nomination for the United States Senate, but lost the election.

I have long pondered the implications for psychiatry of Lincoln's insight. Psychiatry is, as the United States had been, faced with the uneasy coexistence of free and unfree relations between two groups of people of grossly unequal power—psychiatrists and mental patients. The psychiatrist's predicament is embedded in his *professional role*. On the one hand, he is mandated by society to help persons who seek his counsel. On the other hand, he is entrusted by society with the privilege-and-obligation to diagnose individuals against their will and incarcerate them in nominally medical institutions. Thus, some psychiatrists, some times, help their patients, and some psychiatrists, some times, harm them—"help" and "harm" in each case being defined by the patient. The hitch is that psychiatrists qua physicians are not supposed to harm their patients. How did psychiatrists cope with this contradiction? By denying it.

As soon as mad-doctors began to engage in the "restraining" of mad-men and mad women, criticism of the practice arose. Given the nature of their task, the mad-doctors found that they could not abolish the use of restraints. They resolved the problem by declaring that restraint is remedy, coercion is care.[6] That was the official psychiatric position in the 1950s, when I began to address the ethical dilemmas of psychiatry, and it remains the official psychiatric position today. The difference is that, fifty years ago, psychiatrists maintained that they always acted as their patients' agents: they always did good or, at least, intended to. Today, they articulate the same idea in the mind-numbing jargon of "psychiatric ethics." Sidney Bloch, senior author of *Psychiatric Ethics*, a standard work in the field,[7] asks, "Is there an optimal ethical framework for psychiatry?" He answers: "We propose a particular complementarity of principlism [sic]—with its pragmatic focus on respect for autonomy, beneficence, non-maleficence and justice—and care ethics, a variant of virtue theory, which highlights character traits pertinent to caring for vulnerable psychiatric patients."[8] Cardiologists and oncologists also "care for vulnerable patients." Only in psychiatry is the phrase a code for coercion.

Accused of a felony, the defendant—presumed innocent—seeks the assistance of a defense lawyer, not the district attorney. "Accused" of mental illness, the mental patient—presumed "dangerous to himself and others"—has no such choice. *Our society insists that the psychiatrist who deprives a person of liberty in the name of mental health serves the best interests of the imprisoned person, that psychiatric incarceration is preventive and curative medicine.* The legitimacy of psychiatric slavery rests on the fiction that "caring coercion" benefits the coerced, not society. To destroy that pretense would destroy psychiatry as we know it.

The injunction, *Primum non nocere!* (First, do no harm!) may be battered and bruised, but remains the leading moral rule of medical practice. Regardless of how successfully psychiatric coercion masquerades as a "caring" medical treatment, it gnaws at the soul of psychiatry. To be sure, as long as we define psychiatry as a medical specialty, we are compelled to define coercion as care, and the deprivation of liberty under psychiatric auspices as both the prevention of suicide or homicide and the provision of therapy. Abolishing psychiatric slavery—that is, the practice of depriving of persons defined as mental patients of liberty by incarceration in hospitals—requires stripping the psychiatrist of the privilege and power to lock up people. Such a change presupposes recognition and acceptance of the fact that forcibly depriving a person of liberty is not medical care.

Alas, most people feel protected, not oppressed, by psychiatry. We find it difficult to acknowledge that harming patients may be an integral part of the psychiatrist's job description: doing so would bring us back to psychiatry's very origin—the fork in the road where psychiatry took the wrong turn, mistaking disordered behavior for disordered physiology, and defining coercion as care.

2

The Roman playwright Terence (Terentius, c. 190-160 B.C.) remarked, "*Homo sum: humani nil a me alienum puto,*" "I am human: nothing human is alien to me." The theory and practice of psychiatry rest on and embody the opposite principle: "I am human: nothing alien is human to me." Mental illness, psychiatric diagnosis, anosognosia, treatment resistance, suicide prevention, inpatient commitment, outpatient commitment, the insanity defense—each of these ideas and interventions exemplifies treating the "abnormal" as a non-agent, non-person, non-human.

There is nothing new about this sort of division of humanity into "us" versus "them" categories. For example, belief in one true God implies a basic difference between believer and disbeliever, the saved and the damned. History shows that people have resolved this fundamental conflict in three ways—conversion, extermination, and acceptance. It is of no small interest in this connection that the United States was the first country in history explicitly founded on the principle that people of different religious convictions can, and ought to be able to, live together in harmony, as long as they abstain from initiating violence against one another. Ideas, beliefs, thoughts, writings, speech do not injure life, liberty, or property. Only coercion does. Therein lies the uniqueness and splendor of the First Amendment: it decrees tolerance for differing ideas, beliefs, and declarations, and assumes that such tolerance is compatible with harmonious social life. However, there is a notable exception to this tolerance: We are not expected to tolerate ideas, beliefs, and declarations categorized as delusions and hallucinations, that is, as symptoms of mental illnesses.

Fear of the insane and acceptance of the psychiatrist's role as society's protector from the dangers posed by the madman make the mere ascription of the label "insane" a justification for depriving the bearer of liberty—indeed, makes not committing the "dangerous mental patient" an irresponsible dereliction of professional duty. At the same time, the image of the insane as a dangerous madman sets a well-camouflaged trap for the modern, scientifically sophisticated intellectual: he rightly recoils from measures of coercive paternalism presented in religious garb, yet eagerly embraces the same types of measures presented as psychiatric treatment.

The fact that it is coercion that sets psychiatry apart from medicine, and indeed from all other forms of peaceful human endeavors, is obvious. The law prohibits coerced medical treatment, but permits and indeed mandates coerced psychiatric treatment. The psychiatrist says that the mental patient who rejects his help denies that he is ill. I say that the psychiatrist who uses force to impose diagnoses and treatments on a person against his will denies that he practices coercion. The central issue facing psychiatry and our society today is not whether a particular psychiatric intervention works or does not, whether it helps or harms the patient, whether it is therapeutic or toxic, whether it prevents suicide or promotes it. The central issue is whether contact between psychiatrist and patient is voluntary or involuntary, consensual or coercive. All other issues are secondary.

Whether we recognize it or not, the evaluation of the effectiveness or ineffectiveness of psychiatric treatments resembles the evaluation of the truth or falsehood of religious beliefs. After centuries of bitter and bloody debate, we in the modern West have concluded that engaging in that debate is an affront to human decency and dignity, and we abstain from doing so. Instead of distinguishing between true and false religions, we distinguish between religion freely professed and religion forcibly imposed, between choice and coercion. If the history of psychiatry teaches us anything, it teaches us that debating the worth or worthlessness of psychiatric "treatments" leads us down a blind alley at the end of which there is only more conflict and violence.

The institution of psychiatry, like the institution of slavery, consists of a socially sanctioned relationship between a class of superiors coercively controlling a class of inferiors. The system rests on the idea of mental illness, its semantic clones, and their legal implications; it is destined to engender disdain on the one side, and defiance on the other. The juxtaposition of persuasion and coercion lies at the heart of mankind's great moral conflicts—relations between men and women, leaders and followers, capital and labor, expert and lay person. The true healer of the soul is a "doctor" of persuasion, not coercion. Psychiatric peace and tolerance are contingent on the recognition that "mental illness" is a misleading metaphor and on the rejection of psychiatric coercion as a crime against humanity.

I asserted that it is obvious that what sets psychiatry apart from medicine is coercion. This fact was emphasized, under especially dramatic circumstances, by S. Weir Mitchell, founder of the American Neurological Association. In 1894, the American Medico-Psychological Association—now the American Psychiatric Association—invited Mitchell to present a special address at the fiftieth anniversary celebration of the group's first meeting. With grave misgivings, Mitchell agreed. He delivered a scathing lecture, which has been remarkably neglected by psychiatric historians. Here in part is what Mitchell told the assembled mad-doctors:

> You quietly submit to having hospitals called asylums; you are labeled as medical superintendents.... You should urge in every report the stupid folly of this. You... conduct a huge boarding house—what has been called a monastery of the mad.... I presume that you have, through habit, lost the sense of jail and jailor which troubles me when I walk behind one of you and he unlocks door after door. Do you think it is not felt by some of your patients.... *You have for too long maintained the fiction that there is some mysterious therapeutic influence to be found behind your walls and locked doors. We hold the reverse opinion.... Your hospitals are not our hospitals; your ways are not our ways.*[9]

More than ever, the ways of psychiatry are not the ways of medicine.

Notes

Epigraph

1   Nietzsche, F., *Twilight of the Idols or, How to Philosophize with a Hammer* (1895), in *The Portable Nietzsche*, ed. and trans. Walter Kaufman (New York: Viking, 1954), pp. 463-563; p. 505, emphasis in the original.

Preface

1.   Acton, J.E.E.D., *Essays in the Study and Writing of History*, 3 vols., ed. J. Rufus Fears (Indianapolis: Liberty Classics, 1988), p. 624.
2.   Arieti, S., "Preface," in *American Handbook of Psychiatry*, 3 vols., ed. Arieti, S. (New York: Basic Books, 1959-1966), vol. 1, pp. xi-xiii; p. xi.
3.   Kraepelin, E., "The Directions of Psychiatric Research (1886). *History of Psychiatry*, 16: 350-364 (September), 2005, p. 350. Inaugural lecture delivered September 6, 1886 at the Kaiserlichen Universitaet Dorpat.
4.   See Szasz, T., "Psychiatric Training: The Ritualized Indoctrination of the Young Physician into the Theory and Practice of Psychiatric Violence," in Szasz, T., *The Untamed Tongue: A Dissenting Dictionary* (LaSalle, IL: Open Court, 1990), p. 164.
5.   "Psychiatry," http://en.wikipedia.org/wiki/Psychiatr.
6.   Quoted in N. Ridenour, *Mental Health in the United States: A Fifty Year History* (Cambridge: Harvard University Press, 1961), p. 76.
7.   Sharfstein, S. S., "Individual Rights Must be Balanced with 'Caring Coercion," *Psychiatric News*, 40: 3 (September 2), 2005.
8.   Sharfstein, S. S., "Caring versus Coercion: Differences are Clear," *Psychiatric News*, 41: 3 (April 21), 2006, http://pn.psychiatryonline.org/cgi/content/full/41/8/3.
9.   Quoted in http://borntomotivate.com/FamousQuote_Alexander Solzhenitsyn.html.
10.   Whitman, W., "Preface to 'Leaves of Grass' (1855),'" http://bartleby.com/39/45.html.
11.   Ibid.

Introduction

1.   Appelbaum, P. S., "Mental Illness: No Longer a Myth," *The World & I, Washington Times*, November 1987, pp. 607-615; p. 607, http://worldandi.com/specialreport/1987/November/Sa13158.htm.
2.   Locke, J., *The Second Treatise of Government,* in *Two Treatises of Government* [1690], ed. Peter Laslett (New York: New American Library, 1965), pp. 346-350, emphasis in the original. Also http://libertyonline.hypermall.com/Locke/second/second-6.html.

3. Szasz, T., *Insanity: The Idea and Its Consequences* [1987] (Syracuse: Syracuse University Press, 1997), and Szasz, T., *Cruel Compassion: The Psychiatric Control of Society's Unwanted* [1994] (Syracuse: Syracuse University Press, 1998).
4. Ibid.
5. Szasz, T., "The Psychiatric Will: A New Mechanism for Protecting Persons against 'Psychosis' and Psychiatry," *American Psychologist*, 37: 762-770 (July), 1982; "The Psychiatric Will: II. Whose Will is It Anyway?," *American Psychologist*, 38: 344-346 (March), 1983; *Liberation by Oppression: A Comparative Study of Slavery and Psychiatry* (New Brunswick, NJ: Transaction Publishers, 2002).
6. http://brainyquote.com/quotes/quotes/t/thomasjeff132259.html.
7. Szasz, T., *Faith in Freedom: Libertarian Principles and Psychiatric Practices* (New Brunswick, NJ: Transaction Publishers, 2004).
8. Mill, John Stuart, *Utilitarianism* [1863], in *Essential Works of John Stuart Mill*, ed. Max Lerner (New York: Bantam Books, 1961), pp. 183-248; pp. 247-248.
9. Hunter, R., and Macalpine, I., eds., *Three Hundred Years of Psychiatry, 1535-1860: A History Presented in Selected English Texts.* (London: Oxford University Press, 1963), p. ix.
10. Quoted in Porter, R., "Ida Macalpine and Richard Hunter: History Between Psychoanalysis and Psychiatry," in *Discovering the History of Psychiatry*, ed. Micale, M. S., and Porter, R. (New York: Oxford University Press, 1994), pp. 83-94; p. 87.
11. Quoted in ibid., p. 90.
12. Goffman, E., *Asylums: Essays on the Social Situation of Mental Patients and Other Inmates* (Garden City, NY: Doubleday Anchor, 1961), pp. 125-169.
13. Quoted in Skultans, V. *Madness and Morals: Ideas on Insanity in the Nineteenth Century* (London: Routledge & Kegan Paul, 1975), p. 138.
14. Christie, I. R., "Royal Herring" (Letter), *New York Review of Books*, March 8, 1973.
15. Sargant, W., *Battle for the Mind: A Physiology of Conversion and Brainwashing* (1957) (New York: Harper & Row / Perennial Library, 1971), p. 129.
16. Szasz, T. *Pharmacracy: Medicine and Politics in America* [2001] (Syracuse: Syracuse University Press, 2003).
17. Heynick, F., "Sigmund Freud and Emil Kraepelin: 150 Years Old," *Psychiatric News*, 41: 31 (April 21), 2006, http://pn.psychiatryonline.org/cgi/content/full/41/8/31, emphasis added.
18. Sharfstein, S. S., "Caring versus Coercion: Differences are Clear," *Psychiatric News*, 41: 3 (April 21), 2006, http://pn.psychiatryonline.org/cgi/content/full/41/8/3.
19. Dain, N., "Psychiatry and Anti-Psychiatry in the United States," in Micale, M. S., and Porter, R., eds., *Discovering the History of Psychiatry*, pp. 415-444; p. 430.
20. Grob, G. N., "The History of the Asylum Revisited: Personal Reflections," in Micale, M. S., and Porter, R., eds., *Discovering the History of Psychiatry*, pp. 260-281; p. 263.
21. Porter, R., and Micale, M. S., "Reflections on Psychiatry and Its Histories," in Micale, M. S. and Porter, R., eds., *Discovering the History of Psychiatry*, pp. 3-36; pp. 7, 23.
22. Porter, R., "Introduction," in *The Confinement of the Insane: International Perspectives, 1800-1965*, ed. Porter, R., and Wright, D. (Cambridge: Cambridge University Press, 2003); pp. 1-19; p. 2. See also Rogow, A. A., *The Psychiatrists* (New York: G. P. Putnam's Sons, 1970).
23. See Seager, R. H., ed., *The Dawn of Religious Pluralism: Voices from the World's Parliament of Religions, 1893* (LaSalle, IL: Open Court, 1993).

Chapter 1

1. Black, H. C., *Black's Law Dictionary*, rev. 4th ed. (St. Paul: West, 1968), p. 890.
2. Some of the material in this chapter has been adapted from Szasz, T., *Cruel Compassion: The Psychiatric Control of Society's Unwanted* [1994] (Syracuse: Syracuse University Press, 1998), Chapter 6
3. Williams, T., *Memoirs* [1975] (New York: Bantam, 1976), p. 294.
4. Szasz, T., "Defining Disease: The Gold Standard of Disease versus the Fiat Standard of Diagnosis," *The Independent Review*, 10: 325-336 (Winter), 2006.
5. Szasz, T., *Liberation by Oppression: A Comparative Study of Slavery and Psychiatry* (New Brunswick, NJ: Transaction Publishers, 2002).
6. Szasz, T., *Insanity: The Idea and Its Consequences* [1987] (Syracuse: Syracuse University Press, 1997), p. 91.
7. McHugh, P. R., *The Mind Has Mountains: Reflections on Society and Psychiatry* (Baltimore, MD: Johns Hopkins University Press, 2006), p. 5, emphasis added.
8. Bloch, S., and Green, S. A., "An Ethical Framework for Psychiatry," *British Journal of Psychiatry*, 188: 7-12 (January), 2006.
9. Deutsch, A., *The Mentally Ill in America: A History of Their Care and Treatment from Colonial Times*, 2d ed. (New York: Columbia University Press, 1952), p. 2. In this connection, see Hudson, R. P., *Disease and Its Control* (New York: Praeger, 1983).
10. Zilboorg, G., *A History of Medical Psychology*, in collaboration with G. W. Henry (New York: Norton, 1941), pp. 27 and 312-313.
11. Alexander, F. G., and Selesnick, S. T., *The History of Psychiatry: An Evaluation of Psychiatric Thought and Practice from Prehistoric Times to the Present* (New York: Harper & Row, 1966).
12. See Szasz, T., *Pharmacracy: Medicine and Politics in America* [2001] (Syracuse: Syracuse University Press, 2003) and *Liberation by Oppression*.
13. Ibid.
14. Shorter, E., *A History of Psychiatry: From the Era of the Asylum to the Age of Prozac* (New York: Wiley, 1997), p. 1.
15. Ibid.
16. Rothman, D. J., *Conscience and Convenience: The Asylum and Its Alternatives in Progressive America* (Boston: Little, Brown and Company, 1980), p. 21.
17. Beers, C. W., *A Mind That Found Itself: An Autobiography* (1908), 7th ed. (Garden City, NY: Doubleday, 1956).
18. Beers, C. W., quoted in Rothman, D. J., *Conscience and Convenience*, op. cit., pp. 300-301.
19. Ibid., p. 336.
20. Ibid., pp. 347-348.
21. Ibid., pp, 349, 373, 375.
22. Rothman, D. J., *Conscience and Convenience: The Asylum and Its Alternatives in Progressive America*, rev. ed., with a Foreword by Thomas G. Blomberg (New York: Aldine de Gruyter, 2002), p. 10, emphasis added.
23. Blomberg, T., "Foreword," in Rothman, D. J., *Conscience and Convenience*, pp. ix-xiii; p. xi-xii.
24. Quoted in "Brainy Quote," http://205.180.85.40/w/pc.cgi?mid=24098&sid=4345. http://www.losthorizons.com/gq-tyranny.htm.
25. Chesterton, G. K., *Illustrated London News*, 1924, http://quotes.liberty-tree.ca/quote_blog/Gilbert.Keith.Chesterton.Quote.9D5E.
26. La Fond, J. Q., and Durham, M. L., *Back to the Asylum: The Future of Mental Health Law and Policy in the United States* (New York: Oxford University Press, 1992), pp. ix, 3.

27. Grob, G. N., *The Mad Among Us: A History of the Care of America's Mentally Ill* (New York: Free Press, 1994), p. 271.
28. Szasz, T., *The Manufacture of Madness: A Comparative Study of the Inquisition and the Mental Health Movement* [1970] (Syracuse: Syracuse University Press, 1997), pp. xiv-xxv, quoted in Grob, G. N., *The Mad Among Us*, ibid.
29. Sharfstein, S. S., "Individual Rights Must be Balanced with 'Caring Coercion,'" *Psychiatric News*, 40: 3 (September 2), 2005; see also Tannsjo, T., *Coercive Care: The Ethics of Choice in Health and Medicine* (London: Routledge, 1999).
30. Zdanowicz, M. T., "Recovery and Coercion: Reconciling Two Hotbutton Terms," *Catalyst*, Spring 2006, pp. 1 and 4-7; p. 6.
31. Treatment Advocacy Center (TAC), "Briefing Paper," June 2005, http://psychlaws.org/BriefingPapers/BP14.htm.
32. Amador, X., with Johanson, A-L., *I Am Not Sick, I Don't Need Help! Helping the Seriously Mentally Ill Accept Treatment: A Practical Guide for Families and Therapists* (Peconic, NY: Vida Press, 2000), p. 198.
33. Ibid., pp. 40-41, 45, emphasis in the original.
34. Tocqueville, A. de, *The Old Régime and the French Revolution* [1856], trans. Stuart Gilbert (Garden City, NY: Doubleday Anchor, 1955), p. 157. The title of Chapter Three is: "How the desire for reform took precedence over the desire for freedom."
35. Menninger, K., "Reading notes," *Bulletin of the Menninger Clinic*, 53: 350-351 (July), 1989; p. 350.
36. Ibid., p. 351.
37. See, generally, Parry-Jones, W. Ll., *The Trade in Lunacy: A Study of Private Madhouses in England in the Eighteenth and Nineteenth Centuries* (London: Routledge & Kegan Paul, 1976).
38. See Sweetingham, L., "Family Sues after Creative Writing Assignment Lands Teen in Psych Ward," Court TV, February 2, 2006, http://courttv.com/news/2006/0202/riehm_ctv.html?link%20yhlk#continue.
39. Szasz, T., *Cruel Compassion*.
40. Bucknill, J. C., *The Psychology of Shakespeare*, in Hunter, R., and Macalpine, I., *Three Hundred Years of Psychiatry*, pp. 1064-1068.
41. Ibid., p. 1065.
42. Ibid.
43. *Macbeth*, Act V, Scene iii, Lines, 36-39.
44. Ibid., lines 36-44.
45. Ibid., lines 45-46.
46. Engstrom, E. J., *Clinical Psychiatry in Imperial Germany: A History of Psychiatric Practice* (Ithaca, NY: Cornell University Press, 2003), p. 251.
47. Deutsch, A., *The Mentally Ill in America*, op. cit., p. 2.
48. Neugebauer, R., "Diagnosis, Guardianship, and Residential Care of the Mentally Ill in Medieval and Early Modern England," *American Journal of Psychiatry*, 146: 1580-1584 (December), 1989, p. 1580.
49. Ibid., p. 1582.
50. Porter, R., *Mind-Forg'd Manacles: A History of Madness from the Restoration to the Regency* (London: Athlone Press, 1987), pp. 9 and 8, emphasis added.
51. See, Szasz, T., *Law, Liberty, and Psychiatry: An Inquiry into the Social Uses of Psychiatry* [1963] (Syracuse: Syracuse University Press, 1989) and Macalpine, I., and Hunter, R., *George III and the Mad-Business* (New York: Pantheon, 1969).
52. Foucault, M., *Madness and Civilization: A History of Insanity in the Age of Reason* [1961], trans. Richard Howard (New York: Pantheon, 1965).

53. Foucault, M., *Mental Illness and Psychology* (1954), trans. Alan Sheridan (New York: Harper Colophon, 1976), pp. 26, 28.

54. Shorter, E., *A History of Psychiatry*, p. 5. Foucault's thesis remains popular, especially in left-wing circles, because it blames involuntary mental hospitalization on amorphous, capitalist-political forces and thus exonerates psychiatrists.

55. See, generally, Parry-Jones, W. Ll., *The Trade in Lunacy*, op. cit.

56. Ibid., p. 241.

57. Ibid.

58. See Szasz, T., *Liberation by Oppression.*

59. Porter, R., *Mind-forg'd Manacles*, op. cit., p. 88.

60. Quoted in ibid.

61. See Szasz, T., *Cruel Compassion*, chaps. 9 and 10.

62. Hunter, R., and Macalpine, I., *Three Hundred Years of Psychiatry, 1535-1860: A History Presented in Selected English Texts* (New York: Oxford University Press, 1963), p. 196.

63. Cheyne, G., *The English Malady: Or, A Treatise of Nervous Diseases of All Kinds, as Spleen, Vapours, Lowness of Spirits, Hypochondriacal, and Hysterical Distempers, etc.* (London: Strahan & Leake, 1733).

64. Defoe, D., *Augusta Triumphans* (1728), in Hunter, R., and Macalpine, I., *Three Hundred Years*, op. cit., pp. 266-267.

65. Reid, J., *Essays on Insanity, Hypochondriasis, and Other Nervous Affections* (1816), in ibid., pp. 724-725.

66. Szasz, T., *Liberation by Oppression.*

67. Skultans, V., *Madness and Morals: Ideas on Insanity in the Nineteenth Century* (London; Routledge & Kegan Paul, 1975), p. 132.

68. Stevens, J., "The Door in the Wall," http://druglibrary.org/schaffer/lsd/stevens1.htm.

69. Solomon, H., quoted in La Fond, J. Q., and Durham, M. L., *Back to the Asylum: The Future of Mental Health Law and Policy in the United States* (New York: Oxford University Press, 1992), p. 3.

70. 69 Stat. 381 (July 28, 1955), in *U.S. Statutes at Large, 1955*, pp. 381-383; and quoted in Joint Commission on Mental Illness and Health [JCMIH], *Action for Mental Health: Final Report of the Joint Commission on Mental Illness and Health, 1961* (New York: Basic Books, 1961), p. v.

71. JCMIH, *Action for Mental Health*, op. cit., p. 382, emphasis added.

72. See, for example, Langley, M., "Wall Street Star Loses Battle to Depression," *Wall Street Journal*, January 17, 2006.

73. JCMIH, *Action for Mental Health*, op. cit, p. 382. Hereafter also cited as the *Report.*

74. Ibid., p. 277.

75. JCMIH, *Action for Mental Health*, op. cit., p. 39, emphasis added.

76. Ibid., pp. 53-54, emphasis added.

77. Szasz, T. S., *The Myth of Mental Illness,* op. cit.

78. Flynn, L., "The Brain is Back in the Body," *NAMI Advocate*, 13: 16 (July/August) 1992.

79. Sharfstein, S. S., "Privatization: Economic Opportunity and Public Health" (editorial), *American Journal of Psychiatry*, 145: 611-612 (May), 1988; p. 611.

80. Levy, C. J.,"For Mentally Ill, Death and Misery," *New York Times*, April 28, 2002. http://akmhcweb.org/Articles/NYTForMentallyIllDeathandMisery.htm. Subsequent quotes are from this source.

81. State of New York, Department of Health, "State Health Commissioner Announces Further Actions to Protect Residents at Adult Homes in New York State," http://health.state.ny.us/press/releases/2002/adult_homes.htm.

82. Levy, C. J.,"For Mentally Ill, Death and Misery," op. cit.
83. Kissinger, M., "Mentally Ill Suffer Deadly Neglect: With a Promise of Community Care, Psychiatric Wards Were Unlocked 30 Years Ago; Today, the Sickest Patients Live in Squalor," *Milwaukee Journal Sentinel*, March 18, 2006, http://jsonline. com/story/index.aspx?id=409208.
84. Monahan, J., "From the Man Who Brought You Deinstitutionalization," *Contemporary Psychology*, 33: 492 (June), 1988.
85. Bublis, M. D., "Szasz Award" (Letters), *Psychiatric News*, May 15, 1992, p. 16.
86. Isaac, R. J., and Armat, V. C., *Madness in the Streets: How Psychiatry and the Law Abandoned the Mentally Ill* (New York: Free Press, 1990), p. 37.
87. Isaac, R. J., "The Mentally Ill Don't Know They're Sick," *New York Times*, March 2, 1991.
88. Isaac, R. J., and Armat, V. C., *Madness in the Streets*, op. cit., pp. 14-15, 155-156.
89. Regarding the Laing-Szasz linkage, see Szasz, T., "'Knowing What Ain't So': R. D. Laing and Thomas Szasz," *Psychoanalytic Review*, 91: 331-346 (June), 2004; and this volume, chap. 7.
90. Quoted in Schaler, J., "Introduction," in *Szasz Under Fire: The Psychiatric Abolitionist Faces His Critics*, ed. Schaler, J. (Chicago: Open Court, 2004), pp. xiii-xv; pp. xxiii-xxiv.
91. Magnet, M . *The Dream and the Nightmare: The Sixties' Legacy to the Underclass* [1993] (San Francisco: Encounter Books, 2000), pp. 87, 98.
92. Dalrymple, T., "Free to Choose," *City-Journal*, Autumn 1996, http://city-journal. org/html/6_4_oh_to_be.html.
93. Silber, K., "Insight on the News: 1960s AD - Decade," August 30, 1993. http:// findarticles.com/p/articles/mi_m1571/is_n35_v9/ai_13284587.
94. Charen, M., "Lock Up Those Who Need Psychiatric Care," *Jewish World Review*, July 29, 1998. http://jewishworldreview.com/cols/charen072998.html.
95. Charen, M., *Do-Gooders: How Liberals Hurt Those They Claim to Help--and the Rest of Us* (New York: Sentinel, 2004), p. 166.
96. In this connection, see Vatz, R. E., and Weinberg, L. S., "The Rhetorical Paradigm in Psychiatric History: Thomas Szasz and the Myth of Mental Illness," in *Discovering the History of Psychiatry*, ed. Micale, M. S., and Porter, R. (New York: Oxford University Press, 1994), http://szasz.com/vatz2.html.
97. "Frederick Wiseman," http://en.wikipedia.org/wiki/Frederick_Wiseman.
98. "Film on State Hospital Provocative After 20 Years," *New York Times*, May 17, 1987, http://query.nytimes.com/gst/fullpage.html?sec=health&res=9B0DE2DD1 F3DF934A25756C0A961948260, emphasis added.
99. Goodman, W., "An Unhealthy Hospital Stars in 'Titicut Follies'," *New York Times*, April 6, 1993, http://query.nytimes.com/gst/fullpage.html?res=9F0CE3D9173DF 935A35757C0A965958260.
100. Shimkus, J., "Bridgewater State Hospital a Model of Integration," http://ncchc. org/pubs/CC/profiles/17-4.html.
101. Editorial, "How to House the Mentally Ill," *New York Times*, October 26, 1989, emphasis added.
102. Applebaum, P., "Crazy in the Streets," *Commentary*, May 1987, pp. 34-39; p. 38.
103. Ibid., p. 39.
104. Lamb, R., "Will We Save the Homeless Mentally Ill?" *American Journal of Psychiatry*, 147: 649-651 (May), 1990, p. 650; quoted in, Isaac, R. J., and Armat, V. C., *Madness in the Streets*, op. cit., p. 160, emphasis added.

105. Wilson, J. Q., quoted approvingly in Will, G. F., "Nature and the Male Sex," *Newsweek*, June 17, 1991, p. 70.
106. Krauthammer, C., "*Brown v. Board of Re-education*: How to Save the Homeless Mentally Ill," *New Republic*, February 8, 1988, pp. 22-25.
107. Will, G., "Community Has Right to Remove Homeless," *Post-Standard* (Syracuse), November 19, 1987.
108. Olasky, M., *The Tragedy of American Compassion* (Chicago: Regnery, 1992), p. 211, emphasis added.
109. Poole, L., "Developers Turning Lunatic Asylums into Luxury Condos," Associated Press, April 11, 2006, http://articles.news.aol.com/business/article.adp?id=20060 411165809990005&cid=2194.
110. Belli, M. M., "Warning of the Dangerous Patient: A Practical Approach," *American Journal of Forensic Psychiatry*, 2: 6-7, 1981-82; p. 6.
111. Szasz, T., "Szasz on the Dangerous Patient," *American Journal of Forensic Psychiatry*, 2: 6-7 & 17, 1981-82; pp. 6-7.
112. Szasz, T., *Liberation by Oppression*.
113. Leinwand, D., "Secret-telling Sparks Some Ethical Conflicts," *USA Today*, July 30, 2001, Internet edition.
114. Appelbaum, P. S. *Almost a Revolution: Mental Health Law and the Limits of Change*. New York: Oxford University Press, 1994, p. 103.
115. Ibid., p. 100.
116. Jamison, K. R., "Mental illness: End the Stigma, Treat the Disease" (Letter), *New York Times*, December 17, 1999, Internet edition.
117. Jamison, K. R., quoted in Butterfield, F., "Massachusetts Gun Laws Concerning Mentally Ill Are Faulted," *New York Times*, January 14, 2001, Internet edition, and *An Unquiet Mind: A Memoir of Mood and Madness* (New York: Knopf, 1995), p. 113.
118. Satel, S., "For Addicts, Force is the Best Medicine," *Wall Street Journal*, January 7, 1998, p. 6.
119. Satel, S., "Real Help for the Mentally Ill," *New York Times*, January 7, 1999, Internet edition, http://eppc.org/publications/xq/ASP/pubsID.63/qx/pubs_viewdetail.htm, emphasis added.
120. Pekkanen, J., Washington's Best and Brightest: Roots of Mental Illness--E. Fuller Torrey, Psychiatrist, *Washingtonian*, December 2001, http://psychlaws.org/GeneralResources/article65.htm.
121. Szasz, T., *Insanity: The Idea and Its Consequences* [1987] (Syracuse: Syracuse University Press, 1997); *Liberation by Oppression*.
122. The Treatment Advocacy Center, http://psychlaws.org/.
123. Wikipedia, "E. Fuller Torrey," http://en.wikipedia.org/wiki/E._Fuller_Torrey.
124. Torrey, E. F., "A Lesson from Minnesota and California," *The Catalyst*, January-February, 2001, p. 3, http://psychlaws.org/JoinUs/CatalystArchive/CatalystV3N1.pdf.
125. Ibid.
126. Fritz, M., "Strong Medicine: More Forced Care for the Mentally Ill," *Wall Street Journal*, February 1, 2006, p. A1, http://online.wsj.com/article_email/ SB113876185080261746-lMyQjAxMDE2MzA4MTcwNjExWj.html.
127. Stone, A. A., *Law, Psychiatry, and Morality*, (Washington, D.C.: APA Press, 1985), p. 140.
128. Sandford, J. J., "Public Health Psychiatry and Crime Prevention," *British Medical Journal*, May 15, 1999. http://findarticles.com/m0999/7194_318/54851600/p1/article.jhtml.
129. Quoted in Dewey, R., "The Jury Law for Commitment of the Insane in Illinois (1867-1893), and Mrs. E.P.W. Packard, Its Author, also Later Developments in

Lunacy Legislation in Illinois," *American Journal of Insanity,* 69: 571-584 (January), 1913; for details, see Szasz, T. S., *The Manufacture of Madness,* pp. 15, 130-132.

130. *Kansas v. Leroy Hendricks, No. 95-1649.* "Excerpts from Opinions on Status of Sex Offenders," *New York Times,* June 24, 1997, p. B11, emphasis added.

131. Daly, R., "Governor Bypasses Legislature, Orders Commitments," *Psychiatric News,* 40: 5-6 (November 18), 2005, http://pn.psychiatryonline.org/cgi/content/full/40/22/5. Subsequent quotes are from this source.

132. American Psychiatric Association, Council of Psychiatry and Law, "Final Report of the Sub-Committee to Review the Insanity Defense Position," Mimeographed, November 11-13, 1988, pp. 1-11; pp. 3 and 1, emphasis added. I am indebted to Abraham Halpern, M.D. for alerting me to this report and furnishing me with a copy of it.

133. Krupp, B, "A Hospital is Not a Prison," *The Providence (RI) Journal,* November 27, 2005, http://projo.com/opinion/contributors/content/projo_20051127_27krupp.223204b9.html.

134. Ibid.

135. Ibid.

136. Mooney, T., "Doctor Quits over Efforts to Detain Sexual Predator," *The Providence (RI) Journal,* November 8, 2005, http://projo.com/news/content/projo_20051108_krupp8.173eebb9.html.

137. Sharfstein, S., "Hospital or Prison? Psychiatric Care For the Sexual Offender," *Psychiatric News,* 41: 3 (January 20), 2006; in this connection, see Note 68 above and Mansnerus, L, "Unfinished Sentences: Keeping Prisoners as Patients; Questions Rise Over Imprisoning Sex Offenders Past Their Terms," *New York Times,* November 17, 2003, http://query.nytimes.com/gst/fullpage.html?res=9C07E7D71138F934A25752C1A9659C8B63&sec=health&pagewanted=2.

138. See Szasz, T., "Primum nocere." *The Freeman,* 54: 24-25 (December) 2004.

139. Szasz, T., *Liberation by Oppression.*

140. Durham, M. L., "Civil Commitment of the Mentally Ill: Research, Policy, and Practice," in *Mental Health and Law: Research, Policy, and Services,* ed. Sales, Bruce D., and Shah, Saleem A. (Durham, NC: Carolina Academic Press, 1996), pp. 17-40; p. 17.

141. Szasz, T., "Voluntary Mental Hospitalization: An Unacknowledged Practice of Medical Fraud," *New England Journal of Medicine* 287: 277-278 (August 10), 1972.

142. Redlich, F. C., and Freedman, D. X., *The Theory and Practice of Psychiatry* (New York: Basic Books, 1966), p. 781. They refer to my paper, Szasz, T., "Commitment of the Mentally Ill: 'Treatment' or Social Restraint?," *Journal of Nervous and Mental Disease,* 125: 293-307 (April-June), 1957.

143. Jaspers, K., *General Psychopathology* [1913, 1946], 7th ed., Trans. J. Hoenig and M. W. Hamilton (Chicago: University of Chicago Press, 1963), pp. 839-840.

144. Mariner, J., "Prisons as Mental Institutions: The Mass Incarceration of the Mentally Ill," October 23, 2003, http://writ.news.findlaw.com/mariner/20031027.html, emphasis added.

145. Smith, M. B., *For a Significant Social Psychology: The Collected Writings of M. Brewster Smith* (New York: New York University Press, 2003), p. 215.

146. Deutsch, A., *The Shame of the States* (New York: Harcourt, Brace and Company, 1948).

147. Mariner, J., "Prisons as Mental Institutions: The Mass Incarceration of the Mentally Ill," October 23, 2003, http://writ.news.findlaw.com/mariner/20031027.html.

148. Human Rights Watch, "More Mentally Ill in Prison Than in Hospitals," October 22, 2003, http://hrw.org/english/docs/2003/10/22/usdom6472.htm, and Mariner, J., "Prisons as Mental Institutions," op. cit.

149. Martel, N., "Review: The New Asylums: An Image of Prisons as a Warehouse for the Mentally Ill," http://pbs.org/wgbh/pages/frontline/shows/asylums/etc/synopsis. html. "The New Asylums," David Fanning, executive producer; produced, written, and directed by Miri Navasky and Karen O'Connor. Produced by WGBH Boston and co-produced by Mead Street Films, http://movies.nytimes.com/2005/05/10/ arts/television/10mart.html? Subsequent quotes are from this source.

150. Chekhov, A. P., *Ward No. 6*, in Szasz, T., ed., *The Age of Madness: A History of Involuntary Mental Hospitalization Presented in Selected Texts* (Garden City, NY: Doubleday Anchor, 1973), pp. 89-126.

151. Editorial, "Today's 'Snake Pit'," *Westchester Journal News*, September 21, 2002. http://thejournalnews.com/newsroom/092102/21edmentallyill.html.

152. Frueh, B. C., et al., "Special Section on Seclusion and Restraint: Patients' Reports of Traumatic or Harmful Experiences within the Psychiatric Setting," *Psychiatric Services*, 56: 1123-1133 (September) 2005.

153. Frueh, B. C., Grubaugh, A. L., and Robins, C. S., "Elimination of Seclusion and Restraint: A Reasonable Goal?" (Letters) *Psychiatric Services*, 57: 578 (April), 2006.

154. Lieberman, R. P., "Elimination of Seclusion and Restraint: A Reasonable Goal?" (Letters) *Psychiatric Services*, 57: 576 (April), 2006.

155. BBC, "Forced Treatment of Mentally Ill Doubles," October 29, 1999, http://news. bbc.co.uk/hi/english/health/newsid_493000/493643.stm.

156. Healy, D., *The Creation of Psychopharmacology* (Cambridge: Harvard University Press, 2002), p. 329.

157. Ibid., p. 344.

158. See this volume, chap. 8.

159. Healy, D., *The Creation of Psychopharmacology*, op. cit, p. 346.

160. American Psychiatric Association, *Diagnostic and Statistical Manual of Mental Disorders--IV-TR*, 4th ed., text rev. (Washington, D C: American Psychiatric Association, 2000).

161. Sadock, B. J., and Sadock, V. A., *Kaplan and Sadock's Synopsis of Psychiatry: Behavioral Sciences/Clinical Psychiatry,* 9th ed. (Philadelphia: Lippincott Williams & Wilkins, 2003), pp. 999-1000.

162. Cosgrove, L., et al., "Financial Ties between DSM-IV Panel Members and the Pharmaceutical Industry," *Psychotherapy and Psychosomatics*, 75: 154-160 (April), 2006; Vedantam, S., "Experts Defining Mental Disorders Are Linked to Drug Firms," *Washington Post*, April 19, 2006, p. A7, http://washingtonpost. com/wp-dyn/content/article/2006/04/19/AR2006041902560_pf.html.

163. Rothman, D., quoted in Graham, J., "Top Mental Health Guide Questioned," *Chicago Tribune,* April 20, 2006, http://chicagotribune.com/news/nationworld/ chi-0604200194apr20,1,3690657.story?coll=chi-newsnationworld-hed.

164. See Szasz, T., *Ceremonial Chemistry: The Ritual Persecution of Drugs, Addicts, and Pushers* [1976] (Syracuse: Syracuse University Press, 2003); *Our Right to Drugs: The Case for a Free Market* [1992] (Syracuse: Syracuse University Press, 1996); *Pharmacracy: Medicine and Politics in America* [2001] (Syracuse: Syracuse University Press, 2003).

165. Lezon, D., "Bond Set for Andrea Yates," *Houston Chronicle,* February 1, 2006, emphasis added, http://chron.com/disp/story.mpl/front/3628275.html.

166. Lieberman, E. J., "Pharmacracy or Phantom?" in *Szasz Under Fire: The Psychiatric Abolitionist Faces His Critics*, ed. Schaler, J. (Chicago: Open Court, 2004), pp. 225-241; p. 229.

Chapter 2

1. Eliot, T. S., *The Cocktail Party* (London: Faber and Faber, 1974), p. 111.
2. See Szasz, T., *The Myth of Mental Illness: Foundations of a Theory of Personal Conduct* [1961], rev. ed. (New York: HarperCollins, 1974); *The Manufacture of Madness: A Comparative Study of the Inquisition and the Mental Health Movement* [1970] (Syracuse: Syracuse University Press, 1997); *The Myth of Psychotherapy: Mental Healing as Religion, Rhetoric, and Repression* [1978] (Syracuse: Syracuse University Press, 1988); and Zilboorg, G., *A History of Medical Psychology*, in collaboration with G. W. Henry (New York: Norton, 1941).
3. Zilboorg, G. *A History of Medical Psychology*, pp. 216, 226, 230, emphasis added.
4. Quoted in Sartre Online, http://geocities.com/sartresite/articles_praxis_1.html.
5. Szasz, T., *The Myth of Mental Illness*, rev. ed., op. cit., pp. 181-198.
6. Patton, A. S., *A Doctor's Dilemma: William Griggs and the Salem Witch Trials* (Salem, MA: The Salem Witch Museum, 1998), p. 3. See also Linder, D., "Salem Witchcraft Trials, 1692," http://law.umkc.edu/faculty/projects/ftrials/salem/SALEM.HTM.
7. Patton, A. S., *A Doctor's Dilemma*, op. cit., p. 11.
8. Upham, C., quoted in ibid., p. 22.
9. Mackay, C. *Extraordinary Popular Delusions and the Madness of Crowds* [1841, 1852]. With a Foreword by Bernard M. Baruch (New York: Noonday Press, 1962).
10. Patton, A. S., *A Doctor's Dilemma*, op. cit., pp. 43-44.
11. Linder, D., "Salem Witchcraft Trials, 1692," http://law.umkc.edu/faculty/projects/ftrials/salem/SALEM.HTM.
12. Sargant, W., *Battle for the Mind: A Physiology of Conversion and Brainwashing* (1957) (New York: Harper & Row/Perennial Library, 1971), p. 129, emphasis in the original.
13. For a cogent discussion of the modern version of the "sin model of mental illness," see Weckowicz, T., *Models of Mental Illness: Systems and Theories of Abnormal Psychology* (Springfield, IL: Charles C. Thomas, 1984), pp. 312-313.
14. Ward, M. J., *The Snake Pit* (London: Cassel, 1947), http://raintreecounty.com/SnakePit.html.
15. Hunter, R., and Macalpine, I., eds., *Three Hundred Years of Psychiatry, 1535-1860: A History Presented in Selected English Texts* (London: Oxford University Press, 1963), p. 254, emphasis added.
16. Kraepelin, E., "The Directions of Psychiatric Research" (1886), *History of Psychiatry*, 16: 350-364 (September), 2005, p. 356, emphasis in the original.
17. Hunter, R. and Macalpine, I., eds., *Three Hundred Years of Psychiatry*, op. cit., p, 254.
18. Ibid.
19. Van Helmholt, F. M., *The Spirit of Disease; Or, Diseases from the Spirit* (1694), quoted in ibid., pp. 255-256, emphasis added.
20. Philadelphia Hospital: The First Mental Hospital, http://geocities.com/paexplorations/MentalHistory.html.
21. Willis, T., "Of Madness, the Curatory Indications," in Hunter, R. and Macalpine, I., eds. *Three Hundred Years of Psychiatry*, p. 191, emphasis added.
22. Ibid., p. 187.
23. Ibid., p. 192.
24. National Institute of Neurological Disorders and Stroke, "NINDS Shaken Baby Syndrome Information Page," http://ninds.nih.gov/disorders/shakenbaby/shakenbaby.

25. Darwin, E., *Zoonomia* (1801), quoted in Wade, N. J., Norssell, U., and Presly, A., "Cox's Chair: 'Moral and Medical Means in the Treatment of Maniacs,'" *History of Psychiatry*, 16: 73-88 (March), 2005; p. 74.

26. The book was translated into German in 1811, and in 1813 a third edition of it was published in English.

27. Wade, N. J., Norssell, U., and Presly, A., "Cox's Chair," p. 77.

28. Ibid., pp. 78, 80.

29. Rush, B., *Medical Inquiries and Observations upon the Diseases of the Mind* [1812] (New York: Macmillan-Hafner Press, 1962), p. 211.

30. Ibid., pp. 265-266.

31. Brown, E. M., "Who was Benjamin Rush?," Rhode Island District Branch, American Psychiatric Association, *Newsletter,* July 1997, vol.29, no.4, pp. 2-3, http://bms.brown.edu/HistoryofPsychiatry/Rush.html.

32. University of Pennsylvania Health Systems, Dr. Benjamin Rush, http://uphs.upenn.edu/paharc/features/brush.html.

33. Rush, B., "Letter to Granville Sharp" (1774), in Woods, J. A., "The Correspondence of Benjamin Rush and Granville Sharp, 1773–1809," *Journal of American Studies*, 1: 8, 1967.

34. Quoted in Binger, C., *Revolutionary Doctor: Benjamin Rush, 1746–1813* (New York: Norton), p. 281.

35. Rush, B., *Lectures on the Medical Jurisprudence of the Mind* [1810], in *The Autobiography of Benjamin Rush: His 'Travels through Life' Together with His 'Commonplace Book for 1789–1812,'"* ed. Corner, G. W. (Princeton, NJ: Princeton University Press, 1948), p. 350.

36. Rush, B., *Medical Inquiries and Observations upon the Diseases of the Mind*, op. cit., pp. 273-274.

37. Quoted in Boorstin, D. J., *The Lost World of Thomas Jefferson* (Boston: Beacon Press, 1948), p. 182.

38. Quoted in Butterfield, L. H., ed., *Letters of Benjamin Rush* (Princeton, NJ: Princeton University Press, 1951), p. 1092.

39. Rush, B., *Medical Inquiries and Observations upon the Diseases of the Mind*, op. cit., pp. 263-270.

40. Rush, B., *Lectures on the Medical Jurisprudence of the Mind*, op. cit., p. 264.

41. Heinroth, J. C., *Textbook of Disturbances of Mental Life, or Disturbances of the Soul and Their Treatment* [1818], 2 vols., trans. J. Schmorak (Baltimore, MD: Johns Hopkins University Press, 1975).

42. Ibid., vol. 1, p. 25.

43. Ibid., p. 21.

44. Moore, M. S., "Some Myths about 'Mental Illness,'" *Archives of General Psychiatry*, 32: 1483-1497 (December), 1975; p. 1495.

45. *A Midsummer Night's Dream,* V, i-ii.

46. Heinroth, J. C., *Textbook of Disturbances of Mental Life,* op. cit., p. 16, emphasis added.

47. Burke, E., "A Letter from Mr. Burke to a Member of the National Assembly in Answer to Some Objections to His Book on French Affairs" [1791], in Burke, E., *The Works of the Right Honorable Edmund Burke*, 12 vols. (Boston: Wells & Lilly, 1826), vol. 3, p. 315.

48. Szasz, T., *Liberation by Oppression.*

49. Heinroth, J. C., *Textbook of Disturbances of Mental Life,* op. cit., p. 236, emphasis added.

50. Ibid., p. 25.

51. Ibid., p. 413.

52.   Ibid., p. 124. This particular observation of Heinroth's is not without merit. Albeit aphoristically, I have characterized schizophrenia as "the cancer of conceit." Szasz, T., *Words to the Wise: A Medical-Philosophical Dictionary* (New Brunswick, NJ: Transaction, 2003), p. 198.

53.   Heinroth, J. C., *Textbook of Disturbances of Mental Life,* op. cit., p. 28.

54.   Ibid., p. 29.

55.   Ibid., p. 332.

56.   Ibid., p. 415, emphasis added.

57.   Hunter, R. and Macalpine, I., eds., *Three Hundred Years of Psychiatry.*

58.   Heinroth, J. C., *Textbook of Disturbances of Mental Life, or Disturbances of the Soul and Their Treatment* [1818], p. 294, emphasis added.

59.   Several web sites display the picture of this mask and offer copies for sale. See "Kropserkel: Hannibal Lecter restraint mask," http://kropserkel.com/lecter.htm. Lecter's mask was not designed to prevent him from speaking.

60.   Quoted in Kraepelin, E., *One Hunded Years of Psychiatry* [1917] (New York: Philosophical Library, 1962), pp. 70-71.

61.   See http://medizin.uni-tuebingen.de/daten/jubilaeum/Wer_war_eigentlich_Ferdinand_Autenrieth.pdf.

62.   Thompson, S. J., "Friedrich Hölderlin (1770-1843): A Chronology of His Life," http://www.wbenjamin.org/hoelderlin_chron.html.__.

63.   Vida, I., "A pszichiátria Hölderlin korában" ("Psychiatry in Hölderlin's day"), Orvostörténeti Közlemények, 1998, http://members.iif.hu/visontay/ponticulus/limes/hölderlin.html.

64.   Bergmann, H., "Scardanelli--Hölderlin Madman," http://agdok.de/GermanDocumentaries/gD415.htm. For more information about Walser, see Szasz, T., *Liberation by Oppression*, pp. 136-145.

65.   Http://dictionary.reference.com/wordoftheday/archive/2003/12/21.html.

66.   Catholic Encyclopedia, "Anchorites," http://newadvent.org/cathen/01462b.htm.

67.   Aghiorgoussis, M. E., "The Orthodox Monastic Tradition," http://goarch.org/print/en/ourfaith/article7103.asp.

68.   Nietzsche, F., "Letter to Franz Overbeck, March 6, 1883," quoted in Schain, R., *The Legend of Nietzsche's Syphilis* (Westport, CT: Greenwood, 2001), p. 26.

69.   Schain, R., *The Legend of Nietzsche's Syphilis*, op. cit., pp. 25, 49.

70.   Kaufman, W., "Editor's Preface," in *The Portable Nietzsche*, ed. and trans. Walter Kaufman (New York: Viking, 1954), pp. 103-111; p. 103.

71.   Nietzsche, F., "Preface," *Ecce Homo* (1888/1908), compiled from translations by Walter Kaufmann, R. J. Hollingdale, and Anthony M. Ludovici, http://geocities.com/thenietzschechannel/eh.htm, emphasis in the original.

72.   Nietzsche, F., *Thus Spoke Zarathustra*, in Bramann, J. K., "Nietzsche's Zarathustra," http://faculty.frostburg.edu/phil/forum/Zarathustra.htm. Centre Bouddhiste de l'Ile de France, "Thus Spake Zarathustra," http://centrebouddhisteparis.org/En_Anglais/Sangharakshita_en_anglais/Nietzsche_and_Superman/Zarathustra/zarathustra.html.

73.   Nietzsche, F., *Thus Spoke Zarathustra: A Book for One and None* (1883-1885/1891), in *The Portable Nietzsche*, ed. Walter Kaufman (New York: Viking, 1954), pp. 112-439; p.123, emphasis added.

74.   Nietzsche, F., "Letter to Otto Eiser, January 1880," quoted in Schain, R., *The Legend of Nietzsche's Syphilis*, op. cit., p. 26.

75.   Nietzsche, *Ecce Homo*, quoted in ibid., p. 28.

76.   Ozick, C., "Writers Domestic and Demonic," *New York Times*, March 25, 1984, http://dictionary.reference.com/wordoftheday/archive/2003/12/21.html.

77.   Woolf, V., *On Being Ill* (London: Hogarth Press, 1930), p. 18.

Chapter 3

1. Quoted in Engstrom, E. J., *Clinical Psychiatry in Imperial Germany: A History of Psychiatric Practice* (Ithaca, NY: Cornell University Press, 2003), p. 251.
2. University of Toledo Libraries, "Mental Health," http://cl.utoledo.edu/canaday/quackery/quack5.html, emphasis added.
3. *Dorland's Illustrated Medical Dictionary*, http://mercksource.com/pp/us/cns/cns_hl_dorlands.jspzQzpgzEzzSzppdocszSzuszSzcommonzSzdorlandszSzdorlandzSzdmd_i_09zPzhtm, emphasis added.
4. Grob, G. N., *Mental Illness and American Society, 1875-1940* (Princeton, NJ: Princeton University Press, 1983), p. 3.
5. Quoted in Hunter, R., and Macalpine, I., eds., *Three Hundred Years of Psychiatry, 1535-1860: A History Presented in Selected English Texts* (London: Oxford University Press, 1963), p. 685.
6. Ibid.
7. Quoted in ibid., p. 689.
8. Ibid., p. 687, emphasis added.
9. Digby, A., "Moral Treatment at the Retreat, 1796-1846," in *The Anatomy of Madness: Essays in the History of Psychiatry*, 3 vols., ed. Bynum, W. F., Porter, R., and Shepherd, M. (London: Tavistock, 1985-1988), vol. 2, pp. 52-72; p. 53, emphasis added.
10. Conolly, J., quoted in Hunter, R., and Macalpine, I., eds., *Three Hundred Years of Psychiatry,* op. cit, p. 808, emphasis added.
11. Elsewhere, Hunter and Macalpine refer to Conolly's having been able "to abolish all mechanical restraint," ibid., p. 956. However, along with mechanical restraints, mad-doctors were already using chemical restraints as well. For more on this subject, see chap. 5.
12. Quoted in Hunter, R., and Macalpine, I., eds., *Three Hundred Years of Psychiatry,* op. cit., p. 200 (From Booth, W., *Darkest England and the Way Out* [London: The Salvation Army, 1890]).
13. Szasz, T., *The Myth of Mental Illness: Foundations of a Theory of Personal Conduct* [1961], rev. ed. (New York: HarperCollins, 1974).
14. "Pinel," http://en.wikipedia.org/wiki/Philippe_Pinel; http://en.wikipedia.org/wiki/Philippe_Pinel.
15. Ibid. and "Philippe Pinel," http://whonamedit.com/doctor.cfm/1027.html.
16. Deutsch, A., *The Mentally Ill in America: A History of Their Care and Treatment from Colonial Times*, 2d ed. (New York: Columbia University Press, 1952), pp. 88-113.
17. Pinel, P., *A Treatise on Insanity* [1801, 1806], trans. D. D. Davis (New York: Hafner Publishing Company, 1962). Facsimile of the 1806 edition.
18. Ibid., pp. 27-28.
19. Ibid., p. 60.
20. Ibid., p. 69.
21. Ibid., p. 87.
22. Ibid., pp. 187-188.
23. Ibid., p. 288.
24. Ryn, C. G. *The New Jacobinism: Can Democracy Survive?* (Washington, DC: National Humanities Institute, 1991).
25. Szasz, T. *Pharmacracy: Medicine and Politics in America* [2001] (Syracuse: Syracuse University Press, 2003).
26. Lewis, C. S., "The Humanitarian Theory of Punishment" [1953], in Lewis, C. S., *God in the Dock: Essays on Theology and Ethics*, ed. Walter Hooper (Grand Rapids, MI: William B. Eerdmans, 1970), pp. 287-294; p. 293.

27.   "Mental Health (History) Dictionary," http://mdx.ac.uk/www/study/mhhglo. htm#DateOrder.
28.   Zilboorg, G. *A History of Medical Psychology*, in collaboration with G. W. Henry (New York: Norton, 1941), pp. 287-290.
29.   Kraepelin, E., *One Hundred Years of Psychiatry* [1917] (New York: Philosophical Library, 1962), p. 152, emphasis added.
30.   Ibid.
31.   Zilboorg, G. *A History of Medical Psychology*, op. cit., p. 292; Kraepelin, E., *One Hundred Years of Psychiatry*, op. cit., p. 15.
32.   Zilboorg, G., *A History of Medical Psychology*, op. cit., p. 438.
33.   Kraepelin, E., *One Hundred Years of Psychiatry*, op. cit, p. 70.
34.   "Wilhelm Griesinger," http://bms.brown.edu/HistoryofPsychiatry/griesinger. html.
35.   Ibid.
36.   Meynert, T. *Psychiatry: Clinical Treatise on Diseases of the Forebrain* [1884], trans. B. Sachs (New York: G. P. Putnam's Sons, 1885), p. v, emphasis in the original.
37.   Qvarsell, R., "Locked Up or Put to Bed: Psychiatry and the Treatment of the Mentally Ill in Sweden, 1800-1920," in *The Anatomy of Madness: Essays in the History of Psychiatry*, ed. Bynum, W. F., Porter, R., and Shepherd, M. (3 vols., London: Tavistock, 1985-1988), vol. 2, pp. 86-97; p. 93.
38.   Deutsch, A., *The Mentally Ill in America.*, op. cit., p. 90.
39.   Ibid., pp. 91-92, emphasis added.
40.   Zilboorg, G. *A History of Medical Psychology,* op. cit., p. 415.
41.   Deutsch, A., *The Mentally Ill in America.*, op. cit., pp. 132-157.
42.   Ibid., p. 137.
43.   Quoted in ibid., p. 153.
44.   Quoted in ibid., p. 151.
45.   Ibid., p. 151.
46.   Ibid., p, 157.
47.   Bumb, J., "Dorothea Dix," http://civilwarhome.com/dixbio.htm.
48.   Deutsch, A., *The Mentally Ill in America*, op. cit., p. 176.
49.   Dix, D., quoted in ibid., p. 177.
50.   Deutsch, A., ibid.
51.   Emphasis added. For the entire text of "Franklin Pierce's Veto of May 3, 1854," see http://disabilitymuseum.org/lib/docs/682.htm.
52.   Deutsch, A., *The Mentally Ill in America*, op. cit., p. 179.
53.   Ibid., p, 184.
54.   The material in this section is condensed from Szasz, T. *Fatal Freedom: The Ethics and Politics of Suicide* [1999] (Syracuse: Syracuse University Press, 2002), chap. 3.
55.   Szasz, T., "Abortion: Punish the Woman?" *Daily Orange* (Syracuse University), October 19, 1976, p. 3.
56.   Szasz, T., *Pharmacracy: Medicine and Politics in America* [2001] (Syracuse: Syracuse University Press, 2003).

Chapter 4

1.   http://worldofquotes.com/topic/Grave/1/.
2.   See Goodman, L., and Gilman, A., *The Pharmacological Basis of Therapeutics* (New York: Macmillan, 1941).
3.   See Szasz, T., *Ceremonial Chemistry: The Ritual Persecution of Drugs, Addicts, and Pushers* [1976] (Syracuse: Syracuse University Press, 2003); see also this volume, chaps. 7, 8.

4.   Ambien is a product of the Sanofi-Aventis Group, http://arthritis.about.com/b/
     a/201395.htm.
5.   Owens, D.G.C. *A Guide to the Extrapyramidal Side-effects of Antipsychotic Drugs*
     (Cambridge: Cambridge University Press, 1999), p. 11.
6.   Healy, D., *The Creation of Psychopharmacology* (Cambridge, MA: Harvard
     University Press, 2002), p. 50.
7.   Quoted in Pearce, J.M.S., "Silas Weir Mitchell and the 'rest cure,'" *Journal of
     Neurology Neurosurgery and Psychiatry,* 75: 381, 2004, http://jnnp.bmjjournals.
     com/cgi/content/full/75/3/381.
8.   Whonamedit: "Silas Weir Mitchell," http://whonamedit.com/doctor.cfm/959.html.
9.   Mitchell, S. W. *Fat and Blood: Or Hints for the Overworked [Fat and Blood: And
     How to Make Them]* (Philadelphia: J. B. Lippincott Co., 1878), ed. and intro.
     Michael S. Kimmel (Walnut Creek, CA: Altamira Press, 2004), pp. 43-46.
10. Ibid., p. 99, emphasis added.
11. See Gilman, C. P., *The Yellow Wallpaper* [1892], ed. Dale M. Bauer (Boston:
     Belford / St. Martin's, 1998).
12. See Szasz, T., *"My Madness Saved Me": The Madness and Marriage of Virginia
     Woolf* (New Brunswick, NJ: Transaction Publishers, 2006), pp. 103-105.
13. Zilboorg, G. *A History of Medical Psychology,* in collaboration with G. W. Henry
     (New York: Norton, 1941), p. 443.
14. Mitchell, S. W. *Fat and Blood,* op. cit., pp. 28, 37.
15. Szasz, T., *"My Madness Saved Me,"* op. cit.
16. See this volume, chap. 6.
17. Williams, R. L., and Webb, W. B., *Sleep Therapy: A Bibliography and Commentary*
     (Springfield, IL: Charles C. Thomas, 1966), p. 8.
18. Clapp, J. S., and Loomis, E. A., "Continuous Sleep Treatment: Observations on
     the Use of Prolonged, Deep, Continuous Narcosis in Mental Disorders," *American
     Journal of Psychiatry,* 106: 821-829,1950; also this volume, chaps. 5, 6.
19. Williams, R. L., and Webb, W. B., *Sleep Therapy,* op. cit., p. 5.
20. McGraw, R. B., and Oliven, J. F., "Miscellaneous Therapies," in *American Hand-
     book of Psychiatry,* 3 vols., ed. Arieti, S. (New York: Basic Books, 1959-1966);
     vol. 2 (1959), pp. 1552-1582; p. 1572.
21. Freedman, A. M., Kaplan, H. I., and Sadock, B. J., *Modern Synopsis of Compre-
     hensive Textbook of Psychiatry/II,* 2d ed. (Baltimore, MD: Williams & Wilkins,
     1976), p. 1000.
22. Healy, D., *The Creation of Psychopharmacology* (Cambridge, MA: Harvard
     University Press, 2002), pp. 44-45, emphasis added.
23. Kuhn, R., "From Imipramine to Levoprotiline: The Discovery of Antidepressants,"
     in ibid., pp. 93-118.
24. Ellenberger, Henri F., *The Discovery of the Unconscious: The History and Evolu-
     tion of Dynamic Psychiatry* (New York: Basic Books, 1970), p. 642.
25. Ibid., p. 842, emphasis added.
26. Ibid., p. 859.
27. Ibid., p. 856.
28. Ibid., p. 857.
29. Janet, P.M.F, quoted in Williams, R. L., and Webb, W. B., *Sleep Therapy,* op. cit., p. 3.
30. Ibid., p. 7.
31. For a relevant, remarkably naive confusion of diagnosis and disease, see Meador,
     C. K., "The Art and Science of Nondisease," *New England Journal of Medicine,*
     272: 92-95 (January 14), 1965. For clarification, see Szasz, T., "Diagnoses Are
     Not Diseases," *The Lancet* (London), 338: 1574-1576 (December 21-28), 1991.

32.   Delay, J., Deniker, P., and Pauwels, R., *"Cures de sommeil et cures neuroleptique en psychiatrie"* ("Sleep Treatments and Neuroleptic Treatments in Psychiatry"), *L'Encéphale*, 45: 436-439, 1956.

33.   Lempérière, T., "In the Beginning in Paris," in *The Psychopharmacologists—III: Interviews by Dr. David Healy*, ed. Healy, D. (London: Chapman & Hall, 2000), pp. 1-15; p. 2.

34.   Divry, P., Bobon, J., and Collard, J., *"Considérations sur les cures de sommeil potentialisées et les cures neuroleptique en psychiatrie"* (Considerations Concerning Potentialized Sleep Treatments and Neuroleptic Treatments in Psychiatry"), *Acta Neurologica et Psychiatrica Belgica*, 57: 185-201 (March), 1957; p. 201. "Summary" in English.

35.   "Pavlov," http://en.wikipedia.org/wiki/Ivan_Pavlov.

36.   Wortis, J., "Foreword," in Andreev, B. V., *Sleep Therapy in the Neuroses* (1959), translated from the Russian by Basil Haigh (New York: Consultants Bureau, 1960), pp. 3-5; p. 3.

37.   Ibid., p. 4.

38.   Andreev, B. V., *Sleep Therapy in the Neuroses*, pp. 7, 11, 64.

39.   Ibid., p. 95.

40.   Dufresne, T., "An Interview with Joseph Wortis," *Psychoanalytic Review*, 83: 589-610 (August), 1996; pp. 608-609, emphasis added.

41.   Green, C. D., Introduction to "Psychology as the Behaviorist Views It," originally posted 1997. Last revised December 2001, http://psychclassics.yorku.ca/Watson/intro.htm.

42.   Ibid.

43.   Boeree, C. G., "B. F. Skinner," http://ship.edu/~cgboeree/skinner.html, emphasis added.

Chapter 5

1.   Jackson, J. H., *Selected Writings of John Hughlings Jackson*, 2 vols., ed. James Taylor (London: Staples Press, 1958), vol. 2, p. 59.

2.   Pearce, J.M.S., "Positive and Negative Cerebral Symptoms: The Roles of Russell Reynolds and Hughlings Jackson," *Journal of Neurology Neurosurgery and Psychiatry*, 75: 1148, 2004, http://jnnp.bmjjournals.com/cgi/content/full/75/8/1148.

3.   Reynolds, J. R., *Epilepsy,* quoted in, Hunter, R., and Macalpine, I., eds., *Three Hundred Years of Psychiatry, 1535-1860: A History Presented in Selected English Texts* (London: Oxford University Press, 1963), p. 1047.

4.   Maudsley, H., quoted in Hill, D., "Historical Review," in Reynolds, E. H., and Trimble, M. R., eds., *Epilepsy and Psychiatry* (London: Churchill Livingstone, 1981), pp. 1-11; p. 4.

5.   Maudsley, H., *Responsibility in Mental Disease*, 4th ed. (London: Kegan Paul, Trench & Co., 1885), p. 41.

6.   Ibid., pp. 156, 165.

7.   For details, see Szasz, T., *Cruel Compassion: The Psychiatric Control of Society's Unwanted* [1994] (Syracuse: Syracuse University Press, 1998), pp. 43-62.

8.   Shanahan, W. T., "History of the Development of Special Institutions for Epileptics in the United States," *Psychiatric Quarterly*, 2: 422-434, 1928; p. 423, emphasis added.

9.   Ibid., emphasis added.

10.   See, Goodman, L., and Gilman, A., *The Pharmacological Basis of Therapeutics* (New York: Macmillan, 1941), p. 155.

11. Grant, R., "Special Centres," in Reynolds, E. H. and Trimble, M. R., eds., *Epilepsy and Psychiatry,* pp. 347-355, p. 350.

12. Deutsch, A., *The Mentally Ill in America: A History of Their Care and Treatment from Colonial Times,* 2d ed. (New York: Columbia University Press, 1952), pp. 383-384; emphasis added.

13. Zabriskie, E. G., "Epilepsy," in *A Textbook of Medicine,* 5th ed., rev., ed. Cecil, R. L. (Philadelphia: Saunders, 1942), pp. 1626, 1631.

14. Adams, R. D., "Idiopathic Epilepsy," in *Harrison's Principles of Internal Medicine,* 7th ed., ed. Wintrobe, M. M. et al. (New York: McGraw-Hill, 1974), p. 1868.

15. Forster, F. M., and Booker, H. E., "The Epilepsies and Convulsive Disorders," in *Clinical Neurology,* rev. ed., ed. Joynt, R. J. (Philadelphia: Lippincott, 1988), p. 58.

16. Epilepsy Foundation of America, "Protecting Your Legal Rights," in *Living Well with Epilepsy,* ed. Gumnit, R. J. (New York: demos Publications, 1990), pp. 135-141; pp. 135, 139.

17. Trimble, M. R., "Greater Understanding Perceived of Link between Epilepsy and Psychiatry," *Psychiatric Times,* 6: 16 and 25 (February), 1989, p. 16.

18. Livingston, S., "Epilepsy and Murder" (Editorial), *JAMA,* 188: 164 (April 13), 1964.

19. Hamilton, S. W., "The History of American Mental Hospitals," in *One Hundred Years of American Psychiatry, 1844-1944,* ed. Hall, J. K. et al. (New York: Columbia University Press, 1944), pp. 123-124; emphasis added.

20. Ibid., p. 124.

21. http://epilepsyfoundation.org/epilepsyusa/yrc/yrctreating.cfm.

22. Sabbatini, R.M.E., "The History of Shock Therapy in Psychiatry," http://cerebromente.org.br/n04/historia/shock_i.htm. Ibid.

23. Healy, D., *The Creation of Psychopharmacology* (Cambridg, MA: Harvard University Press, 2002), pp. 42, 50.

24. Ibid., p. 53.

25. Ibid., p. 55.

26. Ibid., pp. 53-54.

27. Sabbatini, R.M.E., "The History of Shock Therapy in Psychiatry," op. cit.

28. Lehmann, H., "Psychopharmacotherapy," in *The Psychopharmacologists: Interviews by Dr. David Healy,* ed. Healy, D. (London: Chapman & Hall, 1996), pp. 159-186; pp. 166-167.

29. "Ladislas J. Meduna," http://en.wikipedia.org/wiki/Ladislas_J._Meduna

30. Ibid.

31. Alexander, F. G., and Selesnick, S. T., *The History of Psychiatry: An Evaluation of Psychiatric Thought and Practice from Prehistoric Times to the Present* (New York: Harper & Row, 1966), p. 281.

32. Bleuler, E., *Dementia Praecox, or the Group of Schizophrenias* [1911], trans. Joseph Zinkin (New York: International Universities Press, 1950), p. 175.

33. Bunker, H. A., "American Psychiatric Literature During the Past One Hundred Years," in *One Hundred Years of American Psychiatry,* pp. 258-259.

34. Sabbatini, R.M.E., "The History of Shock Therapy in Psychiatry," http://cerebromente.org.br/n04/historia/shock_i.htm#sakel.

35. Ibid.

36. Rosack, J., "Depression, Epilepsy Link Puzzles Researchers," *Psychiatric News,* 40: 32 (November 4), 2005, http://pn.psychiatryonline.org/cgi/content/full/40/21/32?maxtoshow=&HITS=10&hits=10&RESULTFORMAT=&searchid=1132351973593_6304&stored_search=&FIRSTINDEX=0&sortspec=relevance&volume=40&firstpage=32&journalcode=psychnews.

37.   Szasz, T., *Fatal Freedom: The Ethics and Politics of Suicide* [1999] (Syracuse: Syracuse University Press, 2002).
38.   Cerletti, U., "Old and New Information about Electroshock," *American Journal of Psychiatry*, 1950, http://23nlpeople.com/electroshock_Cerletti.htm, emphasis added.
39.   Ibid., emphasis added.
40.   Cerletti, U., "Electroshock Therapy," in *The Great Physiodynamic Therapies in Psychiatry: An Historical Reappraisal*, ed. Sackler, A. M., Sackler, M. D., Sackler, R. R., and Marti-Ibanez F. (New York, Hoeber-Harper, 1956), pp., 91-120; pp. 92-94, emphasis added.
41.   For further details, see Szasz, T., "From the Slaughterhouse to the Madhouse," *Psychotherapy*, 8:64-67 (Spring), 1971.
42.   Di Cori, F., "In Memoriam (Cerletti)," *Journal of Neuropsychiatry*, 5: 1-2 (September-October), 1963.
43.   Ayd, F. T. Jr., "Guest Editorial: Ugo Cerletti, M.D., 1877-1963," *Psychosomatics*, 4: A6-A7 (November-December), 1963.
44.   Shutts, D., *Lobotomy: Resort to the Knife* (New York: Van Nostrand Reinhold Company, 1982), p. 95.
45.   Kesey, K., "Letter," in *Madness Network News Reader*, ed. Sherry Hirsch et al. (San Francisco: Glide Publications, 1974); also at http://szasz.com/kesey.pdf.
46.   Kneeland, Timothy W., and Carol A. B. Warren. *Pushbutton Psychiatry: A History of Electroshock in America* (Westport, CT: Praeger, 2002), p. 85.
47.   Ibid., pp. 99-100.
48.   Fink, M., *Electroshock: Restoring the Mind* (New York: Oxford University Press, 1999); and "Max Fink, the Grandfather of American ECT," http://healthyplace.com/Communities/Depression/ect/shame/fink.asp.
49.   Fink, M., "A New Appreciation of ECT," *Psychiatric Times*, vol. 23, April 2004. http://psychiatrictimes.com/showArticle.jhtml?articleID=175802377. Subsequent quotes are from this source.
50.   For an understanding of the meaning of Nuland's depression, see Nuland, S. B., *Lost in America: A Journey with My Father* (New York: Knopf, 2003), and especially the review of it by Morris Dickstein, "'Lost in America': The Rise of Shep Nudelman," *New York Times Book Review*, February 9, 2003. http://nytimes.com/2003/02/09/books/review/09DICKSTT.html?ex=1045758573&ei=1&en=b5 6d4ef2d28d36b2.
51.   Fink, M., "A new appreciation of ECT."
52.   Shakespeare, W., *Julius Caesar*, I, ii, 140-141.
53.   "The Journal of ECT," http://ectjournal.com/pt/re/ject/home.htm;jsessionid=D2f9n YM79eYgcuxuALyCF1I0BoFW2QavO697DwfLt5DOSawbE9Qf!1405829113!-949856145!9001!-1.
54.   "Max Fink," http://ect.org/shame/fink.html.
55.   Friedberg, J., *Shock Treatment is Not Good for Your Brain* (San Francisco: Glide Publications, 1976); and "Shock Treatment, Brain Damage, and Memory Loss: A Neurological Perspective," *American Journal of Psychiatry*, 134: 1010-1013 (September), 1977, http://idiom.com/~drjohn/amjpsych.html.
56.   Samant, S., "Brain, Mind, and Language. Shocking Therapy: Electroconvulsive Therapy (ECT) Today," http://23nlpeople.com/ECT.htm.
57.   Quoted in Friedberg, J., "Electroshock: Epitomizing the Myth," 2000, http://idiom.com/~drjohn/maxfink.html; http://mentalhealthconsumers.org/connet/cnn/9910/shock.htm.
58.   Gillmor, D., *I Swear by Apollo: Dr. Ewen Cameron and the CIA-Brainwashing Experiments* (Montreal: Eden Press 1987), p. 1; Charron, M., "Ewen Cameron

and The Allan Memorial Psychiatric Institute: A Study in Research and Treatment Ethics," http://sfu.ca/~wwwpsyb/issues/2000/summer/charron.htm; and Collins, A., *In the Sleep Room: The Story of the CIA Brainwashing Experiments in Canada* (Toronto: Lester & Orpen Dennys, 1988).

59. Canadian Broadcasting Corporation, "MKULTRA, 'Dr.' Ewen Cameron Psychiatrist and Torturer," Documentary, "The Fifth Estate," January 6, 1998, http://mk.net/~mcf; http://raven1.net/cameron.htm; all further quotes are from this source.

60. Marks, J., *The Search for the "Manchurian Candidate": The CIA and Mind Control* (New York: Times Books, 1979), pp. 137, 214.

61. Marks, J., *The Search for the "Manchurian Candidate,"* op. cit., p. 141, emphasis added.

62. Ban, T. A., "They Used to Call It Psychiatry," in *The Psychopharmacologists: Interviews by Dr. David Healy*, pp. 587-620; p. 601.

63. Ibid.

64. Ibid., pp. 604, 605, emphasis added.

65. Ibid.

66. Marks, J., *The Search for the "Manchurian Candidate,"* op. cit., p. 140.

67. Paris, J., "History of the McGill Department of Psychiatry," May 1, 1998. http://medicine.mcgill.ca/psychiatry/history.htm.

68. Szasz, T., "Patriotic Poisoners," *Humanist*, 36: 5-7 (November-December), 1976; reprinted in Szasz, T., *The Therapeutic State: Psychiatry in the Mirror of Current Events* (Buffalo: Prometheus Books, 1984), pp. 170-174.

69. "History of Magnetism and Electricity," http://rare-earth-magnets.com/magnet_university/history_of_magnetism.htm.

70. For an in-depth review and discussion of Mesmer's work and its historical significance, see Szasz, T., *The Myth of Psychotherapy: Mental Healing as Religion, Rhetoric, and Repression* [1978] (Syracuse: Syracuse University Press, 1988), pp. 43-66.

71. Ellenberger, Henri F., *The Discovery of the Unconscious: The History and Evolution of Dynamic Psychiatry* (New York: Basic Books, 1970), p. 53 ff; Zilboorg, G. *A History of Medical Psychology,* in collaboration with G. W. Henry (New York: Norton, 1941), p. 347 ff.

72. Szasz, T. *Pharmacracy: Medicine and Politics in America* [2001] (Syracuse: Syracuse University Press, 2003); *The Theology of Medicine: The Political-Philosophical Foundations of Medical Ethics* [1977] (Syracuse: Syracuse University Press, 1988); *The Therapeutic State: Psychiatry in the Mirror of Current Events.*

73. "Vagus Nerve Stimulation," http://emedicine.com/neuro/topic559.htm; "Vagus Nerve Stimulation for Treating Depression," http://healthyplace.com/communities/depression/treatment/vns/index.asp.

74. Ibid.

75. Columbia University Medical Center, "Nerve-Stimulation Therapy for Patients with Treatment-Resistant Depression Now Available in New York," http://cumc.columbia.edu/news/press_releases/VNS_therapy.html.

76. Harris, G., "Device Won Approval though F.D.A. Staff Objected," *New York Times*, February 17, 2006, http://nytimes.com/2006/02/17/politics/17fda.html, emphasis added.

77. Ibid.

78. "Expanding Horizons: Vascular Surgeons Train in New York on Vagus Nerve Stimulation," http://emediawire.com/releases/2005/11/emw310623.htm.

79. Fischman, J., "Fixing Your Brain: When Pills Fail, Electrical Iimplants Can Mend Brains Damaged by Parkinson's, Stroke, and Depression," *U. S. News & World*

Report, February 20, 2006, http://usnews.com/usnews/health/articles/060220/20brain.htm.

80. Dobbs, D., "A Depression Switch?," *New York Times Magazine,* April 2, 2006.http://nytimes.com/2006/04/02/magazine/02depression.html?pagewanted=7&_r=1.

81. "Brain 'Pacemaker' for Depression Sufferers," http://technovelgy.com/ct/Science-Fiction-News.asp?NewsNum=345.

82. Dobbs, D., "A Depression Switch?," op. cit. Subsequent quotes are from this source.

83. "Deep Impact: A Way of Switching Depression Off," *Economist,* March 3, 2005, http://wireheading.com/brainstim/antidepressant.html.

84. "Transcranial Magnetic Stimulation," BlueCross BlueShield Association, Medical Policy Reference Manual, April 2, 2002, http://regence.com/trgmedpol/mental-Health/mh17.html.

85. Gershon, A. A., Dannon, P. N., and Grunhaus, L., "Transcranial Magnetic Stimulation in the Treatment of Depression," *American Journal of Psychiatry,* 160: 835-45 (May), 2003, http://biopsychiatry.com/tms.htm.

86. Foreman, J., "New Depression Therapy Intriguing," *Boston Globe,* June 8, 1998, p. C1, http://boston.com/globe/search/stories/health/health_sense/060898.htm.

87. Travis, J., "Snap, Crackle, and Feel Good? Magnetic Fields That Map the Brain May also Treat Its Disorders," *Science News,* week of September 23, 2000; vol. 158, no. 13, p. 204, http://sciencenews.org/articles/20000923/bob10.asp.

88. Quoted in ibid.

89. Rosch, P. J., "International Congress on 'Stress': How It All Began," http://newmediaexplorer.org/chris/2004/09/16/bioelectromagnetic_medicine_the_book.htm.

90. Antonioli, C., and Reveley, M. A., "Randomised Controlled Trial of Animal Facilitated Therapy with Dolphins in the Treatment of Depression," *British Medical Journal,* 331: 1231 (November 26), 2005, http://bmj.bmjjournals.com/cgi/content/full/331/7527/1231, emphasis added.

91. Goldsmith, M., *Franz Anton Mesmer: A History of Mesmerism* (New York: Doubleday, 1934), p. 148.

92. Ibid., p. 151.

93. Ibid., p. 153.

94. Ibid.

95. James, W., "A Plea for Psychology as a 'Natural Science,'" *Philosophical Reviews,* 1: 146-153, 1892.

Chapter 6

1. Quoted in Arendt, H. *Eichmann in Jerusalem: A Report on the Banality of Evil* (New York: Viking, 1963), p. 64.

2. El-Hai, J., *The Lobotomist: A Maverick Medical Genius and His Tragic Quest to Rid the World of Mental Illness* (Hoboken, NJ: Wiley, 2005); Scull, A., "A Monster or a Medical Genius?," *Los Angeles Times,* April 24, 2005, http://latimes.com/\features/health/medicine/la-bk-scull24apr24,1,7980705.story?coll=la-health-medicine.

3. Valenstein, E. S., *Great and Desperate Cures: The Rise and Decline of Psychosurgery and Other Radical Treatments for Mental Illness* (New York: Basic Books, 1986).

4. "The Nobel Assembly at Karolinska Institutet awards the Nobel Prize in Physiology and Medicine," http://mednobel.ki.se/.

5. Szasz, T., *The Theology of Medicine: The Political-Philosophical Foundations of Medical Ethics* [1977] (Syracuse: Syracuse University Press, 1988).

6. Weil, M., "Rosemary Kennedy, 86; President's Disabled Sister," *Washington Post,* January 8, 2005, p. B6.

7.   Leamer, L., *The Kennedy Men, 1901-1963: The Laws of the Father* (New York: William Morrow, 2001), p. 168.
8.   Ibid., pp. 168-169.
9.   Leamer, L., *The Kennedy Women: The Saga of an American Family* (New York: Villard Books/Random House, 1994), p. 319.
10. Leamer, L., *The Kennedy Men,* op. cit., p. 169, and *The Kennedy Women,* p. 321.
11. Ibid., p. 170.
12. Leamer, L., *The Kennedy Women,* p. 323.
13. Leamer, L., *The Kennedy Men,* op. cit., p. 170.
14. http://kennedyinstitute.georgetown.edu/site/index.htm.
15. Weil, M., "Rosemary Kennedy, 86; President's Disabled Sister," p. B6, emphasis added.
16. El-Hai, Jack. *The Lobotomist,* p. 173, emphasis added.
17. Leamer, L., *The Kennedy Men,* op. cit., pp. 171, 279.
18. Leamer, L., *The Kennedy Women,* op. cit., p. 412.
19. Ibid.
20. Ibid., pp. 573-574.
21. Kennedy, J. F., quoted in, Torrey, E. F., *Nowhere to Go: The Tragic Odyssey of the Homeless Mentally Ill* (New York: Harper & Row, 1988), p. 108.
22. Ibid.
23. From Kennedy's "Inaugural Address," January 20, 1961, http://www.arlingtocem-etery.net/jfk.htm.
24. Leamer, L., *The Kennedy Men,* op. cit., p. 170.
25. Ibid.
26. Leamer, L., *The Kennedy Women,* op. cit., p. 574.
27. Weil, M., "Rosemary Kennedy, 86; President's Disabled Sister," p. B6.
28. Leamer, L., *The Kennedy Women,* op. cit., pp. 319, 364, emphasis added.
29. Ozarin, L. D., "William A. White, M.D.: A Distinguished Achiever," *Psychiatric News,* January 1, 1999, http://psych.org/pnews/99-01-01/hx.html.
30. Valenstein, E. S., *Great and Desperate Cures,* op. cit., p. 145.
31. Nuland, S., "'Killing Cures': An Exchange," *New York Review of Books,* November 3, 2005, p. 73.
32. El-Hai, J., *The Lobotomist,* p. 168.
33. Http://amazon.com/exec/obidos/tg/detail/-/0471232920/qid=1115084754/sr=8-1/ref=sr_8_xs_ap_i1_xgl14/103-1292605-5023862?v=glance&s=books&n=507846.
34. Valenstein, E. S., *Great and Desperate Cures,* op. cit., p. 218.
35. El-Hai, J., *The Lobotomist,* op. cit, p. 71, emphasis added.
36. Scull, A., "A Monster or a Medical Genius?," op. cit.
37. El-Hai, J., *The Lobotomist,* op. cit, p. 168.
38. Ibid., p. 77.
39. Ibid., op. 118.
40. El-Hai, J., *The Lobotomist,* op. cit, p. 116.
41. Ibid., p. 77.
42. Jacobson, P., "Sweden is Rocked by Scandal of Forced Lobotomies," *Sunday Telegraph* (London), April 12, 1998.
43. See Szasz, T., "In the Church of America, Psychiatrists are Priests," *Hospital Physician,* October, 1971, pp. 44-46.
44. Sargant, W., *The Unquiet Mind: The Autobiography of a Physician in Psychological Medicine* (London: Pan Books, 1967), p. 64.
45. Sargant, W., *The Unquiet Mind,* op. cit., p, 59.

46. Ibid., p. 93.
47. Quoted in "William Sargant," http://en.wikipedia.org/wiki/William_Sargant.
48. Sargant, W.,*The Unquiet Mind,* op. cit., pp. 107, 152.
49. Ibid., p. 161.
50. There is a vast literature on this subject. See for example, Centers for Disease Control and Prevention, "The Tuskegee Syphilis Study," http://cdc.gov/nchstp/od/tuskegee/time.htm.
51. American Scientist, http://americanscientist.org/template/SiteOfTheWeekType-Detail/assetid/21792;jsessionid=aaa5wXlGe31xoy.
52. Jansson, B., "Controversial Psychosurgery Resulted in a Nobel Prize," http://nobelprize.org/medicine/articles/magnets/. Originally published October 29,1998; reprinted December 29, 2004. Subsequent quotes refer to this source.
53. See, for example, Gordon, R., *Great Medical Disasters* (New York: Stein & Day, 1983).
54. Lothane, Z., *In Defense of Schreber: Soul Murder and Psychiatry* (Hillsdale, NJ: Analytic Press, 1992); and Schatzman, M., *Soul Murder: Persecution in the Family* (London: Allen Lane, 1973).
55. "At 100, Alfred Nobel's Legacy Retains Its Luster," *Science,* 294: 291 (October) 2001, http://sciencemag.org.
56. Http://psychosurgery.org/index_files/Page2782.htm.
57. Ibid., emphasis added.
58. Sutherland, J., "Should They De-Nobel Moniz? What Happens When a Nobel Prize Winner is Subsequently Exposed as a Fraud? Nothing, apparently," *The Guardian,* August 2, 2004, http://education.guardian.co.uk/higher/columnist/story/0,9826,1274355,00.html.
59. McGrath, C., "A Lobotomy That He Says Didn't Touch His Soul," *New York Times,* November 16, 2005, http://nytimes.com/2005/11/16/arts/16lobo.html.
60. National Public Radio (NPR), "All Things Considered: 'My Lobotomy:' Howard Dully's Journey," November 16, 2005, http://npr.org/templates/story/story.php?storyId=5014080; further quotes about the story are from this source.
61. Szasz, T., *Fatal Freedom: The Ethics and Politics of Suicide* [1999] (Syracuse: Syracuse University Press, 2002).
62. Valenstein, E. S., *Great and Desperate Cures: The Rise and Decline of Psychosurgery and Other Radical Treatments for Mental Illness* (New York: Basic Books, 1986).
63. Ibid., p. 3.
64. Shutts, D., *Lobotomy: Resort to the Knife* (New York: Van Nostrand Reinhold Company, 1982), p. 112.
65. Quoted in Frank, L. R., ed., *The Random House Webster's Quotationary* (New York: Random House, 1999), p. 786. *Inter alia,* Hoch poisoned patients with psychoactive drugs on behalf of the CIA. See Szasz, T., "Patriotic Poisoners," *Humanist,* 36: 5-7 (November-December), 1976. Reprinted in Szasz, T., *The Therapeutic State: Psychiatry in the Mirror of Current Events* (Buffalo: Prometheus Books, 1984), pp. 170-174.
66. Ibid., p. 154.
67. Valenstein, E. S., *Great and Desperate Cures,* op. cit., p. 45, emphasis added.
68. Quoted in Halgin, R. P., "Taking Sides," http://dushkin.com/text-data/catalog/0072917091.mhtml?SECTION=TOC.
69. "Undaunted by Mistakes of the Past, a New Generation of Brain Surgeons is Ready to Step in When Pills and Therapy Fail," *Chicago Tribune Magazine,* April 24, 2005, p. 16, and Alliance for Human Research Protection, "A Come Back for Psychosurgery?," August 6, 2003, http://ahrp.org/infomail/03/08/06.php, emphasis added; http://cornellphysicians.com/jfins/biography.html.

70. Szasz, T., "Voluntary Mental Hospitalization: An Unacknowledged Practice of Medical Fraud," *New England Journal of Medicine*, 287: 277-278 (August 10), 1972; and *Liberation by Oppression: A Comparative Study of Slavery and Psychiatry* (New Brunswick, NJ: Transaction Publishers, 2002).

71. Szasz, T., *Sex By Prescription* [1980] (Syracuse: Syracuse University Press, 1990); "Self-Mutilation," http://wso.williams.edu/~atimofey/self_mutilation/.

72. Szasz, T., *Fatal Freedom: The Ethics and Politics of Suicide* [1999] (Syracuse: Syracuse University Press, 2002).

73. Herbert, W., "Psychosurgery Redux," *U.S .News & World Report*, November 3, 1997. http://findarticles.com/p/articles/mi_m1218/is_n17_v123/ai_n12437986.

74. Ibid.

Chapter 7

1. Pauling, L., "Academic address," in *Biological Treatment of Mental Illness*, ed. Rinkel, M. (New York: L. C. Page/Farrar, Straus and Giroux, 1966), pp. 30-39; p. 32.

2. Ban, T. A., "Pharmacotherapy of Mental Illness: A Historical Analysis," *Progress in Neuro-Psychopharmacology & Biological Psychiatry*, 25: 709-727 (2001); p. 712.

3. See Szasz, T., *Ceremonial Chemistry: The Ritual Persecution of Drugs, Addicts, and Pushers* [1976] (Syracuse: Syracuse University Press, 2003).

4. Zweig, S., *Master Builders* (1936), http://historyguide.org/europe/zweig.html, emphasis added.

5. See, for example, Ginsberg, T., "Donations Tie Drug Firms and Nonprofits: Many Patient Groups Reveal Few, If Any, Details on Relationships with Pharmaceutical Donors," *Philadelphia Inquirer*, May 28, 2006, http://philly.com/mld/inquirer/14687073.htm.

6. See Szasz, T., *Ceremonial Chemistry*; *Our Right to Drugs: The Case for a Free Market* [1992] (Syracuse: Syracuse University Press, 1996).

7. Szasz, T., *Pharmacracy: Medicine and Politics in America* [2001] (Syracuse: Syracuse University Press, 2003).

8. Robitscher, J., "The Impact of New Legal Standards on Psychiatry, or Who Are David Bazelon and Thomas Szasz and Why Are They Saying Such Terrible Things about Us? or Authoritarianism versus Nihilism in Legal Psychiatry," *Journal of Psychiatry and Law*, 3: 151-174 (Summer), 1975; see also Robitscher, J., *The Powers of Psychiatry* (Boston: Houghton Mifflin, 1980).

9. See Owens, D.G.C., *A Guide to the Extrapyramidal Side-effects of Antipsychotic Drugs* (Cambridge: Cambridge University Press, 1999), and Kleinfield, N. R., "In Diabetes, One More Burden for the Mentally Ill," *New York Times,* June 12, 2006, http://nytimes.com/2006/06/12/health/12diabetes.html?

10. Ban, T. A., "Pharmacotherapy of Mental Illness: A Historical Analysis," p. 718.

11. Ibid., p. 720.

12. Healy, D., "Contra Pfizer," *Ethical Human Psychology & Psychiatry*, 7: 181-195 (Fall-Winter), 2005, http://springerpub.com/journalsamples/contra_Pfizer.pdf.

13. For an early, perceptive critique of the fakeries of the psychiatrist in the courtroom, see the writings of Karl Kraus (1874-1936). Szasz, T., *Anti-Freud: Karl Kraus's Criticism of Psychoanalysis and Psychiatry* [1976] (Syracuse: Syracuse University Press, 1990), chap. 7.

14. Healy, D., "Contra Pfizer," *Ethical Human Psychology & Psychiatry*, pp. 194, 181.

15. The State of New Mexico, 42nd Legislature, First Session (1995), Senate Bill 459, March 24, 1995. Copyright © 1995 by Information for Public Affairs, Inc.,

http://dtek.chalmers.se/~d3rebas/humor/archive/11.txt. I thank my friend Robert Spillane for providing this story, and my daughter Susan Szasz Palmer for verifying its authenticity.

16. Thuillier, J., "Ten Years that Changed Psychiatry," in *The Psychopharmacologists—II: Interviews by Dr. David Healy*, ed. Healy, D. (London: Chapman & Hall, 2000), pp. 543-559; p. 544.

17. Domino, E. F., "History of Modern Psychopharmacology: A Personal View with an Emphasis on Antidepressants," *Psychosomatic Medicine*, 61:591-598, 1999, http://psychosomaticmedicine.org/cgi/content/full/61/5/591; Boeree, C. G., "A Brief History of Psychopharmacology," http://ship.edu/~cgboeree/psychopharm.html.

18. Laborit, H., quoted in, Johnson, A. B., *Out of Bedlam: The Truth About Deinstitutionalization* (New York: Basic Books, 1990), p. 40.

19. Cohen, S., and Scull, A., eds., *Social Control and the State* (New York: St. Martin's Press, 1983), p. 80.

20. PBS, "People and Discoveries,"1998, http://pbs.org/wgbh/aso/databank/entries/dh52dr.html. Also at http://pbs.org/wgbh/aso/ontheedge/pill/indext.html.

21. Comité Lyonnais de Recherches Thérapeutiques en Psychiatrie, "The Birth of Psychopharmacotherapy: Explorations in a New World, 1952-1968,"in *The Psychopharmacologists—III: Interviews by Dr. David Healy*, ed. Healy, D. (London: Chapman & Hall, 2000), pp. 1-53; p. 29.

22. Ibid.

23. Ibid., p. 26.

24. Thuillier, J., "Ten Years That Changed Psychiatry," pp. 543-559; pp. 556-557, emphasis added.

25. Healy, D., "Preface," in *The Psychopharmacologists—III: Interviews by Dr. David Healy*, ed. Healy, D. (London: Chapman & Hall, 2000), pp. xiii-xxiii; p. xix.

26. Szasz, T., *The Manufacture of Madness: A Comparative Study of the Inquisition and the Mental Health Movement* [1970] (Syracuse: Syracuse University Press, 1997).

27. Healy, D., "Psychopharmacology and the Government of the Self," http://pharmapolitics.com/feb2healy.html; also at http://academyanalyticarts.org/healy.htm, emphasis added.

28. Ibid., emphasis added.

29. Healy, D., *The Creation of Psychopharmacology* (Cambridge, MA: Harvard University Press, 2002), dust jacket.

30. Ibid., p. 4.

31. Healy, D., *The Psychopharmacologists—III*, p. xxxiv.

32. Massachusetts Mental Health Center, "Psychobiology of Major Affective Disorders," http://massmentalhealthcenter.org/research/programs-programpages-majoraffective.htm.

33. "Chemical Imbalance Theory," http://en.wikipedia.org/wiki/Chemical_imbalance_theory.

34. Kleinfield, N. R., "In Diabetes, One More Burden for the Mentally Ill," *New York Times*, June 12, 2006, http://nytimes.com/2006/06/12/health/12diabetes.html? Subsequent quotes are from this source.

35. Szasz, T., *Schizophrenia: The Sacred Symbol of Psychiatry* [1976] (Syracuse: Syracuse University Press, 1988).

36. Tamminga, C., "Practical Treatment Information for Schizophrenia"(Editorial), *American Journal of Psychiatry*, 163: 563-565 (April) 2006, http://ajp.psychiatryonline.org/cgi/content/full/163/4/563.

37. http://quotations.home.worldnet.att.net/johannwolfgangvongoethe.html.
38. Cole, Jonathan. "The Evaluation of Psychotropic Drugs," in *The Psychopharmacologists: Interviews by Dr. David Healy*, ed. Healy, D. (London: Chapman & Hall, 1996), pp. 239-263; p. 241.
39. Klein, D., "Reaction Patterns to Psychotropic Drugs and the Discovery of Panic Disorder," in Healy, D., *The Psychopharmacologists: Interviews by Dr. David Healy*, pp. 329-352; p. 344.
40. Szasz, T. S., "Some Observations on the Use of Tranquilizing Agents," *A.M.A. Archives of Neurology and Psychiatry*, 77: 86-92 (January), 1957; p. 91.
41. Finn, S. E., et al., "Subjective Utility Ratings of Neuroleptics in Treating Schizophrenia," *Psychological Medicine*, 20: 843-848, 1990, p. 848, emphasis added. And, generally, see Langreth, R., and Herper, M., "Pill Pushers: How the Drug Industry Abandoned Science for Salesmanship," *Forbes*, May 8, 2006, pp. 94-102, http://forbes.com/business/forbes/2006/0508/094a.html?_requestid=5098.
42. Wikipedia, "Prohibition in the United States," http://en.wikipedia.org/wiki/Prohibition#Prohibition_in_the_United_States.
43. See Szasz, T., *Liberation by Oppression: A Comparative Study of Slavery and Psychiatry* (New Brunswick, NJ: Transaction Publishers, 2002).
44. Olfson, M., et al., "Awareness of Illness and Nonadherence to Antipsychotic Medications among Persons with Schizophrenia," *Psychiatric Services*, 57: 205-211 (February) 2006.
45. Klein, D., "Reaction Patterns to Psychotropic Drugs and the Discovery of Panic Disorder," in Healy, D., *The Psychopharmacologists: Interviews by Dr. David Healy*, pp. 329-352; p. 344.
46. Cole, J., "The Evaluation of Psychotropic Drugs," in Healy, D., *The Psychopharmacologists: Interviews by Dr. David Healy*, pp. 239-263; p. 250.
47. Ibid., pp. 246, 241.
48. Ibid., p. 246, emphasis added.
49. Praag, H. Van, "Psychiatry and the March of Folly?" in Healy, D., *The Psychopharmacologists: Interviews by Dr. David Healy*, pp. 353-379; p. 357.
50. Ibid., pp. 367, 368.
51. Ibid., p. 372.
52. Proctor, R. N., *The Nazi War on Cancer* (Princeton, NJ: Princeton University Press, 1999), p. 46.
53. Praag, H. Van, "Psychiatry and the March of Folly?" in Healy, D., *The Psychopharmacologists*, op. cit., p. 378.
54. Ibid., pp. 375, 376.
55. National Institute of Psychobiology in Israel, "Founding Chairman: Prof. Joel Elkes,"http://psychobiology.org.il/hibol/elkes.html.
56. Elkes, J., "Towards Footings in a New Science: Psychopharmacology, Receptors, and the Pharmacy Within," in Healy, D., *The Psychopharmacologists—II*, pp. 183-213; p. 194, emphasis added.
57. Lasagna, L., "Back to the Future: Evaluation and Drug Development, 1948-1998,"in Healy, D., *The Psychopharmacologists—II*, pp. 135-165; p. 153.
58. Sandler, M., "The Place of Chemical Pathology in Psychopathology," in Healy, D., *The Psychopharmacologists*, pp. 383-400; p. 385.
59. Kline, N., quoted in, Brody, J.,"A Simple Salt Promises Relief of Mania," *New York Times*, April 2, 1970.
60. "The Nathan S. Kline Institute for Psychiatric Research," http://rfmh.org/nki.
61. Orwell, G., *The Collected Essays, Journalism and Letters of George Orwell*, 4 vols., ed. Sonia Orwell and Ian Angus (Harmondsworth: Penguin, 1970), vol. 4, p. 145.

62. See Szasz, T., "Patriotic Poisoners," *Humanist,* 36: 5-7 (November-December), 1976; reprinted in Szasz, T., *The Therapeutic State: Psychiatry in the Mirror of Current Events* (Buffalo: Prometheus Books, 1984), pp. 170-174.

63. See, Schaler, J., ed., *Szasz Under Fire: The Psychiatric Abolitionist Faces His Critics* (Chicago: Open Court, 2004), pp. xix-xxi, 396-397.

64. Quoted in Marks, John. *The Search for the "Manchurian Candidate": The CIA and Mind Control* (New York: Times Books, 1979), p. 67. See Hoch, P. H., Cattell, J. P., and Pennes, H. H., "Effects of Mescaline and Lysergic Acid (d-LSD-25)," *American Journal of Psychiatry,* 108: 579-584 (February), 1952.

65. Kalinowsky, L. B., "In Memoriam, Paul H. Hoch," *Proceedings of the Annual Meeting of the American Psychopathological Association,* 55: 326-329, 1967.

66. See also, for example, Healy, D., *The Creation of Psychopharmacology* (Cambridge, MA: Harvard University Press, 2002).

67. "Prisons in the United States," http://en.wikipedia.org/wiki/United_States_prison_population.

68. Wilkinson, R. A., "Testimony on Offenders with Mental Illness in the Criminal Justice System," September 21, 200, http://drc.state.oh.us/web/Articles/article70.htm. Subsequent quotations are from this source.

69. Johnson, K., "TV Screen, Not Couch, is Required for this Session," *New York Times,* June 8, 2006, http://nytimes.com/2006/06/08/us/08teleshrink.html.

70. Butterfield, F., "Prisons: The Nation's New Mental Institutions," *New York Times,* reprinted in *CAPT Outreach Magazine,* February 2000, http://psych-health.com/mental8.htm. Subsequent quotes are from this source.

71. Rehnquist, J., Inspector General, *Psychotropic Drug Use in Nursing Homes.* U.S. Department of Health and Human Services, November 21, 2001, http://hhs.gov/oig/oei.

72. Hilton, C., "The Origin of Old Age Psychiatry in Britain in the 1940s,"*History of Psychiatry,* 16: 267-289, 2005; p. 268.

73. Ibid., p. 273.

74. Ban, T. A., "Pharmacotherapy of Mental Illness: A Historical Analysis," p. 720.

75. See Obey, M., "Bipolar Disorder is a Physical Ill, U.S. Judge Rules," *Wall Street Journal,* March 12, 2002, pp. B1 and B4.

76. "AGS Position Statement," January 1997, http://americangeriatrics.org/products/positionpapers/psychot.shtml.

77. Espinoza, R. T., and Unützer, J., "Diagnosis and Management of Late-Life Depression," September 1, 2005, https://store.utdol.com/app/index.asp. Subsequent quotes refer to this source.

78. Steck, M., et al., "Natural History of Depression in the Oldest Old: Population-based Prospective Study," *British Journal of Psychiatry,* 188: 65-69, 2006. Also at http://psychiatrymatters.md/International/News/2006/Week_02/Day_1/Depression__frequent_and_persistent__in_over-85s.asp?C=5789438732993.

79. Gurwich, T., and Cunningham, J. A., "Appropriate Use of Psychotropic Drugs in Nursing Homes," http://medicarenhic.com/whats_new/archive2002/psychodrug_1002.htm, emphasis added.

80. Ancelin, M. L., et al., "Non-Degenerative Mild Cognitive Impairment in Elderly People and Use of Anticholinergic Drugs: Longitudinal Cohort Study," *British Medical Journal,* 332: 455-459 (February 25), 2006, http://bmj.bmjjournals.com/cgi/content/full/332/7539/455; Rosack, J., "FDA Orders New Warning on Atypical Antipsychotics," *Psychiatric News,* 40: 1 (May 6), 2005.

81. Espinoza, R. T., and Unützer, J., "Diagnosis and Management of Late-Life Depression," op. cit.

82. Ibid.
83. Rehnquist, J., Inspector General, *Psychotropic Drug Use in Nursing Homes*, op. cit.
84. Ibid.
85. Academy of Psychosomatic Medicine, "Position Statement: Psychiatric Aspects of Excellent End-of-Life Care," http://apm.org/papers/eol-care.shtml, emphasis added.
86. Shanfield, S. B., "Some Observations of a Psychiatric Consultant to a Hospice," *Hillside Journal of Clinical Psychiatry*, 5: 31-42, 1983, http://ncbi.nlm.nih.gov/entrez/query.fcgi?cmd=Retrieve&db=PubMed&list_uids=6662494&dopt=.
87. Ibid.
88. Szasz, T., *Cruel Compassion*, op. cit., and *Pharmacracy*, op. cit.
89. Martin, A., et al., "Multiple Psychotropic Pharmacotherapy among Child and Adolescent Enrollees in Connecticut Medicaid Managed Care," *Psychiatric Services*, 54:72-77 (January), 2003, http://ps.psychiatryonline.org/cgi/content/full/54/1/72, emphasis added.
90. Vascellaro, J. E., "Prevalence of Drugs for DSS Wards Questioned," *Boston Globe*, August 9, 2004, http://boston.com/news/local/articles/2004/08/09/prevalence_of_drugs_for_dss_wards_questioned?mode=PF.
91. Garrett, R. T., "Drug Fraud Alleged in Foster Care: Strayhorn Believes Kids Are Getting Unnecessary Psychiatric Medication," *The Dallas Morning News*, November 12, 2004, http://woai.com/troubleshooters/story.aspx?content_id=168321B6-DF50-4A2F-83D1-1789D8F2A18A, emphasis added.
92. Harper, J., "Prescriptions of Mind-Altering Drugs for Teens Rise," *Washington Times*, January 4, 2006, http://washingtontimes.com/national/20060104-122700-9017r.htm, emphasis added.
93. Jackson, M., "Police Fight Attention Disorder," BBC News, March 15, 2005. http://news.bbc.co.uk/2/hi/health/4347991.stm, emphasis added.
94. Miller, L. M., "Drugged into Submission: Forced Medication Straitjackets Kids," *Columbus Dispatch,* April 25, 2005, http://dispatch.com/reports-story.php?story=dispatch/2005/04/24/20050424-A1-00.html, emphasis added.
95. Ibid.
96. Tanner, L., "More Kids are Getting Anti-Psychotic Drugs," *South Florida Sun-Sentinel*, March 16, 2006, http://sun-sentinel.com/news/nationworld/ats-ap_health-12mar16,1,3869296.story?ctrack=1&cset=true.
97. Associated Press, "Antipsychotic Drug Use among Kids Soars: Report Raises Concerns That Mind-Altering Pills Are Being Overprescribed," May 3, 2006, http://msnbc.msn.com/id/12616864/from/ET/.
98. Smidebush, A., "Happy Pills Don't Make Me Happy," *New America Media*, Youth Commentary, January 20, 2006. http://news.ncmonline.com/news/view_alt-category.html?category_id=50
99. See Szasz, T., "The psychiatrist: A policeman in the schools," *This Magazine Is About Schools*, October, 1967, pp. 114-134; "The psychiatrist as double agent," *Transaction*, 4: 16-24 (October), 1967; *Cruel Compassion*, op. cit., Chapter 4; Platt, A. M., *The Child Savers: The Invention of Delinquency* (Chicago: University of Chicago Press, 1969); and Schrag, P. and Dioky, D., *The Myth of the Hyperactive Child and Other Means of Child Control* (New York: Pantheon, 1975

Chapter 8

1. Szasz, T., *Words to the Wise: A Medico-Philosophical Dictionary* (New Brunswick, NJ: Transaction Publishers, 2004), p. 31.

2. See Szasz, T., *Ceremonial Chemistry: The Ritual Persecution of Drugs, Addicts, and Pushers* [1976] (Syracuse: Syracuse University Press, 2003).
3. "LSD," http://coolnurse.com/lsd.ht.
4. Stevens, J., "History of the Psychedelic Rediscovery: The Door in the Wall," http://druglibrary.or/schaffer/lsd/stevens1/htm.
5. Hofmann, http://hallucinogens.com/hofmann/albert-hofmann.html.
6. Hofmann, A., *LSD: My Problem Child* (New York: McGraw-Hill, 1980). "LSD: My Problem Child," http://hallucinogens.com/hofmann/albert-hofmann.html.
7. Based on "A Who's Who of Acid Dreams," http://levity.com/aciddreams/whoswho.html. See also Marks, J., *The Search for the "Manchurian Candidate": The CIA and Mind Control* (New York: Times Books, 1979).
8. Sigal, C. *Zone of the Interior* [1976] (Hebden Bridge, West Yorkshire, UK: Pomona, 2005).
9. Laing, R. D., *Wisdom, Madness, and Folly* (New York: McGraw-Hill, 1985), pp. 5-6. See also Szasz, T., "'Knowing What Ain't So': R. D. Laing and Thomas Szasz," *Psychoanalytic Review*, 91: 331-346 (June), 2004.
10. Clay, J. R., *D. Laing: A Divided Self* (London: Hodder & Staughton, 1996), p. 79.
11. Ibid., pp. 96, 97, emphasis added.
12. Quoted in ibid., p. 114, emphasis added.
13. Ibid., pp. 118-119.
14. Laing, A. C., *R. D. Laing: A Biography* (London: Peter Owen, 1994), pp. 71, 91.
15. Ibid., pp. 108, 109.
16. Ibid., p. 128.
17. Kramer, P. D. *Listening to Prozac* (New York: Viking, 1993); *Listening to Prozac: The Landmark Book About Antidepressants and the Remaking of the Self*, rev. ed. (New York: Penguin, 1997).
18. Laing, A. C., *R. D. Laing*, op. cit., p. 131.
19. Sigal, C., "A Trip to the Far Side of Madness," *The Guardian* (UK), December 3, 2005, http://books.guardian.co.uk/departments/politicsphilosophyandsociety/story/0,6000,1656440,00.html. See also Sigal, C., *Zone of the Interior*.
20. Laing, R. D., *The Politics of Experience and the Bird of Paradise* (Harmondsworth: Penguin, 1967), p. 156. For details, see Szasz, T., *Schizophrenia: The Sacred Symbol of Psychiatry* [1976] (Syracuse: Syracuse University Press, 1988), chap. 2.
21. Lemov, R., *World as Laboratory: Experiments with Mice, Mazes, and Men* (New York: Hill and Wang, 2005), p. 188.
22. Ibid., pp. 199-200.
23. West, L. J., Pierce, C. M., and Thomas, W. D., "Lysergic Acid Diethylamide: Its Effect on a Male Asiatic Elephant," *Science*, 138, 1100-1102 (December 7), 1962. For details, see Jensen, J., "The Anti-Cultist and the Elephant: 'A Dose of Madness'—Forty Years Ago, Two Psychiatrists Administered History's Largest Dose of LSD," *The Guardian* (UK), August 8, 2002, http://cesnur.org/2002/brain_aug.htm.
24. Ibid., p. 200.
25. Quoted in ibid., p. 202.
26. Ibid., pp. 230-231.
27. Weyburn Mental Hospital, "The Journey In," http://saskurbex.prairiepast.com/main/weyburn/weyburn.htm. See also http://city.w heyburn.sk.ca/modules.php?name=Sections&op=viewarticle&artid=98.
28. Stevens, J., "History of the Psychedelic Rediscovery: The Door in the Wall," http:\\druglibrary.or/schaffer/lsd/stevens1/htm.
29. "Humphry Osmond," http://en.wikipedia.org/wiki/Humphry_Osmond.
30. Hoffer, A., "Orthomolecular Psychiatry in Theory and Practice," http://laleva.cc/choice/orthomolecolar_psychiatry.html, emphasis added.

31.   "Abram Hoffer, "http://en.wikipedia.org/wiki/Abram_Hoffer; and Stevens, J., "History of the Psychedelic Rediscovery: The Door in the Wall," http:\\druglibrary. or/schaffer/ lsd/stevens 1 /htm.

Conclusion

1.   Swift, J., *The Examiner*, no. 15, November 9, 1710, http://jaffebros.com/lee/ gulliver/quotes/other_swift.html.

2.   For an extended comparison of involuntary psychiatry with involuntary servitude, see Szasz, T., *Liberation by Oppression: A Comparative Study of Slavery and Psychiatry* (New Brunswick, NJ: Transaction Publishers, 2002); see also *Psychiatric Slavery: When Confinement and Coercion Masquerade as Cure* [1977] (Syracuse: Syracuse University Press, 1998).

3.   Trujillo, M., "Deinstitutionalizing the Mentally Ill,"*City Journal*, Spring 1993. http://city-journal.org/article01.php?aid=1503.

4.   See Stone, A., "Psychiatry and the Law,"Class Notes, January 2001, http://law. harvard.edu/academics/registrar/exams/2000-01/html/stone1.html.

5.   Lincoln, A., "'House Divided'Speech,"http://historyplace.com/lincoln/divided. htm.

6.   See Szasz, T., *Law, Liberty, and Psychiatry: An Inquiry into the Social Uses of Psychiatry* [1963] (Syracuse: Syracuse University Press, 1989).

7.   Bloch, S., Chodoff, P., and Green, S. A., *Psychiatric Ethics* (New York: Oxford University Press, 1999).

8.   Bloch, S., and Green, S. A., "An Ethical Framework for Psychiatry,"*British Journal of Psychiatry*, 188: 7-12 (January), 2006.

9.   Mitchell, S. W., "Address before the Fiftieth Annual Meeting of the American Medico-Psychological Association, held in Philadelphia, May 16, 1894,"*Journal of Nervous and Mental Disease,* 21: 413-437 (July), 1894, pp. 414, 427, emphasis added.

Bibliography

Alexander, F. G., and Selesnick, S. T. *The History of Psychiatry: An Evaluation of Psychiatric Thought and Practice from Prehistoric Times to the Present.* New York: Harper & Row, 1966.

Amador, X., with Johanson, A-L. *I Am Not Sick, I Don't Need Help! Helping the Seriously Mentally Ill Accept Treatment: A Practical Guide for Families and Therapists.* Peconic, NY: Vida Press, 2000.

American Psychiatric Association. *Diagnostic and Statistical Manual of Mental Disorders—IV-TR,* 4th ed. text revision. Washington, DC: American Psychiatric Association, 2000.

Andreev, B. V. *Sleep Therapy in the Neuroses* (1959). Translated from the Russian by Basil Haigh. New York: Consultants Bureau, 1960.

Andrews, R., ed. *The Columbia Dictionary of Quotations.* New York: Columbia University Press, 1993.

Appelbaum, P. S. *Almost a Revolution: Mental Health Law and the Limits of Change.* New York: Oxford University Press, 1994.

Arendt, H. *Eichmann in Jerusalem: A Report on the Banality of Evil.* New York: Viking, 1963.

Arieti, S., ed. *American Handbook of Psychiatry,* 3 vols. New York: Basic Books, 1959-1966.

Bean, P. *Compulsory Admissions to Mental Hospitals.* New York: Wiley, 1980.

Beers, C. W. *A Mind That Found Itself: An Autobiography* [1908], 7th ed. Garden City, NY: Doubleday, 1956.

Berrios, G. E., and Porter, R. *A. History of Clinical Psychiatry.* London: Athlone Press, 1995.

Binger, C. *Revolutionary Doctor: Benjamin Rush, 1746-1813.* New York: Norton, 1966.

Binswanger, L. *Freud: Reminiscences of a Friendship.* Trans. Norbert Guterman. New York: Grune & Stratton, 1957.

Bird, K., and Sherwin, M. J., *American Prometheus: The Triumph and Tragedy of J. Robert Oppenheimer.* New York: Knopf, 2005.

Black, E. *War Against the Weak: Eugenics and America's Campaign to Create a Master Race.* New York: Four Walls Eight Windows, 2003.

Black, H. C. *Black's Law Dictionary.* Rev. 4th ed. St. Paul: West, 1968.

Bleuler, E. *Dementia Praecox, or the Group of Schizophrenias* [1911]. Trans. Joseph Zinkin. New York: International Universities Press, 1950.

Bloch, S., Chodoff, P., and Green, S. A. *Psychiatric Ethics*. New York: Oxford University Press, 1999.

Boorstin, D. J. *The Lost World of Thomas Jefferson*. Boston: Beacon Press, 1948.

Bulwer-Lytton, R. *A Blighted Life: A True Story* (1880). Bristol, UK: Thoemmes Press, 1994.

Burke, E. *The Works of the Right Honorable Edmund Burke*, 12 vols. Boston: Wells & Lilly, 1826.

Burrell, B. *Postcards from the Brain Museum: The Improbable Search for Meaning in the Matter of Famous Minds*. New York: Broadway, 2005.

Bynum, W. F., Porter, R., and Shepherd, M., eds. *The Anatomy of Madness: Essays in the History of Psychiatry*, 3 vols. London: Tavistock, 1985-1988.

Campbell, A. V. *Health as Liberation: Medicine, Theology, and the Quest for Justice*. Cleveland, OH: Pilgrim Press, 1995.

Camus, A. *The Rebel: An Essay on Man in Revolt* [1951]. Trans. Anthony Bower. New York: Vintage Books, 1956.

Camus, A. *Resistance, Rebellion, Death*. Trans. Justin O'Brien. New York: Knopf, 1961.

Cecil, R. L., ed. *A Textbook of Medicine*, 5th ed. rev. Philadelphia: Saunders, 1942.

Charen, M. *Do-Gooders: How Liberals Hurt Those They Claim to Help—and the Rest of Us*. New York: Sentinel, 2004.

Chekhov, A. *Seven Short Stories by Chekhov*. Trans. Barbara Makanowitzky. New York: Bantam Books, 1963.

Chesterton, G. K. *Orthodoxy*. London: John Lane, 1909.

Chesterton, G. K. *The Everlasting Man*. New York: Dodd, Mead & Company, 1926.

Clay, J. *R. D. Laing: A Divided Self*. London: Hodder & Staughton, 1996.

Cohen, S., and Scull, A., eds. *Social Control and the State*. New York: St. Martin's Press, 1983.

Collingwood, R. G. *An Autobiography* [1939]. With a new Introduction by Stephen Toulmin. Oxford: Clarendon Press/Oxford University Press, 1978.

Collingwood, R. G. *The New Leviathan, or Man, Society, Civilization and Barbarism* [1942]. Oxford: Clarendon Press/Oxford University Press, 1947.

Collins, A. *In the Sleep Room: The Story of the CIA Brainwashing Experiments in Canada*. Toronto: Lester & Orpen Dennys, 1988.

Cooper, D. *The Death of the Family*. New York: Pantheon, 1970.

Deutsch, A. *The Shame of the States*. New York: Harcourt, Brace and Company, 1948.

Deutsch, A. *The Mentally Ill in America: A History of Their Care and Treatment from Colonial Times*, 2d ed. New York: Columbia University Press, 1952.

Dudman, C. *98 Reasons for Being*. London: Sceptre/Hodder and Stoughton, 2004.

El-Hai, J. *The Lobotomist: A Maverick Medical Genius and His Tragic Quest to Rid the World of Mental Illness*. Hoboken, NJ: Wiley, 2005.

Eliot, T. S. *The Cocktail Party*. London: Faber and Faber, 1974.

Ellenberger, H. F. *The Discovery of the Unconscious: The History and Evolution of Dynamic Psychiatry.* New York: Basic Books, 1970.

Engstrom, E. J. *Clinical Psychiatry in Imperial Germany: A History of Psychiatric Practice.* Ithaca, NY: Cornell University Press, 2003.

Fink, M. *Electroshock: Restoring the Mind.* New York: Oxford University Press, 1999.

Forrest, D. *Hypnotism: A History.* Harmondsworth: Penguin, 1999.

Foucault, M. *Mental Illness and Psychology* (1954). Trans. Alan Sheridan. New York: Harper Colophon, 1976.

Foucault, M. *Madness and Civilization: A History of Insanity in the Age of Reason* [1961]. Trans. Richard Howard. New York: Pantheon, 1965.

Freedman, A. M., Kaplan, H. I., and Sadock, B. J. *Modern Synopsis of Comprehensive Textbook of Psychiatry/II,* 2d ed. Baltimore, MD: Williams & Wilkins, 1976.

Freud, S. *The Standard Edition of the Complete Psychological Works of Sigmund Freud,* 24 vols. Trans. James Strachey. London: Hogarth Press, 1953-1974. Cited as *SE.*

Friedberg, J. *Shock Treatment is Not Good for Your Brain.* San Francisco: Glide Publications, 1976.

Friedman, M. *Capitalism and Freedom.* Chicago: University of Chicago Press, 1962.

Gaylin, W. *Hatred: The Psychological Descent Into Violence.* New York: Public Affairs, 2003.

Gilman, C. P. *The Yellow Wallpaper* [1892]. Ed. Dale M. Bauer. Boston: Belford/St. Martin's, 1998.

Gillespie, C. C., ed. *Dictionary of Scientific Biography.* New York: Scribner's, 1971.

Gillmor, D. *I Swear by Apollo: Dr. Ewen Cameron and the CIA-Brainwashing Experiments.* Montreal: Eden Press 1987).

Goffman, E. *Asylums: Essays on the Social Situation of Mental Patients and Other Inmates.* Garden City, NY: Doubleday Anchor, 1961.

Goldsmith, M. *Franz Anton Mesmer: A History of Mesmerism.* New York: Doubleday, 1934.

Goldstein, J. *Console and Classify: The French Psychiatric Profession in the Nineteenth Century.* New York: Cambridge University Press, 1987.

Goodman, L., and Gilman, A. *The Pharmacological Basis of Therapeutics.* New York: Macmillan, 1941.

Gordon, R. *Great Medical Disasters.* New York: Stein & Day, 1983.

Grob, G. N. *Mental Illness and American Society, 1875-1940.* Princeton, NJ: Princeton University Press, 1983.

Grob, G. N., *The Mad Among Us: A History of the Care of America's Mentally Ill.* New York: Free Press, 1994.

Hall, J. K., et al., eds. *One Hundred Years of American Psychiatry.* New York: Columbia University Press, 1944.

Halperin, D. M. *Saint Foucault: Towards a Gay Hagiography.* New York: Oxford University Press, 1995.

Healy, D. *The Psychopharmacologists: Interviews by Dr. David Healy*. London: Chapman & Hall, 1996.

Healy, D. *The Antidepressant Era*. Cambridge, MA: Harvard University Press, 1997.

Healy, D. *The Psychopharmacologists—II: Interviews by Dr. David Healy*. London: Chapman & Hall, 1998.

Healy, D. *The Psychopharmacologists—III: Interviews by Dr. David Healy*. London: Chapman & Hall, 2000.

Healy, D. *The Creation of Psychopharmacology*. Cambridge, MA: Harvard University Press, 2002.

Heinroth, J. C. *Textbook of Disturbances of Mental Life, or Disturbances of the Soul and Their Treatment* [1818], 2 vols. Trans. J. Schmorak. Baltimore, MD: Johns Hopkins University Press, 1975.

Hoch, P., ed. *Failures in Psychiatric Treatment*. New York: Grune & Stratton, 1948.

Hoffmann, H. *Struwwelpeter: Fearful Stories & Vile Pictures to Instruct Good Little Folks* (1845). Introduction by Jack Zipes. Venice, CA: Feral House, 1999.

Horgan, J. *The Undiscovered Mind: How the Human Brain Defies Replication, Medication, and Explanation*. New York: Simon and Schuster, 1999.

Hudson, R. P. *Disease and Its Control*. New York: Praeger, 1983.

Hunter, R., and Macalpine, I., eds. *Three Hundred Years of Psychiatry, 1535-1860: A History Presented in Selected English Texts*. London: Oxford University Press, 1963.

Huxley, A. *After Many a Summer Dies the Swan*. New York: Harper & Brothers, 1939.

Huxley, A. *Brave New World Revisited* [1958]. New York: HarperPerennial, 1989.

Isaac, R. J., and Armat, V. C. *Madness in the Streets: How Psychiatry and the Law Abandoned the Mentally Ill*. New York: Free Press, 1990.

Jackson, J. H. *Selected Writings of John Hughlings Jackson*, 2 vols. Ed. James Taylor. London: Staples Press, 1958.

Jamison, K. R. *An Unquiet Mind: A Memoir of Mood* and *Madness*. New York: Knopf, 1995.

Jaspers, K. *General Psychopathology* [1913, 1946], 7th ed. Trans. J. Hoenig and M. W. Hamilton. Chicago: University of Chicago Press, 1963.

Johnson, A. B. *Out of Bedlam: The Truth About Deinstitutionalization*. New York: Basic Books, 1990.

Joint Commission on Mental Illness and Health. *Action for Mental Health: Final Report of the Joint Commission on Mental Illness and Health, 1961*. New York: Basic Books, 1961.

Joynt, R. J., ed. *Clinical Neurology*, rev. ed. Philadelphia: Lippincott, 1988.

Kaplan, H. I., and Sadock, B. J. *Comprehensive Textbook of Psychiatry/VI*, vol. 2. Baltimore, MD: Williams & Wilkins, 1995.

Kasper, D. L., et al., eds. *Harrison's Principles of Internal Medicine*, 16th ed. New York: McGraw-Hill, 2005.

Kaufman, W., ed. *The Portable Nietzsche*. Trans. Walter Kaufman. New York: Viking, 1954.

Kesey, K. *One Flew Over the Cuckoo's Nest*. New York: Viking, 1962.

Kneeland, T. W., and Warren, C.A.B. *Pushbutton Psychiatry: A History of Electroshock in America*. Westport, CT: Praeger, 2002.

Kotowicz, Z. R. D. *Laing and Paths of Anti-Psychiatry*. London: Routledge, 1997.

Kramer, P. D. *Listening to Prozac*. New York: Viking, 1993.

Kramer, P. D. *Listening to Prozac: The Landmark Book About Antidepressants and the Remaking of the Self*. New York: Penguin, 1997.

La Fond, J. Q., and Durham, M. L. *Back to the Asylum: The Future of Mental Health Law and Policy in the United States*. New York: Oxford University Press, 1992.

Laing, A. C. *R. D. Laing: A Biography*. London: Peter Owen, 1994.

Laing, R. D. *The Politics of Experience and the Bird of Paradise*. Harmondsworth: Penguin, 1967.

Laing, R. D. *Wisdom, Madness, and Folly*. New York: McGraw-Hill, 1985.

Lawford, C. K. *Symptoms of Withdrawal: A Memoir of Snapshots and Redemption*. New York: William Morrow, 2005.

Leamer, L. *The Kennedy Women: The Saga of an American Family*. New York: Villard Books/Random House, 1994.

Leamer, L. *The Kennedy Men, 1901-1963: The Laws of the Father*. New York: William Morrow, 2001.

Leary, T. The *Politics of Psychopharmacology*. Berkeley, CA: Ronin Publishing, 2001.

Lee, H. *To Kill A Mockingbird*. Philadelphia: J. B. Lippincott, 1960.

Lemov, R. *World as Laboratory: Experiments With Mice, Mazes, and Men*. New York: Hill and Wang, 2005.

Lewis, C. S. *Mere Christianity*. New York: Macmillan, 1952.

Lewis, C. S. *God in the Dock: Essays on Theology and Ethics*. Ed. Walter Hooper. Grand Rapids, MI: William B. Eerdmans, 1970.

Locke, J. *An Essay Concerning Human Understanding* [1690]. Chicago: Regnery/Gateway, 1956.

Locke, J. *Two Treatises of Government* [1690]. Ed. Peter Laslett. New York: New American Library, 1965.

Lothane, Z. *In Defense of Schreber: Soul Murder and Psychiatry*. Hillsdale, NJ: Analytic Press, 1992.

Lytton, R. B. *A Blighted Life: A True Story* (1880). Bristol, UK: Thoemmes Press, 1994.

Mackay, C. *Extraordinary Popular Delusions and the Madness of Crowds* [1841, 1852]. Foreword by Bernard M. Baruch. New York: Noonday Press, 1962.

Magnet, M. *The Dream and the Nightmare: The Sixties' Legacy to the Underclass* [1993]. San Francisco: Encounter Books, 2000.

Mahoney, J. M. *Schizophrenia: The Bearded Lady Disease*. Bloomington, IN: Authorhouse, 2003.

Marks, J. *The Search for the "Manchurian Candidate": The CIA and Mind Control.* New York: Times Books, 1979.

Maudsley, H. *Responsibility in Mental Disease*, 4th ed. London: Kegan Paul, Trench & Co., 1885.

McHugh, P. R., *The Mind Has Mountains: Reflections on Society and Psychiatry.* Baltimore, MD: Johns Hopkins University Press, 2006.

Meduna, L. J., ed. *Carbon Dioxide Therapy: A Neurophysiological Treatment of Nervous Disorders* [1955], 2d ed. Springfield, IL: Charles C. Thomas, 1958.

Menninger, K. *The Crime of Punishment.* New York: Viking, 1968.

Meynert, T. *Psychiatry: Clinical Treatise on Diseases of the Forebrain* [1884]. Trans. B. Sachs. New York: G. P. Putnam's Sons, 1885.

Micale, M. S., and Porter, R., eds. *Discovering the History of Psychiatry.* New York: Oxford University Press, 1994.

Mill, J. S. *On Liberty* [1859]. Chicago: Regnery, 1955.

Mill, J. S. *Utilitarianism* [1863], in *Essential Works of John Stuart Mill.* Ed. Max Lerner. New York: Bantam Books, 1961.

Millon, T. *Masters of the Mind: Exploring the Story of Mental Illness from Ancient Times to the New Millennium.* Hoboken, NJ: Wiley, 2004.

Mises, L. von. *Human Action: A Treatise on Economics.* New Haven, CT: Yale University Press, 1949.

Mitchell, S. W. *Fat and Blood: Or Hints for the Overworked* [*Fat and Blood: And How to Make Them.* Philadelphia: J. B. Lippincott Co., 1878]). Ed. and intro. Michael S. Kimmel. Walnut Creek, CA: Altamira Press, 2004.

Munthe, A. *The Story of San Michele* [1929]. New York: Dutton, 1957.

Nietzsche, F. *Twilight of the Idols or, How to Philosophize with a Hammer* (1895), in *The Portable Nietzsche.* Ed. and trans. Walter Kaufman. New York: Viking, 1954.

Nietzsche, F. *Ecce Homo: How One Becomes What One Is* (1888/1908). Extracts in *The Portable Nietzsche.* Ed. and trans. Walter Kaufman. New York: Viking, 1954.

Olasky, M. *The Tragedy of American Compassion.* Chicago: Regnery, 1992.

Orwell, G. *The Collected Essays, Journalism and Letters of George Orwell,* 4 vols. Ed. Sonia Orwell and Ian Angus. Harmondsworth: Penguin, 1970.

Owens, D.G.C. *A Guide to the Extrapyramidal Side-effects of Antipsychotic Drugs.* Cambridge: Cambridge University Press, 1999.

Parry-Jones, W. Ll. *The Trade in Lunacy: A Study of Private Madhouses in England in the Eighteenth and Nineteenth Centuries.* London: Routledge & Kegan Paul, 1976.

Patton, A. S. *A Doctor's Dilemma: William Griggs and the Salem Witch Trials.* Salem, MA: The Salem Witch Museum, 1998.

Pinel, P. *A Treatise on Insanity* [1801, 1806]. Trans. D. D. Davis. New York: Hafner Publishing Company, 1962. Facsimile of the 1806 edition: *A Treatise on Insanity, in Which Are Contained the Principles of a New and More Practical Nosology of Maniacal Disorders than Has Yet Been Offered to the Public, etc.* London: Cadell and Davies, 1806.

Platt, A. M. *The Child Savers: The Invention of Delinquency*. Chicago: University of Chicago Press, 1969.

Pols, J. *The Politics of Mental Illness: Myth and Power in the Works of Thomas S. Szasz*. Trans. Mira de Vries (1984/2005). Http://janpols.jconserv. net/index.php.

Porter, R. *Mind-Forg'd Manacles: A History of Madness from the Restoration to the Regency*. London: Athlone Press, 1987.

Porter, R. *A Social History of Madness: The World Through the Eyes of the Insane*. New York: Weidenfeld & Nicolson, 1987.

Porter, R. *Flesh in the Age of Reason: The Modern Foundations of Body and Soul*. New York: Norton, 2004.

Porter, R., ed. *The Faber Book of Madness*. London: Faber and Faber, 1991.

Porter, R., and Wright, D., eds. *The Confinement of the Insane: International Perspectives, 1800-1965*. Cambridge: Cambridge University Press, 2003.

Proctor, R. N. *The Nazi War on Cancer*. Princeton, NJ: Princeton University Press, 1999.

Redlich, F. C., and Freedman, D. X. *The Theory and Practice of Psychiatry*. New York: Basic Books, 1966.

Reynolds, J. R. *Epilepsy: Its Symptoms, Treatment, and Relation to Other Chronic Convulsive Diseases*. London: Churchill Livingstone, 1861.

Reynolds, E. H., and Trimble, M. R., eds. Epilepsy and Psychiatry. London: Churchill Livingstone, 1981.

Ridenour, N. *Mental Health in the United States: A Fifty Year History*. Cambridge, MA: Harvard University Press, 1961.

Rinkel, M., ed. *Biological Treatment of Mental Illness: Proceedings of the II International Conference of the Manfred Sakel Foundation, held October 31 to November 3, 1962, at the New York Academy of Medicine, New York*. New York: L. C. Page/Farrar, Straus and Giroux, 1966.

Robitscher, J. *The Powers of Psychiatry*. Boston: Houghton Mifflin, 1980.

Rogow, A. A. *The Psychiatrists*. New York: G. P. Putnam's Sons, 1970.

Rosen, G. *Madness in Society: Chapters in the Historical Sociology of Mental Illness*. Chicago: University of Chicago Press, 1968.

Rothman, D. J. *The Discovery of the Asylum: Social Order and Disorder in the New Republic*. Boston: Little, Brown, 1971.

Rothman, D. J. *Conscience and Convenience: The Asylum and Its Alternatives in Progressive America*. Boston: Little, Brown, 1980.

Rothman, D. J. *Conscience and Convenience: The Asylum and Its Alternatives in Progressive America*, rev. ed. With a Foreword by Thomas G. Blomberg. New York: Aldine de Gruyter, 2002.

Rush, B. *Medical Inquiries and Observations upon the Diseases of the Mind* (1812). New York: Macmillan-Hafner Press, 1962.

Russell, B. *Sceptical Essays*. London: Allen & Unwin, 1928.

Russell, B. *A History of Western Philosophy: And Its Connection with Political and Social Circumstances from the Earliest Times to the Present Day*. New York: Simon and Schuster, 1945.

Ryn, C. G. *The New Jacobinism: Can Democracy Survive?* Washington, DC: National Humanities Institute, 1991.

Sackler, A. M., Sackler, M. D., Sackler, R. R., and Marti-Ibanez, F., eds. *The Great Physiodynamic Therapies in Psychiatry: An Historical Reappraisal.* New York: Hoeber-Harper, 1956.

Sadock, B. J., and Sadock, V. A. *Kaplan and Sadock's Synopsis of Psychiatry: Behavioral Sciences/Clinical Psychiatry*, 9th ed. Philadelphia: Lippincott Williams & Wilkins, 2003.

Sargant, W. *Battle for the Mind: A Physiology of Conversion and Brainwashing* (1957). New York: Harper & Row/Perennial Library, 1971.

Sargant, W. *The Unquiet Mind: The Autobiography of a Physician in Psychological Medicine.* London: Pan Books, 1967.

Satel, S. *Drug Treatment: The Case for Coercion.* Washington, DC: American Enterprise Institute for Public Policy Research, 1999.

Schain, R. *The Legend of Nietzsche's Syphilis.* Westport, CT: Greenwood, 2001.

Schaler, J., ed. *Szasz Under Fire: The Psychiatric Abolitionist Faces His Critics.* Chicago: Open Court, 2004.

Schama, S. *Citizens: A Chronicle of the French Revolution.* New York: Vintage/ Random House, 1990.

Schatzman, M. *Soul Murder: Persecution in the Family.* London: Allen Lane, 1973.

Schumpeter, J. A. *History of Economic Analysis.* New York: Oxford University Press, 1954.

Schrag, P., and Dioky, D. *The Myth of the Hyperactive Child and Other Means of Child Control.* New York: Pantheon, 1975.

Seager, R. H., ed. *The Dawn of Religious Pluralism: Voices from the World's Parliament of Religions, 1893.* LaSalle, IL: Open Court, 1993.

Shorter, E. *A History of Psychiatry: From the Era of the Asylum to the Age of Prozac.* New York: Wiley, 1997.

Shutts, D. *Lobotomy: Resort to the Knife.* New York: Van Nostrand Reinhold Company, 1982.

Sigal, C. *Zone of the Interior* [1976]. Hebden Bridge, West Yorkshire, UK: Pomona, 2005.

Simon, L. *Dark Light: Electricity and Anxiety from the Telegraph to the X-Ray.* New York: Harcourt, 2004.

Skultans, V. *Madness and Morals: Ideas on Insanity in the Nineteenth Century.* London; Routledge & Kegan Paul, 1975.

Smith, M. B. *For a Significant Social Psychology: The Collected Writings of M. Brewster Smith.* New York: New York University Press, 2003.

Stillman, E., and Pfaff, W. *The Politics of Hysteria: The Sources of Twentieth-Century Conflict.* New York: Harper & Row, 1964.

Stone, A. A. *Law, Psychiatry and Morality.* Washington, DC: American Psychiatric Press, 1985.

Szasz, T. *Pain and Pleasure: A Study of Bodily Feelings* [1957], 2d expanded ed. [1975]. Syracuse: Syracuse University Press, 1988.

Szasz, T. *The Myth of Mental Illness: Foundations of a Theory of Personal Conduct* [1961], rev. ed. New York: HarperCollins, 1974.

Szasz, T. *Law, Liberty, and Psychiatry: An Inquiry into the Social Uses of Psychiatry* [1963]. Syracuse: Syracuse University Press, 1989.

Szasz, T., *The Ethics of Psychoanalysis: The Theory and Method of Autonomous Psychotherapy* [1965]. Syracuse: Syracuse University Press, 1988.

Szasz, T. *Psychiatric Justice* [1965]. Syracuse: Syracuse University Press, 1988.

Szasz, T. *Ideology and Insanity: Essays on the Psychiatric Dehumanization of Man* [1970]. Syracuse: Syracuse University Press, 1991.

Szasz, T. *The Manufacture of Madness: A Comparative Study of the Inquisition and the Mental Health Movement* [1970]. Syracuse: Syracuse University Press, 1997.

Szasz, T. *The Second Sin*. Garden City, NY: Doubleday Anchor, 1973.

Szasz, T. *Ceremonial Chemistry: The Ritual Persecution of Drugs, Addicts, and Pushers* [1976]. Syracuse: Syracuse University Press, 2003.

Szasz, T. *Anti-Freud: Karl Kraus's Criticism of Psychoanalysis and Psychiatry* [1976]. Syracuse: Syracuse University Press, 1990.

Szasz, T. *Schizophrenia: The Sacred Symbol of Psychiatry* [1976]. Syracuse: Syracuse University Press, 1988.

Szasz, T. *Psychiatric Slavery: When Confinement and Coercion Masquerade as Cure* [1977]. Syracuse: Syracuse University Press, 1998.

Szasz, T. *The Theology of Medicine: The Political-Philosophical Foundations of Medical Ethics* [1977]. Syracuse: Syracuse University Press, 1988.

Szasz, T. *The Myth of Psychotherapy: Mental Healing as Religion, Rhetoric, and Repression* [1978]. Syracuse: Syracuse University Press, 1988.

Szasz, T. *Sex by Prescription* [1980]. Syracuse: Syracuse University Press, 1990.

Szasz, T. *The Therapeutic State: Psychiatry in the Mirror of Current Events*. Buffalo: Prometheus Books, 1984.

Szasz, T. *Insanity: The Idea and Its Consequences* [1987]. Syracuse: Syracuse University Press, 1997.

Szasz, T. *The Untamed Tongue: A Dissenting Dictionary*. LaSalle, IL: Open Court, 1990.

Szasz, T. *Our Right to Drugs: The Case for a Free Market* [1992]. Syracuse: Syracuse University Press, 1996.

Szasz, T. *A Lexicon of Lunacy: Metaphoric Malady, Moral Responsibility, and Psychiatry*. New Brunswick, NJ: Transaction Publishers, 1993.

Szasz, T. *Cruel Compassion: The Psychiatric Control of Society's Unwanted* [1994]. Syracuse: Syracuse University Press, 1998.

Szasz, T. *The Meaning of Mind: Language, Morality, and Neuroscience* [1996]. Syracuse: Syracuse University Press, 2002.

Szasz, T. *Fatal Freedom: The Ethics and Politics of Suicide* [1999]. Syracuse: Syracuse University Press, 2002.

Szasz, T. *Pharmacracy: Medicine and Politics in America* [2001]. Syracuse: Syracuse University Press, 2003.

Szasz, T. *Liberation by Oppression: A Comparative Study of Slavery and Psychiatry*. New Brunswick, NJ: Transaction Publishers, 2002.

Szasz, T. *Words to the Wise: A Medical-Philosophical Dictionary.* Brunswick, NJ: Transaction Publishers, 2003.

Szasz, T. *Faith in Freedom: Libertarian Principles and Psychiatric Practices.* New Brunswick, NJ: Transaction Publishers, 2004.

Szasz, T. *"My Madness Saved Me": The Madness and Marriage of Virginia Woolf.* New Brunswick, NJ: Transaction, 2006.

Szasz, T., ed. *The Age of Madness: A History of Involuntary Mental Hospitalization Presented in Selected Texts.* Garden City, NY: Doubleday Anchor, 1973.

Tannsjo, T. *Coercive Care: The Ethics of Choice in Health and Medicine.* London: Routledge, 1999.

Tocqueville, A. de. *The Old Régime and the French Revolution* [1856]. Trans. Stuart Gilbert. Garden City, NY: Doubleday Anchor, 1955.

Todorov, T. *Mikhail Bakhtin: The Dialogical Principle* [1981]. Trans. Wlad Godzich. Minneapolis: University of Minnesota Press, 1984.

Torrey, E. F. *Nowhere to Go: The Tragic Odyssey of the Homeless Mentally Ill.* New York: Harper & Row, 1988.

Torrey, E. F., et al. *Criminalizing the Seriously Mentally Ill: The Abuse of Jails as Mental Hospitals.* Washington, DC: The National Alliance for the Mentally Ill and Public Citizen's Health Research Group, 1992.

Valenstein, E. S. *Great and Desperate Cures: The Rise and Decline of Psychosurgery and Other Radical Treatments for Mental Illness.* New York: Basic Books, 1986.

Weckowicz, T., Thaddeus, E. *Models of Mental Illness; Systems and Theories of Abnormal Psychology.* Springfield, IL: Charles C. Thomas, 1984.

Wexler, D. B., and Winick, B. J., eds. *Essays in Therapeutic Jurisprudence.* Durham, NC: Carolina Academic Press, 1991.

Wexler, D. B., and Winick, B. J., eds. *Law in a Therapeutic Key: Developments in Therapeutic Jurisprudence.* Durham, NC: Carolina Academic Press, 1996.

Williams, R. L., and Webb, W. B. *Sleep Therapy: A Bibliography and Commentary.* Springfield, IL: Charles C. Thomas, 1966.

Williams, T. *Memoirs* [1975]. New York: Bantam, 1976.

Wintrobe, M. M., et al., eds. *Harrison's Principles of Internal Medicine*, 7th ed. New York: McGraw-Hill, 1974.

Wortis, J. *Soviet Psychiatry.* Baltimore, MD: Williams and Wilkins, 1950.

Zilboorg, G. *A History of Medical Psychology.* New York: Norton, 1941.

Zweig, S. *Master Builders: A Typology of the Spirit* 1920-1928). Trans. Eden and Cedar Paul. New York: Viking Press, 1939.

Zweig, S. *Mental Healers: Franz Anton Mesmer, Mary Baker Eddy, Sigmund Freud* [1931]. Trans. Eden and Cedar Paul. New York: Frederick Ungar, 1962.

Acknowledgments

Once again, I am pleased to acknowledge my gratitude to Peter Uva and his colleagues at the library of the Upstate Medical University of the State University of New York in Syracuse for their unceasingly generous and devoted help.

I owe special thanks to Mira de Vries and Elizabeth Daly for their careful reading of the manuscript and countless helpful suggestions, and also to Roger Yanow for his reading and critiquing still another one of my books. Words cannot express my gratitude to my brother George.

Index